T0263161

Technical Advances in Mediastinal Surgery

Guest Editor

TOMMASO C. MINEO, MD

THORACIC SURGERY CLINICS

www.thoracic.theclinics.com

Consulting Editor
MARK K. FERGUSON, MD

May 2010 • Volume 20 • Number 2

SAUNDERS an imprint of ELSEVIER, Inc.

W.B. SAUNDERS COMPANY
A Division of Elsevier Inc.

1600 John F. Kennedy Boulevard • Suite 1800 • Philadelphia, Pennsylvania 19103-2899

http://www.theclinics.com

THORACIC SURGERY CLINICS Volume 20, Number 2
May 2010 ISSN 1547-4127, ISBN-13: 978-1-4377-1880-5

Editor: Catherine Bewick
Developmental Editor: Donald Mumford

Thoracic Surgery Clinics (ISSN 1547-4127) is published quarterly by Elsevier Inc., 360 Park Avenue South, New York, NY 10010-1710. Months of publication are February, May, August, and November. Business and editorial offices: 1600 John F. Kennedy Boulevard, Suite 1800, Philadelphia, PA 19103-2899. Periodicals postage paid at New York, NY, and additional mailing offices. Subscription prices are $269.00 per year (US individuals), $367.00 per year (US institutions), $134.00 per year (US students), $343.00 per year (Canadian individuals), $464.00 per year (Canadian institutions), $183.00 per year (Canadian and foreign students), $365.00 per year (foreign individuals), and $464.00 per year (foreign institutions). Foreign air speed delivery is included in all Clinics' subscription prices. All prices are subject to change without notice. **POSTMASTER:** Send address changes to Thoracic Surgery Clinics, Elsevier Health Sciences Division, Subscription Customer Service, 3251 Riverport Lane, Maryland Heights, MO 63043. **Customer Service (orders, claims, online, change of address): Telephone: 1-800-654-2452 (U.S. and Canada); 314-447-8871 (outside U.S. and Canada). Fax: 314-447-8029. Email: journalscustomerservice-usa@elsevier.com (for print support); journalsonlinesupport-usa@elsevier.com (for online support).**

Reprints. For copies of 100 or more, of articles in this publication, please contact Commercial Rights Department, Elsevier Inc., 360 Park Avenue South, New York, NY 10010-1710. Tel: (212) 633-3812; Fax: (212) 462-1935; E-mail: reprints@elsevier.com.

Thoracic Surgery Clinics is covered in *MEDLINE/PubMed (Index Medicus)* and *EMBASE/Excerpta Medica*.

Printed and bound in the United Kingdom
Transferred to Digital Print 2011

Contributors

CONSULTING EDITOR

MARK K. FERGUSON, MD
Professor of Surgery, Section of Cardiac and Thoracic Surgery, The University of Chicago Medical Center, Chicago, Illinois

GUEST EDITOR

TOMMASO C. MINEO, MD
Professor and Head, Department of Thoracic Surgery, Fondazione Policlinico Tor Vergata, Tor Vergata University, Rome, Italy

AUTHORS

JOHANNES BODNER, MD
Department of Visceral, Transplant and Thoracic Surgery, Innsbruck Medical University, Innsbruck, Austria

JAMES I. COHEN, MD, PhD
Professor, Otolaryngology Head and Neck Surgery; Section Chief, Otolaryngology, Department of Surgery, Portland Veterans Affairs Medical Center, Oregon Health and Sciences University, Portland, Oregon

W. COOSEMANS, MD, PhD
Professor of Surgery, Clinical Head, Department of Thoracic Surgery, University Hospitals Leuven, Leuven, Belgium

THOMAS A. D'AMICO, MD
Professor, Department of Surgery, Duke University Medical Center, Durham, North Carolina

ANTONIO D'ANDRILLI, MD
Assistant Professor, Department of Thoracic Surgery, Sant'Andrea Hospital, University of Rome La Sapienza, Via di Grottarossa, Rome, Italy

VINCENT C. DANIEL, MD
Resident, Division of Thoracic Surgery, Massachusetts General Hospital, Boston, Massachusetts

H. DECALUWÉ, MD
Staff Surgeon, Department of Thoracic Surgery, University Hospitals Leuven, Leuven, Belgium

G. DECKER, MD
Attending Surgeon, Department of Thoracic Surgery, University Hospitals Leuven, Leuven, Belgium

P. DE LEYN, MD, PhD
Professor of Surgery, Clinical Head, Department of Thoracic Surgery, University Hospitals Leuven, Leuven, Belgium

TETSUHIKO GO, MD
General Thoracic and Breast-Endcrinological Surgery, Faculty of Medicine, Kagawa University Miki-Cho, Kita-gun, Kagawa, Japan

ERNESTO IPPOLITO, MD
Professor and Head, Department of Orthopedic Surgery, Fondazione Policlinico Tor Vergata, Tor Vergata University, Rome, Italy

CHRISTOPHER B. KOMANAPALLI, MD
Chief Resident, General Surgery, Department of Surgery, Oregon Health and Sciences University, Portland Veterans Affairs Medical Center, Portland, Oregon

MARK J. KRASNA, MD
Program in Health Policy, St Joseph Cancer Institute, University of Maryland, Towson, Maryland

T. LERUT, MD, PhD
Chairman, Professor of Surgery, Department of Thoracic Surgery, University Hospitals Leuven, Leuven, Belgium

PAOLO MACCHIARINI, MD, PhD
Honorary Professor, University College London; Consultant Thoracic Surgeon, The London Clinic; Honorary Consultant Thoracic Surgeon, Great Ormond Street Hospital, London, United Kingdom; Director, Department of General Thoracic and Regenerative Surgery and Intrathoracic Biotransplantation, University Hospital Careggi, Florence, Italy

FEDERICO MANCINI, MD
Associate Professor, Department of Orthopedic Surgery, Fondazione Policlinico Tor Vergata, Tor Vergata University, Rome, Italy

TOMMASO C. MINEO, MD
Professor and Head, Department of Thoracic Surgery, Fondazione Policlinico Tor Vergata, Tor Vergata University, Rome, Italy

P.H. NAFTEUX, MD
Fockt Clinical Head, Department of Thoracic Surgery, University Hospitals Leuven, Leuven, Belgium

CALVIN S.H. NG, BSc (Hons), MBBS (Hons) (Lon), MD (Lon), FRCS(Edin) (CTh)
Associate Consultant, Division of Cardiothoracic Surgery, Department of Surgery, The Chinese University of Hong Kong, Prince of Wales Hospital, Shatin, N.T. Hong Kong SAR, China

EUGENIO POMPEO, MD
Associate Professor, Department of Thoracic Surgery, Fondazione Policlinico Tor Vergata, Tor Vergata University, Rome, Italy

D. VAN RAEMDONCK, MD, PhD
Clinical Head, Department of Thoracic Surgery, University Hospitals Leuven, Leuven, Belgium

ERINO A. RENDINA, MD
Professor and Chief, Department of Thoracic Surgery, Sant'Andrea Hospital, University of Rome La Sapienza, Via di Grottarossa, Rome, Italy

MITHRAN S. SUKUMAR, MD
Section Chief, Thoracic Surgery, Associate Professor, Division of Cardiothoracic Surgery, Department of Surgery, Portland Veterans Affairs Medical Center, Oregon Health and Sciences University, Portland, Oregon

FEDERICO TACCONI, MD
Assistant Professor, Department of Thoracic Surgery, Fondazione Policlinico Tor Vergata, Tor Vergata University, Rome, Italy

FEDERICO VENUTA, MD
Associate Professor, Division of Thoracic Surgery, University of Rome La Sapienza, Policlinico Umberto I, Rome, Italy

ANNEMARIE WEISSENBACHER, MD
Department of Visceral, Transplant and Thoracic Surgery, Innsbruck Medical University, Innsbruck, Austria

CAMERON D. WRIGHT, MD
Associate Professor, Division of Thoracic Surgery, Massachusetts General Hospital, Boston, Massachusetts

ANTHONY P.C. YIM, MA (Cantab), DM (Oxon), FRCS (Eng, Edin, Glas), FACS
Professor, Department of Surgery, Division of Cardiothoracic Surgery, The Chinese University of Hong Kong, Prince of Wales Hospital; Director, Minimally Invasive Centre, Union Hospital, Shatin, N.T. Hong Kong SAR, China

MARCIN ZIELIŃSKI, MD, PhD
Department of Thoracic Surgery, Pulmonary Hospital, Zakopane, Poland

Contents

Thoracic Surgery Clinics

Preface
Technical Advances in Mediastinal Surgery

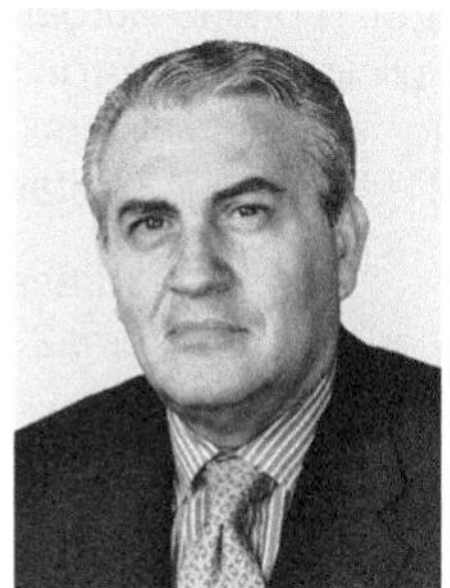

Tommaso C. Mineo, MD
Guest Editor

When nature accomplished its task, the mediastinum resulted as one of the most anatomically complex regions of the human body. A real Pandora's box, it is a relatively inaccessible area containing different structures whose surgical dominium represented a long-lasting challenge. The multiplicity of conditions and diseases that afflict the mediastinal organs adds to the challenge when considering surgical therapeutic solutions.

Over time, different surgical approaches and techniques have been developed and many of these have benefited from continuing refinements and improvements, mainly related to the ability and creativity of surgeons themselves. In this light, cervical mediastinoscopy introduced in 1959 by Carlens, can be considered the very first minimally invasive diagnostic-endoscopic surgical technique, whereas transcervical thymectomy, popularized by Papatestas in 1975, was the first minimally invasive mediastinal major surgical procedure.

It was necessary to wait several decades before relevant technologic advances could favor a real jump ahead in surgical evolution that culminated in the development of video-assisted thoracic surgery (VATS). This advance has been rapidly supported by technical innovations in radiologic diagnostic tools culminating in CT imaging. Hence, several minor and major thoracic procedures could be performed safely by mini-invasive surgery.

Classic open surgery as well has continued to develop new frontiers and improved results taking advantage mainly of significant developments in surgical technology, anesthesiology, and intensive care.

As a result, all mediastinal surgery has greatly profited from these advances, which increased the possibility of successfully performing aggressive demolitive-reconstructive operations. At the same time, video-assisted surgery has rendered many procedures safer, less traumatic, and more effective with improved surgical and cosmetic results and relevant benefits in cost-effectiveness. In addition, VATS has allowed patients and referring physicians to be more participative and less reluctant to accept surgery.

Since my first surgical steps, surgery of the mediastinum has fascinated me and continues to do so thanks to the continuing technical improvements, many of which I have had the opportunity to use during my 40 years of surgical activity.

For these reasons I was delighted to accept the invitation to edit this issue of the *Thoracic Surgery Clinics* devoted to technical advances in mediastinal surgery.

I would like to address special thanks to all the distinguished colleagues who have participated in this project by submitting their outstanding contributions. They are all surgeons with highly consolidated experience in mediastinal surgery whom I asked to give overviews in their fields of specific expertise and ability.

I have no doubt that all of the contributors undertook their assignments with particular

Thorac Surg Clin 20 (2010) xi–xii
doi:10.1016/j.thorsurg.2010.02.009
1547-4127/10/$ – see front matter

energy and enthusiasm. I was sure that texts would provide not only excellent state-of-the-art information but also a strong stimulus for further investigation in this evolving field of thoracic surgery.

I would also like to express my gratitude to Dr Mark Ferguson, consulting editor, for his decision to revisit this fascinating topic of thoracic surgery and for having entrusted me for this most pleasant task.

I am very grateful to Mrs Catherine Bewick and appreciate her discreet promptness, vivid attention, and constant support that greatly facilitated our job.

Thanks to everybody.

Tommaso C. Mineo, MD
Department of Thoracic Surgery
Fondazione Policlinico Tor Vergata
Tor Vergata University
Viale Oxford 81, Rome 00133, Italy

E-mail address:
mineo@med.uniroma2.it

Cervical Videomediastinoscopy

T. Lerut, PhD, MD*, P. De Leyn, PhD, MD,
W. Coosemans, PhD, MD, H. Decaluwé, MD, G. Decker, MD,
Ph. Nafteux, MD, D. Van Raemdonck, PhD, MD

KEYWORDS

- Videomediastinoscopy • Cervical mediastinoscopy
- Non–small cell lung cancer • Cancer staging

Cervical mediastinoscopy is widely used to explore the upper part of the mediastinum in patients with suspicion of mediastinal disease or presenting with mediastinal lymphadenopathy. Cervical mediastinoscopy is mainly used, however, as an invasive staging procedure in non–small cell lung cancer (NSCLC). The history of mediastinoscopy goes back to over half a century ago, when Harken and colleagues[1] first described the technique in 1954. Over time the procedure underwent several refinements, and the technique as it is still used today has to be credited to the Swedish ear, nose, and throat surgeon Carlens.[2] However, cervical mediastinoscopy through a pretracheal suprasternal approach became popular within the thoracic surgical community mainly through the efforts of F.G. Pearson in Toronto.[3] He proved that the presence of involved mediastinal lymph nodes in patients with lung cancer resulted in a dismal prognosis, and suggested the abandonment of resectional surgery in such cases. This pioneering work on the prognostic importance of mediastinal lymph node involvement in NSCLC laid the basis of the subsequent development of an internationally accepted lymph node map by Mountain and Dressler,[4] which is still used today.

CERVICAL VIDEOMEDIASTINOSCOPY

One of the drawbacks of mediastinoscopy is that it obliges the surgeon to work in an uncomfortable position. Only the surgeon has a view through the instrument. Teaching therefore is extremely difficult because of the danger of damaging vital organs. The development of videoscopic and video-assisted technology in the last decade of the twentieth century opened new perspectives in surgical practice, initially in abdominal surgery but later also in thoracic surgery. The senior author of this article (T.L.) is credited for developing in 1989 the concept of what is now called videomediastinoscopy. A right-angled scope containing a working channel used by gynecologists for sterilization through tubal ligation was assembled into a classic mediastinoscope, allowing not only the surgeon but also the assisting surgeon and theater nurses to watch the intervention. After some further tests, a first model of videomediastinoscope was developed in cooperation with the Storz company (**Fig. 1**A). This concept of videomediastinoscopy was brought to the attention of the international thoracic surgical community at the First International Symposium on thoracoscopic surgery in San Antonio, Texas in January 1993 and subsequently published in *Annals of Thoracic Surgery* in the same year.[5] Later on, the instrumentation of the videomediastinoscope was further developed and refined by different researchers and companies.[6–9]

Because the working channel of the mediastinoscope remains unchanged, the surgical procedure can be performed under direct vision as usual, but the build-in options can be connected to a video camera, allowing simultaneous video recording and viewing on a TV monitor (see **Fig. 1**B).

Department of Thoracic Surgery, University Hospitals Leuven, Herestraat 49, 3000 Leuven, Belgium
* Corresponding author.
E-mail address: Toni.Lerut@uzleuven.be

Thorac Surg Clin 20 (2010) 195–206
doi:10.1016/j.thorsurg.2010.01.006
1547-4127/10/$ – see front matter

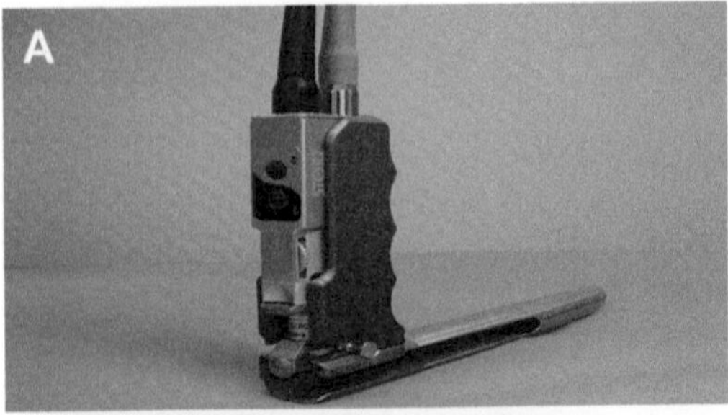

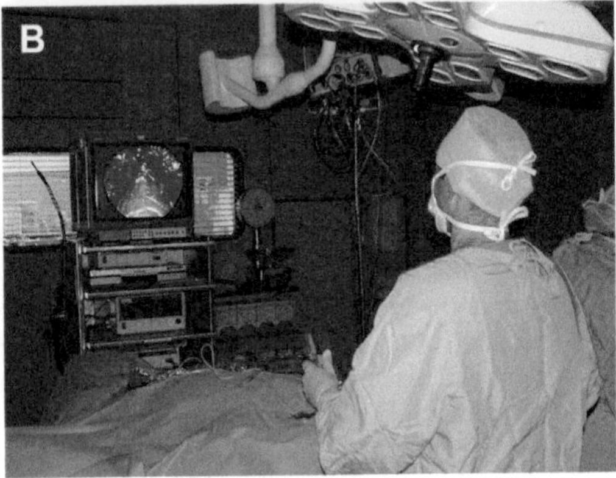

Fig. 1. (*A*) The Lerut scope (K. Storz, Tüttlingen, Germany) resembles the normal mediastinoscope with light optics built into the framework of the scope. (*B*) Operation room setup for videomediastinoscopy. (*From* De Leyn P, Lerut T. Videomediastinoscopy. Multimedia Man Cardiothorac Surg doi:10.1510/mmcts.2004.000166. Copyright © European Association for Cardiothoracic Surgery.)

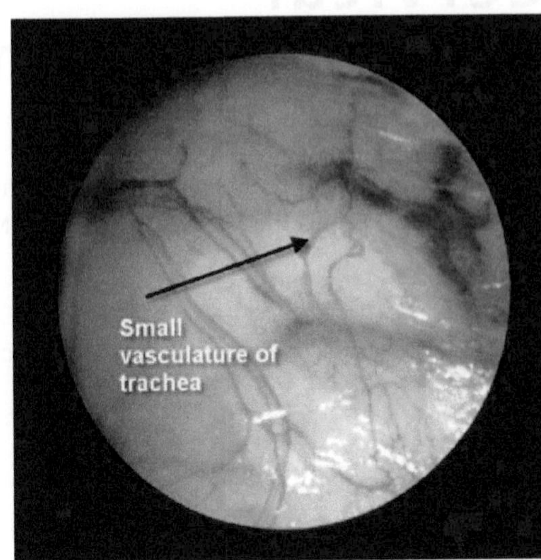

Fig. 2. Improved visualization y the use of the videomediastinoscopy. The magnification on the screen offers a much more detailed image. Even the small vascularization of the trachea is clearly visible at this level of magnification. (*From* De Leyn P, Lerut T. Videomediastinoscopy. Multimedia Man Cardiothorac Surg doi:10.1510/mmcts.2004.000166. Copyright © 2005 European Association for Cardiothoracic Surgery.)

The advantages are the following:

1. The operation can still be performed under direct vision, even when the telescope is inserted and a video camera is connected. However, the magnified image on the screen offers a highly detailed image. As a result, a more accurate and extensive dissection is possible[6,7] (**Fig. 2**).
2. Classic mediastinoscopy is a difficult procedure to teach, because the working channel is narrow. With direct and simultaneous video recording on a TV monitor, several people can watch the operation. Thus, this technique offers greater teaching capabilities. A recent paper has shown that the learning curve of videomediastinoscopy is low compared with conventional mediastinoscopy. This study reported that after a short learning curve, trainees were able to identify all stations, obtain adequate histologic samples, and perform the procedure without direct assistance in more than 20% of the cases.[10]
3. Mediastinoscopy is accepted worldwide as a key procedure for the staging of lung cancer. However, there seems to be great variation in the way that biopsies are sampled. Recording the surgical procedure on videotape may result in greater accuracy of judgment during clinicopathological discussions.
4. Widespread international use of videotaped mediastinoscopy may lead to better understanding and standardization of this procedure.
5. Videomediastinoscopy has generated new refinements and variations on the existing technique of mediastinoscopy.

SURGICAL TECHNIQUE OF VIDEOMEDIASTINOSCOPY

The technique and approach of cervical videomediastinoscopy is not different from that of conventional mediastinoscopy. The patient is brought under general anesthesia with the endotracheal tube positioned on the left corner of the mouth (or for the left-handed surgeon at the right corner) (**Fig. 3**).

The neck is extended by placing a shoulder roll behind the shoulders but avoiding “floating” of the head. The patient is then draped in such a way that the anterior part of the chest is also

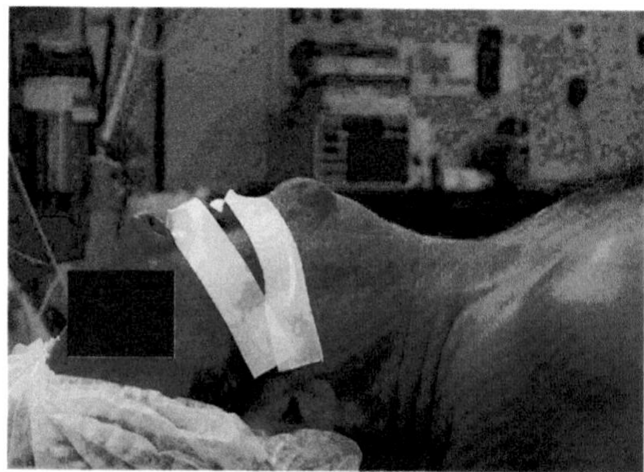

Fig. 3. The endotracheal tube is positioned at the left corner of the mouth, with the anesthesia equipment at the patients left side. The table should be horizontal or slightly tilted foot downwards to reduce venous congestion. For left-handed surgeons, the installation may be mirrored to the right side. (*From* De Leyn P, Lerut T. Conventional mediastinoscopy. Multimedia Man Cardiothorac Surg doi:10.1510/mmcts.2004.000158; with permission. Copyright © 2005 European Association for Cardio-thoracic Surgery.)

part of the operative field, in case an urgent median sternotomy should be necessary. A transverse incision, 1 finger breadth proximal from the manubrium sternum, is made. The pretracheal muscles are separated vertically in the midline to expose the anterior surface of the trachea, and the isthmus of the thyroid is retracted superiorly. The trachea is now exposed and the pretracheal fascia incised, and the dissection is now continued (**Fig. 4**).

The surgeon's index finger is advanced along the pretracheal plane, and the mediastinum is carefully palpated for the presence of nodal disease. This palpation is of extreme importance, because pretracheal nodes are more easily palpated than visualized. The finger is withdrawn then the mediastinoscope is introduced and advanced. The plane in front of the mediastinoscope is developed with the use of blunt dissection, using a metal sucker through the channel of the mediastinoscope (**Fig. 5**).

Small bleeding vessels can be coagulated. One has to be very careful with coagulation at the left paratracheal side because of the presence of the left recurrent nerve (**Fig. 6**).

Bleeding at this side is best handled with hemostatic gauze introduced through the mediastinoscope. Before taking a biopsy from a lymph node, the node should be mobilized as much as possible to ensure that the structure under view is a lymph node and not a major vessel. This mobilization is usually performed easily by the use of a suction device. In case of doubt, the lymph node can be punctured by a long aspiration needle under negative suction to ensure that the structure to be biopsied is not a vessel. However, with adequate mobilization and clear identification of the anatomic landmark structures, such a maneuver will rarely be necessary. The lymph node is grasped by a biopsy forceps (**Fig. 7**).

In case of resistance while exerting traction, one has to be aware of the possible adherence of the node to an adjacent vessel, for example, azygos vein, first branch of the pulmonary artery, or the innominate artery. Pulling too strong may result in a vascular tear and major bleeding.

Usually the node stations along the trachea are the first to be biopsied, the subcarinal nodes being biopsied last (**Fig. 8**). This order is followed because the subcarinal nodes are surrounded by a denser vascularization, more easily causing bleeding and thus hampering the surgeon's view.

When substantial bleeding occurs, packing should be done immediately. Packing for at least 10 minutes causes most—even seemingly dramatic—bleeding to stop. Through the mediastinoscope, vascular clips can be placed easily. If packing and vascular clips have no effect, right thoracotomy (for bleeding of the azygos vein, caval vein, or right pulmonary artery) or median sternotomy (for bleeding from the aorta or innominate artery and vein) may be necessary.

Using cervical mediastinoscopy, the following nodal stations (according to the Mountain/Dressler modification[4] from the Naruke/American Thoracic Society-North American Lung Cancer Study Group [ATS-LCSG][11] map) can be sampled: the highest mediastinal nodes (level 1), left and right upper paratracheal nodes (levels 2L and 2R), left and right lower paratracheal nodes (levels 4L and 4R), and subcarinal nodes (level 7). The posterior subcarinal nodes (level 3), paraesophageal nodes (level 8), inferior pulmonary ligament nodes (level 9), subaortic nodes (level 5), and para-aortic nodes (level 6) cannot be biopsied using standard cervical mediastinoscopy (**Fig. 9**).

COMPLICATIONS

Complications are rare and usually not life threatening. Unless additional or more extensive procedures are performed under the same general anesthesia and provided the patient's condition permits, the procedure can be performed on an outpatient basis.[12] In experienced hands, cervical mediastinoscopy has no mortality and minimal morbidity. In a review by Kirschner[13] of more than 20,000 cases, complications did not surpass

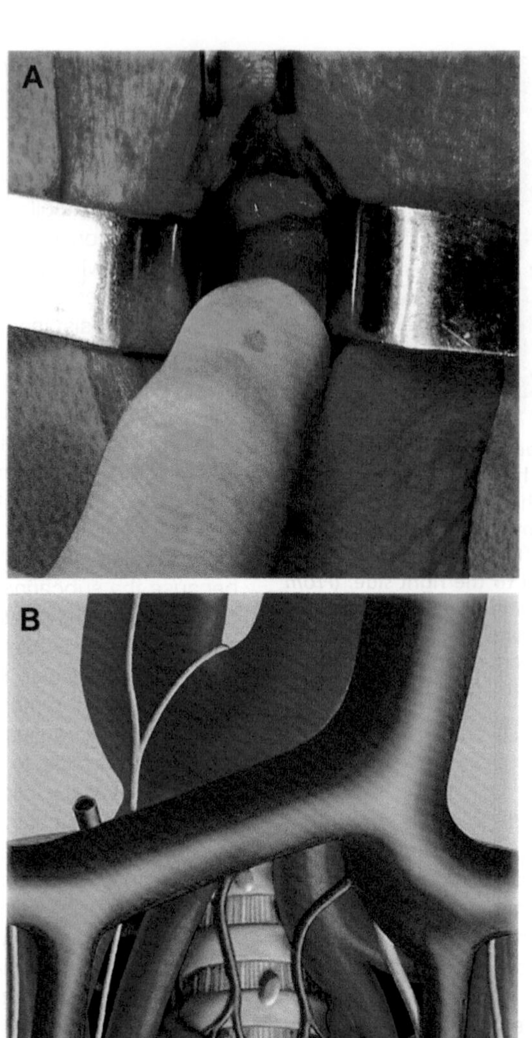

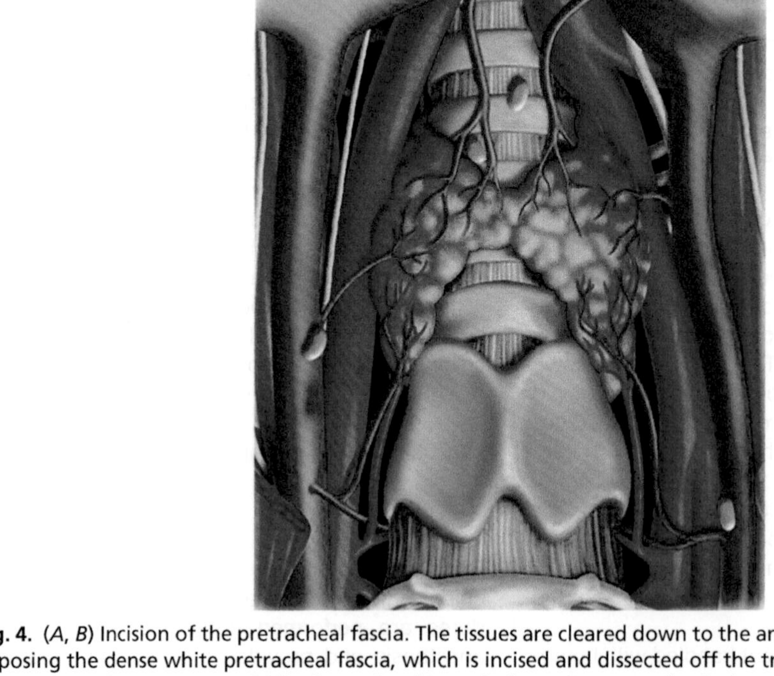

Fig. 4. (*A*, *B*) Incision of the pretracheal fascia. The tissues are cleared down to the anterior surface of the trachea exposing the dense white pretracheal fascia, which is incised and dissected off the trachea exposing the cartilaginous rings. The surgeon's middle finger is advanced along the pretracheal plane and blunt dissection is performed along the anterior surface of the trachea down to the carina. (*From* De Leyn P, Lerut T. Conventional mediastinoscopy. Multimedia Man Cardiothorac Surg doi:10.1510/mmcts.2004.000158; with permission. Copyright © 2005 European Association for Cardio-thoracic Surgery)

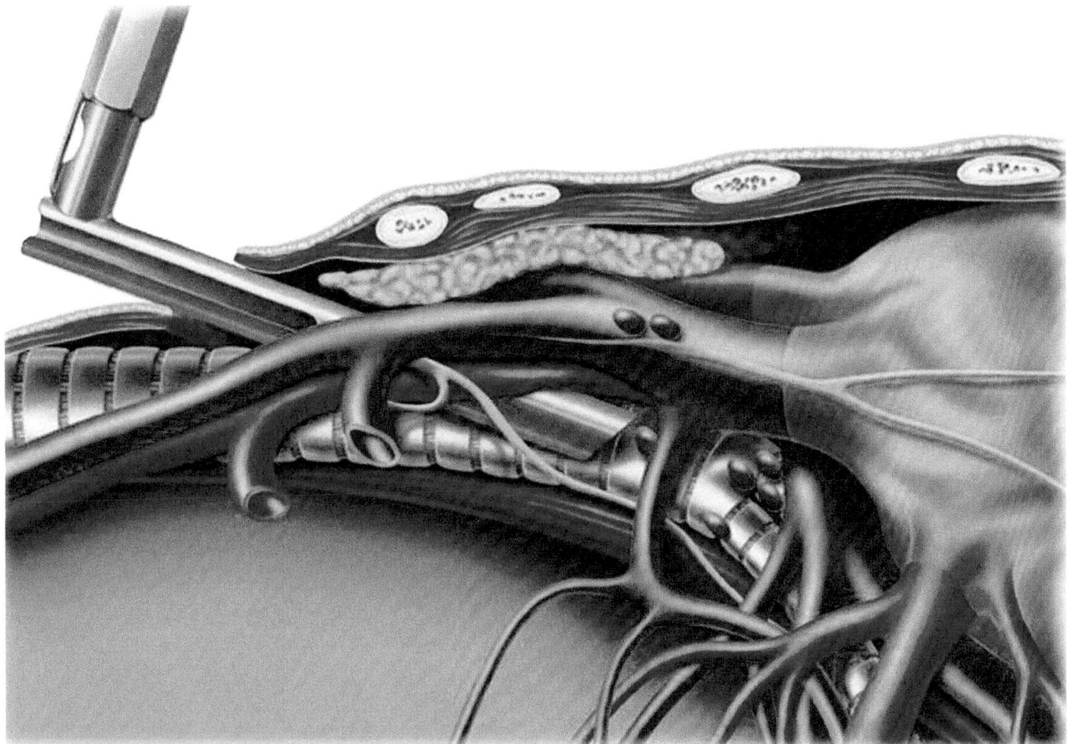

Fig. 5. The mediastinoscope is further advanced. (*From* De Leyn P, Lerut T. Conventional mediastinoscopy. Multimedia Man Cardiothorac Surg doi:10.1510/mmcts.2004.000158; with permission. Copyright © 2005 European Association for Cardio-thoracic Surgery)

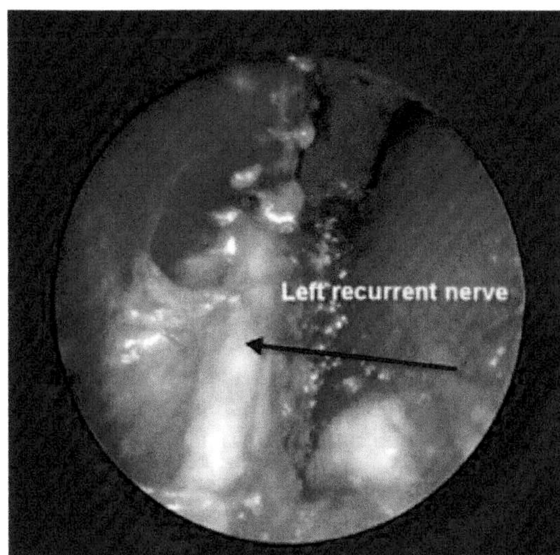

Fig. 6. The left recurrent nerve lies approximately 1 cm lateral to the trachea and can usually be visualized in the midtracheal plane. From there it can be followed more distally. (*From* De Leyn P, Lerut T. Videomediastinoscopy. Multimedia Man Cardiothorac Surg doi:10.1510/mmcts.2004.000166. Copyright © 2005 European Association for Cardio-thoracic Surgery)

2.5% and mortality was less than 0.5%, with only 0.1% to 0.5% of all complications considered as major. The most important major complication is severe bleeding.

The most frequent cause of bleeding is caused by damage to the branches of the bronchial arteries that run through the subcarinal region. By taking advantage of the magnification effect of videomediastinoscopy, these vessels can easily be seen and "biopsying" them avoided. If they are damaged, applying some pressure temporarily, for example, using the suction device or by temporarily packing the space for 5 to 10 minutes using a narrow-gauze pad, will suffice to stop the bleeding. After removing the gauze, the vessel can be clipped to secure permanent hemostasis. Other vessels that may be injured are the azygos vein or the right upper lobe branch of the pulmonary artery. Again, gauze packing may stop the bleeding if the azygos vein has been injured, and subsequent clipping will permanently stop further bleeding. However, in some instances packing may not solve the problem. In such a case the easiest way to proceed is to firmly pack the mediastinum and to turn the patient for a thoracotomy to repair the

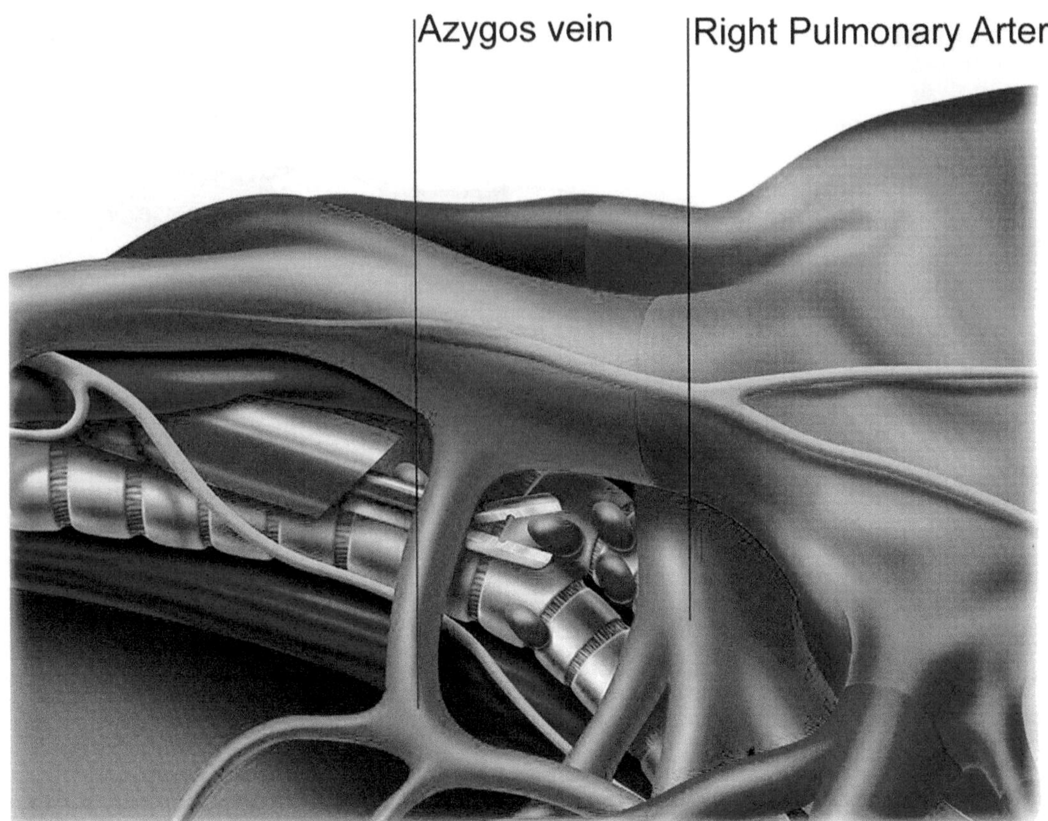

Fig. 7. To avoid and to handle major complications, it is important to visualize the anatomic landmarks such as the azygos vein, the right and left main bronchus, and the first branch of the right pulmonary artery before biopsies are taken. (*From* De Leyn P, Lerut T. Conventional mediastinoscopy. Multimedia Man Cardiothorac Surg doi:10.1510/mmcts.2004.000158; with permission. Copyright © 2005 European Association for Cardio-thoracic Surgery)

vessel. If a left-sided resection was planned, a median sternotomy is the preferred approach, although exposure is less optimal and one may consider separate bilateral thoracotomy to solve the problem. Injury to the aorta or innominate artery is extremely rare unless the sight is obscured by extensive tumor mass or when the space is obliterated as a result of radiotherapy. The best way to avoid injury to these vessels is to make sure to keep the trachea and bronchus visible.

Another structure at risk for injury is the left recurrent nerve. Vocal cord paralysis may result in hoarseness and poor cough, thus increasing the risk for postoperative pulmonary infection.

Injury can be avoided by visualizing the nerve, being extremely cautious when taking biopsies at the level of the left tracheobronchial angle, and avoiding by all means the use of electrocautery in this particular area. If a permanent lesion of the nerve is anticipated, thyroplasty to avoid further pulmonary complications should be considered.

Injury to the trachea or main stem bronchus is possible, and can be managed by leaving a small drain behind.

Injury of the esophagus is possible when dissecting the subcarinal or left tracheobronchial space. Pain and mediastinal emphysema in the immediate postoperative period should alert the surgeon if the injury was not detected at the time of mediastinoscopy. If the tear is small and detected at the time of surgery, simple drainage, and nil by mouth and antibiotic treatment for a few days may solve the problem. If the injury to the esophagus is suspected in the immediate postoperative period, endoscopy or water-soluble contrast study has to be performed to confirm diagnosis. A small contained leak can be treated conservatively, but if there is a free leak into the mediastinum, prompt repair through a right thoracotomy or video-assisted thoracoscopic surgery (VATS) approach is the therapy of choice.

An analysis of a cohort of 4000 consecutive mediastinoscopies from the authors' own center

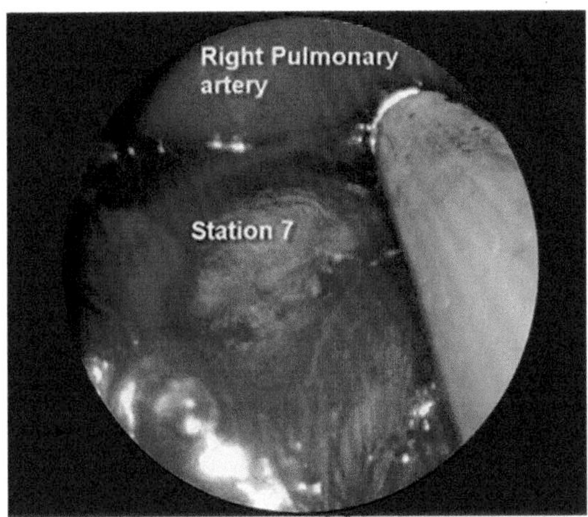

Fig. 8. Stepwise, the paratracheal tissues are entered to expose the lymph nodes at the various stations. The lymph nodes lie outside of the fascial envelope (as in this illustration in the subcarinal area and the lower paratracheal area). When the mediastinoscope reaches the subcarinal area, a thin layer of firm fibrous tissue has to be broken to visualize the subcarinal nodes. Beneath the subcarinal nodes, the esophagus can be visualized. (*From* De Leyn P, Lerut T. Conventional mediastinoscopy. Multimedia Man Cardiothorac Surg doi:10.1510/mmcts.2004.000158; with permission. Copyright © 2005 European Association for Cardiothoracic Surgery)

revealed no hospital mortality.[14] Major bleeding requiring immediate intervention occurred in 4 patients. Injury of the esophagus was seen in 1 patient in whom the mediastinum was drained through the mediastinoscopy incision, and the fistula dried up after a few days of conservative treatment. In 1 patient a tear of the left main stem bronchus was successfully repaired by endoscopic suturing through the videomediastinoscope.

PLACE OF CERVICAL MEDIASTINOSCOPY IN THE DIAGNOSTIC ALGORITHM OF NSCLC

For decades cervical mediastinoscopy was the gold standard for staging of patients with operable NSCLC. In a recent review it appeared that sensitivity of cervical mediastinoscopy varies between 72% and 89%, the average being 81%, and with a negative predictive value (NPV) of 91%.[15] Videomediastinoscopy, through improved visualization of the operative field, definitely has the potential to lead to an even higher accuracy.[7]

Positron emission tomography (PET) scanning, introduced in the late 1990s, as well as the more recently integrated PET/computed tomography (CT), have enhanced the diagnostic accuracy of mediastinal lymph node involvement in comparison with CT alone. Sensitivity of 84% and NPV of 93% for PET are comparable with those of mediastinoscopy but the positive predictive value and specificity of PET appear to be lower than those of mediastinoscopy[15] (**Table 1**). Because of the high NPV of PET, in particular in peripheral tumors, it is now accepted that mediastinoscopy can generally be omitted in patients with clinical stage I NSCLC in peripheral tumors with negative PET images, sufficient fluorodeoxyglucose uptake in the primary tumor, and a diameter of the largest lymph nodes of less than 16 mm. As a result, the number of mediastinoscopies has gone down by more than 50% in centers that have PET or PET/CT at their disposal.[16]

A new "player in the field" is the recent introduction of endobronchial ultrasound (EBUS) and endoesophageal ultrasound (EUS) combined with fine-needle aspiration (FNA) as an invasive nonsurgical staging of the mediastinal nodes in NSCLC. A recent review of the literature has indicated a pooled sensitivity of 88%, a specificity of 91%, a positive predictive value of 98%, and NPV of 77%[15] for EUS. Annema and colleagues[17] showed that the combination of mediastinoscopy and EUS-FNA significantly improved sensitivity and NPV because EUS + FNA reaches stations 5 and 8, which are not accessible to mediastinoscopy. For EBUS a recent review of 8 publications revealed a sensitivity of 90% and a specificity of 100%, with an NPV of 76%.[18]

An advantage of EBUS is that it also reaches stations 10 to 12. Herth and colleagues[19] recently demonstrated an impressive sensitivity of 89% for EBUS in suspected malignant lymph nodes in patients with normal radiological staging on CT and PET.

The downside of this technology is that it is very much operator dependent. Nevertheless, it appears that EBUS/EUS + FNA is increasingly replacing mediastinoscopy in provision of histologic proof of suspicious mediastinal lymph nodes, albeit there is consensus that it cannot be used to exclude mediastinal lymph node disease because of the lower NPV. For this reason mediastinoscopy remains indicated if EBUS and/or EUS + FNA yield negative results in the presence of otherwise suspicious nodes on CT or PET (**Fig. 10**).[20]

For left upper lobe tumors, the subaortic nodes (level 5) and para-aortic nodes (level 6) are frequently involved. These nodes cannot be biopsied by routine cervical mediastinoscopy. Ginsberg and colleagues[21] described a technique to explore these levels through the cervical incision. After the cervical mediastinoscopy is completed, blunt dissection is performed between the innominate and carotid arteries, and the mediastinoscope is

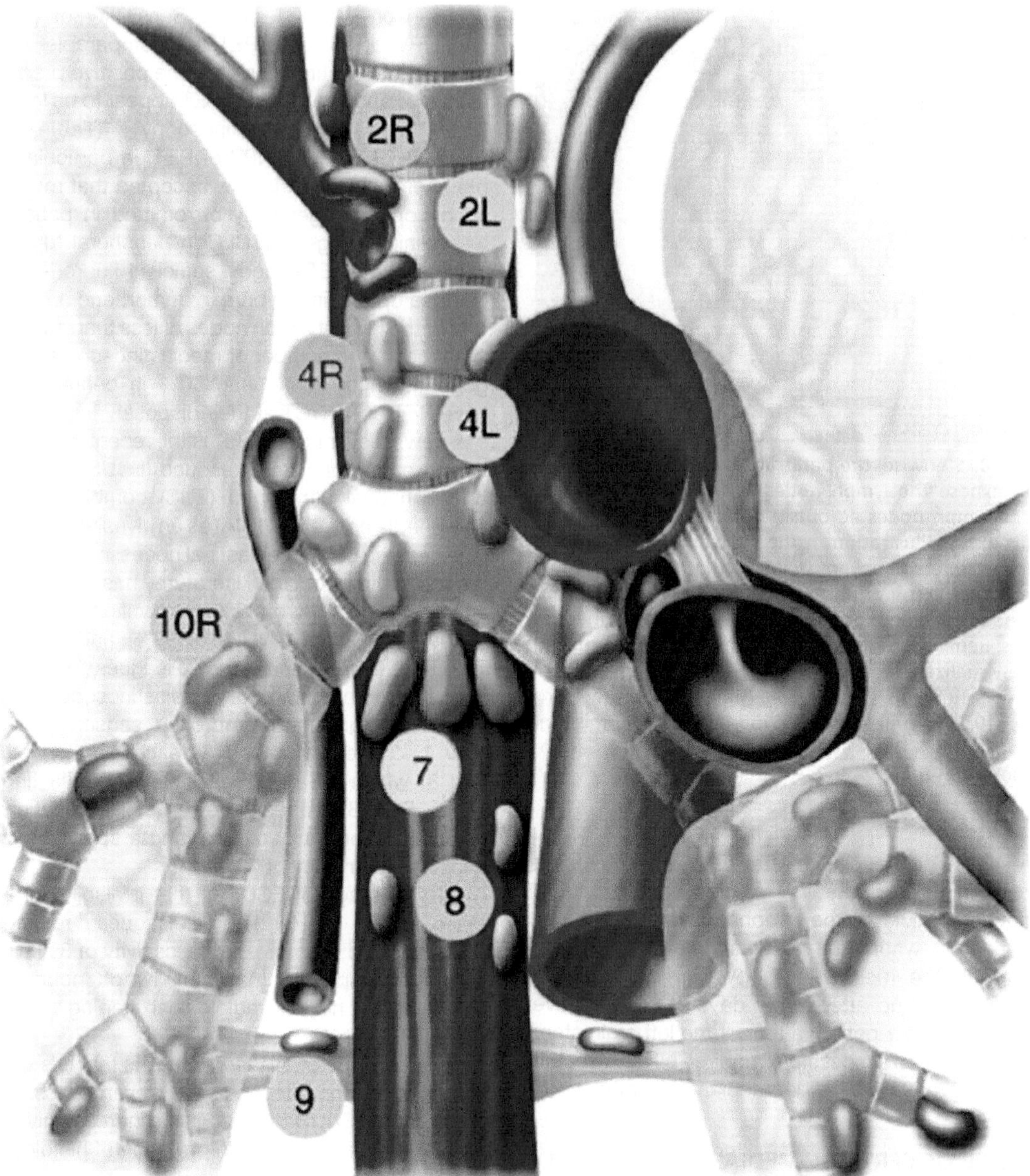

Fig. 9. Mountain/Dressler map showing nodal stations used in staging of NSCLC. By cervical mediastinoscopy the following nodal stations (according to the Mountain/Dressler modification, 1997 from Naruke/ATS-LCSG map[11]) can be searched for and biopsied: the left and right upper paratracheal nodes (stations 2L and 2R), left and right lower paratracheal nodes (stations 4L and 4R), and the subcarinal nodes (station 7). In the mean time the AJCC cancer staging manual 7th edition has adopted a new proposal by the International Association for the Study of Lung Cancer (IASLC) on mapping of nodal status. (*From* De Leyn P, Lerut T. Conventional mediastinoscopy. Multimedia Man Cardiothorac Surg doi:10.1510/mmcts.2004.000158; with permission. Copyright © 2005 European Association for Cardio-thoracic Surgery)

introduced above the aortic arch. In experienced hands, this technique has a high level of accuracy and minimal morbidity.[21,22]

However, a valid alternative that may be preferred by most surgeons is the anterior mediastinoscopy (Chamberlain procedure) or VATS.

VIDEO-ASSISTED MEDIASTINOSCOPIC LYMPHADENECTOMY AND TRANSCERVICAL EXTENDED MEDIASTINAL LYMPHADENECTOMY

The introduction of the videomediastinoscopy has resulted in further development in techniques to

Table 1
Performance of different staging technique

Technique	Sensitivity, %	Specificity, %	NPV, %	PPV, %	Prevalence, %
CT	57	82	83	56	28
PET	84	89	93	79	32
EUS + FNA	88	91	77	98	69
EBUS + FNA	90	100	76	NA	68
Mediastinoscopy	81	100	91	100	87

Data from Toloza E, Harpole L, Detterbeck F, et al. Invasive staging of non-small cell lung cancer: a review of the current evidence. Chest 2003;123(1):157S–66S; and Detterbeck F, Jantz M, Wallace M, et al. Invasive mediastinal staging of lung cancer. Chest 2007:132;202S–20S.

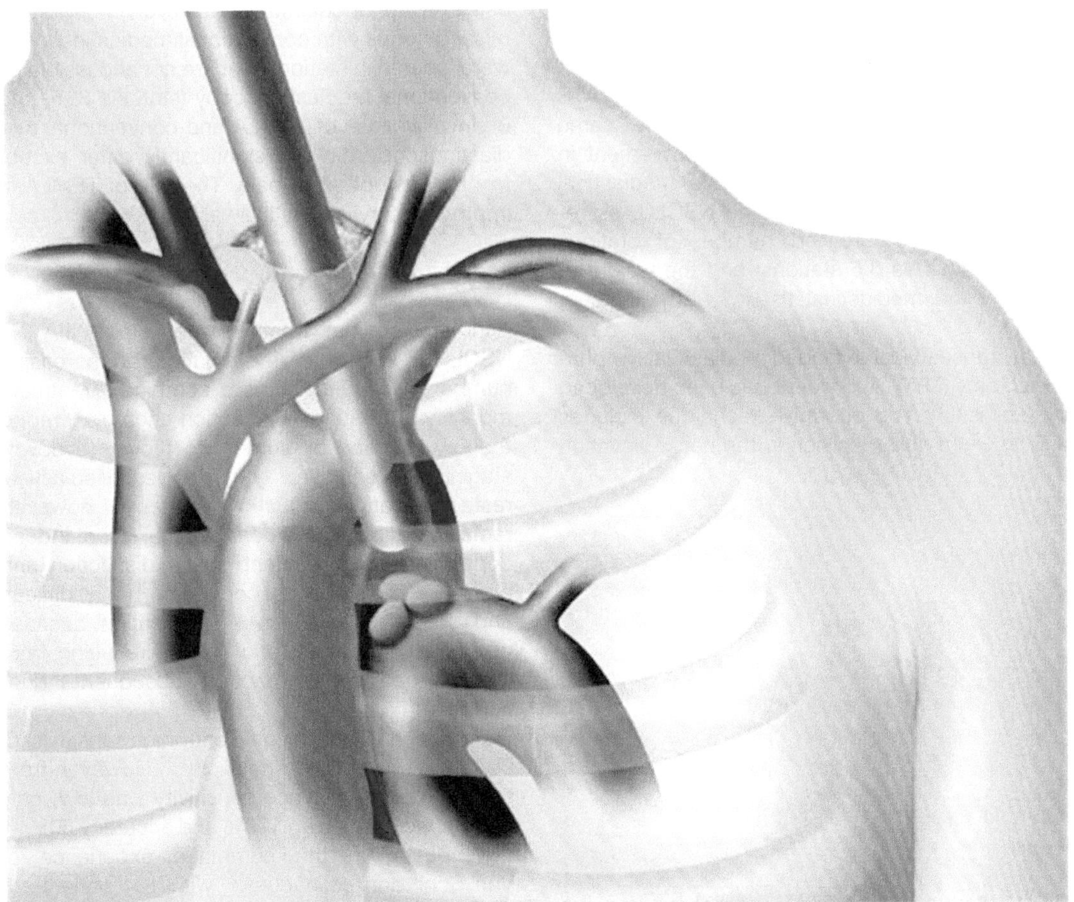

Fig. 10. Extended cervical mediastinoscopy. If the standard cervical mediastinoscopy is negative, a plane can be developed anterior to the aortic arch, down to the subaortic space. To do so, blunt dissection is performed with the finger anterior to the innominate artery, between the innominate artery and the innominate vein. The mediastinoscope is introduced through the cervical incision above the aortic arch. The scope is advanced over the top of the aortic arch down to the aortopulmonary window for biopsy of the lymph nodes. Biopsies of lymph nodes in the aortopulmonary window are taken. (*From* De Leyn P, Lerut T. Conventional mediastinoscopy. Multimedia Man Cardiothorac Surg doi:10.1510/mmcts.2004.000158; with permission. Copyright © 2005 European Association for Cardio-thoracic Surgery)

explore the mediastinum. Hürtgen and colleagues[23] published the concept of video-assisted mediastinoscopic lymphadenectomy (VAMLA). Introduction and positioning of the videomediastinoscope is the same as used in conventional mediastinoscopy. The tracheal bifurcation, the main stem bronchi, and left recurrent nerve are first identified. Bimanual instrumentation through the mediastinoscope allows for bimanual preparation and dissection of the tissues (**Fig. 11**).

The optical enlargement of the videomediastinoscope facilitates the subsequent dissection and removal of the lymph nodes alongside the left recurrent nerve. The next step is the dissection of the subcarinal region. The subcarinal nodes are dissected away from the right and the left main stem bronchus and removed, exposing the esophagus between the 2 main stem bronchi. Finally, the right paratracheal nodes are removed mostly en bloc, visualizing the right mediastinal pleura, the azygos vein, and its confluence with the vena cava. In combining VAMLA with VATS lobectomy and lymphadenectomy, the same investigators claim a significant improvement in the radicality of minimally invasive mediastinal lymphadenectomy in early stage NSCLC, as reflected by the increased number of stations dissected (6.4 vs 3.6 stations) and the weight of the removed mediastinal tissue (11.2 vs 5.5 g; $P<.05$).[24]

The transcervical extended mediastinal lymphadenectomy (TEMLA) concept has been developed by Zielinski.[25] The operative technique includes a 5- to 8-cm collar incision in the neck, elevation of the manubrium sterni with a retractor specially designed for this operation, and bilateral visualization of the laryngeal recurrent nerve and both vagal nerves. All mediastinal lymph node stations can be dissected except for the pulmonary ligament nodes (station 9) and the most distal left paratracheal nodes (station 4L). Most of the procedure is open, but the subcarinal and periesophageal nodes (stations 7 and 8) are removed using the videomediastinoscope. The para-aortic and pulmonary window nodes are removed with the aid of the introduction of the videomediastinoscope. In a prospective study, the same group[26] claimed a significantly higher sensitivity and NPV in detecting unforeseen mediastinal metastasis in NSCLC compared with conventional mediastinoscopy (100% and 100% vs 37.5% and 66.7%) after performing pulmonary resection and extensive mediastinal lymphadenectomy. However, most of the missed nodes with conventional mediastinoscopy were located in stations that are not accessible by conventional mediastinoscopy (stations 8, 5, and 6). Invasiveness of TEMLA and conventional mediastinoscopy did not significantly differ except for the postoperative pain. The role of TEMLA in improving survival is still awaited.

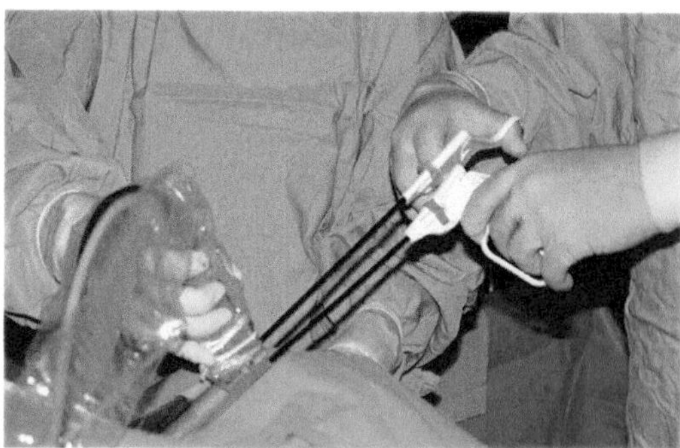

Fig. 11. Because the working channel is somewhat broader and because the instruments do not obscure the view, bimanual dissection is feasible. The scope (here the Storz scope) can be held by an assistant who can also follow the intervention. (*From* De Leyn P, Lerut T. Videomediastinoscopy. Multimedia Man Cardiothorac Surg doi:10.1510/mmcts.2004.000166. Copyright © 2005 European Association for Cardio-thoracic Surgery)

REMEDIASTINOSCOPY

Although optimal treatment for stage IIIA N2 NSCLC is still under investigation, an increasing number of centers favors a combined treatment modality consisting of induction chemo- ± radiotherapy followed by surgery to provide a downstaging of mediastinal lymph nodes. Mediastinal restaging after induction therapy, however, remains a difficult and controversial issue. Indeed depending on the extent of the dissection and biopsies, remediastinoscopy can be a difficult and potentially dangerous intervention because of extensive scarring and fibrosis resulting from the first mediastinoscopy and subsequent induction therapy.

Proponents claim a sufficiently high sensitivity of up to 70% and 100% specificity.[27] However, from the authors' experience sensitivity was low, only 29%, specificity being 100% and accuracy 60%.[28]

Moreover, in the combined experience of Van Schil and colleagues[29] with 104 patients, 3 patients developed severe bleeding during the intervention, resulting in 1 mortality and 1 thoracotomy with pneumonectomy. One can assume that if such events occur in high-volume centers, further diffusion in centers with less experience may result in even more catastrophes. Therefore, consideration must be given to the alternative methods for restaging, in particular PET/CT combined with EBUS and EUS. It might well be that in the future EBUS/EUS may become the first step in confirming the diagnosis of N2 disease, reserving mediastinoscopy for the assessment of the mediastinal lymph node status after the induction therapy.

SUMMARY

Cervical mediastinoscopy is a frequently used technique for assessment of the mediastinum, in particular the mediastinal lymph nodes, in patients presenting with NSCLC. The introduction of videomediastinoscopy has proven to be superior to conventional mediastinoscopy, and has made teaching of this operation much easier. Videomediastinoscopy has also generated further refinements in the technique of mediastinal exploration, in particular technical aspects of the more extensive lymphadenectomy.

However, imaging modalities, in particular PET scanning, have substantially decreased the need for mediastinoscopy in early stage NSCLC. In the more advanced stage IIIA-N2 the indication for primary staging and/or restaging after induction therapy is now challenged by the increasing experience with EBUS/EUS and FNA. Further careful study will redefine the place of cervical mediastinoscopy in the staging of NSCLC.

REFERENCES

1. Harken D, Black H, Clauss R, et al. A simple cervicomediastinal exploration for tissue diagnosis of intrathoracic disease. N Engl J Med 1954;251:1041.
2. Carlens E. Mediastinoscopy: a method for inspection and tissue biopsy in the superior mediastinum. Dis Chest 1959;36:343–52.
3. Pearson FG, Delarue NC, Ilves R, et al. Significance of positive superior mediastinal nodes identified at mediastinoscopy in patients with respectable cancer of the lung. J Thorac Cardiovasc Surg 1982;83:1–11.
4. Mountain C, Dressler C. Regional lymph node classification for lung cancer staging. Chest 1997;111: 1718–23.
5. Coosemans W, Lerut T, Van Raemdonck D. Thoracoscopic surgery: the Belgian experience. Ann Surg 1993;56:721–30.
6. De Leyn P, Lerut T. Videomediastinoscopy. Minimal access in cardiothoracic surgery, vol. 22. Philadelphia: WB Saunders Company; 2000. p. 169–174.
7. De Leyn P, Lerut T. Videomediastinoscopy. Multimedia manual Cardiothoracic Surgery. 2004. DOI:10.1510/mmcts.2004.000166. Available at: http://mmcts.ctsnetjournals.org/cgi/collection/standard_lung_resections?page=2. Accessed January, 2005.
8. Lardinois D, Schallberger A, Betticher D, et al. Postinduction video-mediastinoscopy is as accurate and safe as video-mediastinoscopy in patients without pre-treatment for potentially operable non-small cell lung cancer. Ann Thorac Surg 2003;75: 1102–6.
9. Leschber G, Sperling D, Klemm W, et al. Does videomediastinoscopy improve the results of conventional mediastinoscopy? Eur J Cardiothorac Surg 2008;33(2):289–93.
10. Martin-Ucar AE, Chetty GK, Vaughan R, et al. A prospective audit evaluating the role of video-assisted cervical mediastinoscopy as a training tool. Eur J Cardiothorac Surg 2004;26:393–5.
11. Naruke T, Suemasu K, Ishikawa S. Lymph node mapping and curability at various levels of metastasis in resected lung cancer. J Thorac Cardiovasc Surg 1978;76:832–7.
12. Bonadies J, D'Agostino R, Ruskis A, et al. J Thorac Cardiovasc Surg 1993;106(4):686–8.
13. Kirschner P. Cervical mediastinoscopy. Chest Surg Clin N Am 1996;6(1):1–20.
14. De Leyn P, Lerut T. Conventional mediastinoscopy. Multimedia Manual Cardio thoracic Surgery. DOI:10.1510/mmcts.2004.000158. Available at: http://mmcts.ctsnetjournals.org/cgi/content/full/2005/0324/mmcts.2004.000158. Accessed March, 2005.
15. Toloza E, Harpole L, Detterbeck F, et al. Invasive staging of non-small cell lung cancer: a review of the current evidence. Chest 2003;123(1):157S–66S.
16. De Leyn P, Lardinois D, Van Schil P, et al. ESTS guidelines for preoperative lymph node staging for non-small cell lung cancer. Eur J Cardiothorac Surg 2007;32:1–8.
17. Annema J, Versteegh M, Veselic M, et al. Endoscopic ultrasound added to mediastinoscopy for preoperative staging of patients with lung cancer. JAMA 2005;294(8):931–6.
18. Detterbeck F, Jantz M, Wallace M, et al. Invasive mediastinal staging of lung cancer. Chest 2007; 132:202S–20S.
19. Herth F, Annema J, Eberhardt R, et al. Endobronchial ultrasound with transbronchial needle aspiration for restaging the mediastinum in lung cancer. J Clin Oncol 2008;26(20):3346–50.
20. Medford A, Bennett J, Free C, et al. Mediastinal staging procedures in lung cancer: EBUS, TBNA and mediastinoscopy. Curr Opin Pulm Med 2009; 15:334–42.
21. Ginsberg RJ, Rice TW, Goldberg M, et al. Extended cervical mediastinoscopy. A single procedure for bronchogenic carcinoma of the left upper lobe. J Thorac Cardiovasc Surg 1984;94:673–8.
22. Lopez L, Varela A, Freixinet J, et al. Extended cervical mediastinoscopy: Prospective study of fifty cases. Ann Thorac Surg 1994;7:555–8.
23. Hürtgen M, Friedel G, Toomes H, et al. Radical video-assisted mediastinoscopic lymphadenectomy

(VAMLA)—technique and first results. Eur J Cardiothorac Surg 2002;21:348–51.
24. Witte B, Messerschmidt A, Hillebrand H, et al. Combined videothoracoscopic and videomediastinoscopic approach improves radicality of minimally invasive mediastinal lymphadenectomy for early stage lung carcinoma. Eur J Cardiothorac Surg 2009;35:343–7.
25. Zielinski M. Transcervical extended mediastinal lymphadenectomy: results of staging in two hundred fifty-six patients with non-small cell lung cancer. J Thorac Oncol 2007;2(4):370–2.
26. Kuzdzal J, Zielinski M, Papla B, et al. The transcervical extended mediastinal lymph-adenectomy versus cervical mediastinoscopy in non-small cell lung cancer staging. Eur J Cardiothorac Surg 2007;31:88–94.
27. Van Schil P, van der Schoot J, Poniewierski J, et al. Remediastinoscopy after neoadjuvant therapy for non-small cell lung cancer. Lung Cancer 2002;37(3):281–5.
28. De Leyn P, Stroobants S, De Wever W, et al. Prospective comparative study of integrated positron emission tomography-computed tomography scan compared with remediastinoscopy in the assessment of residual mediastinal lymph node disease after induction chemotherapy for mediastinoscopy-proven stage IIIA-N2 non-small cell lung cancer: a Leuven Lung Cancer Group Study. J Clin Oncol 2006;24(21):3333–9.
29. De Waele M, Serra-Mitjans M, Hendriks J, et al. Accuracy and survival of repeat mediastinoscopy after induction therapy for non-small cell lung cancer in a combined series of 104 patients. Eur J Cardiothorac Surg 2008;33:824–8.

Videothoracoscopic Mediastinal Lymphadenectomy

Thomas A. D'Amico, MD

KEYWORDS

- Videothoracoscopic dissection
- Non–small cell lung cancer
- Thoracoscopic mediastinal lymphadenectomy
- Thoracoscopic lobectomy

Mediastinal lymph node assessment is an integral component of a resection for all stages of non–small cell lung cancer (NSCLC).[1,2] There is argument as to whether there is a therapeutic benefit to complete mediastinal lymph node dissection (MLND) when compared with mediastinal lymph node sampling,[2–4] a question that is answered by the American College of Surgeons Oncology Group (ACOSOG) Z0030 study.[5] Nevertheless, there is no debate that MLND improves the staging of patients with NSCLC at the time of resection by appropriately upstaging patients without clinically obvious lymph node involvement and enabling the use of adjuvant therapy, which may improve survival.[6,7]

Thoracoscopic lobectomy has emerged as an effective strategy for the management of patients with early-stage lung cancer.[1,8–10] When compared with lobectomy by thoracotomy, thoracoscopic lobectomy is associated with shorter hospital stay,[8,9] less postoperative pain,[11,12] superior compliance with adjuvant chemotherapy,[13,14] and fewer overall postoperative complications.[15–17] Concerns regarding oncologic effectives are focused on the ability to achieve complete MLND using the minimally invasive technique.[18,19] The technique and results of thoracoscopic mediastinal lymphadenectomy are reviewed.

TECHNIQUE

Effective thoracoscopic lymphadenectomy depends on a comprehensive understanding of the anatomy (**Fig. 1**), including the correct nomenclature as defined by staging[20,21] and treatment[1] guidelines. Although complete MLND may include all ipsilateral N2 stations, current guidelines recommend that at least 3 stations be included in the resection.[1] For a right upper lobectomy, the most important lymph node stations are the right paratracheal stations, 2R and 4R. For lower lobectomy, the critical station is level 7. Level 5 and level 6 are the key stations for a left upper lobectomy.

The technique of thoracoscopic lymphadenectomy does not differ from the conventional approach using thoracotomy: any maneuver that can be performed during open lymph node dissection may be performed using the minimally invasive strategy, although instrumentation may differ. Although surgeons may use different combinations of ports and access incisions to achieve anatomic pulmonary resection, the incisions used for completion of thoracoscopic lobectomy are enough to complete the lymphadenectomy. In the author's experience, 2 precisely placed incisions, in the eighth intercostal space posterior to the midaxillary line and in the fifth intercostal space anteriorly, facilitate resection in most patients.[22] Although some surgeons perform MLND after the completion of lobectomy, others prefer to begin with lymphadenectomy, using frozen section analysis to determine respectability. Although there is no consensus regarding the 2 strategies, nodal dissection before hilar vascular dissection improves exposure. Lymph node dissection may

Department of Surgery, Duke University Medical Center, Box 3496, Duke South, White Zone, Room 3589, Durham, NC 27710, USA
E-mail address: damic001@mc.duke.edu

Thorac Surg Clin 20 (2010) 207–213
doi:10.1016/j.thorsurg.2010.02.001
1547-4127/10/$ – see front matter

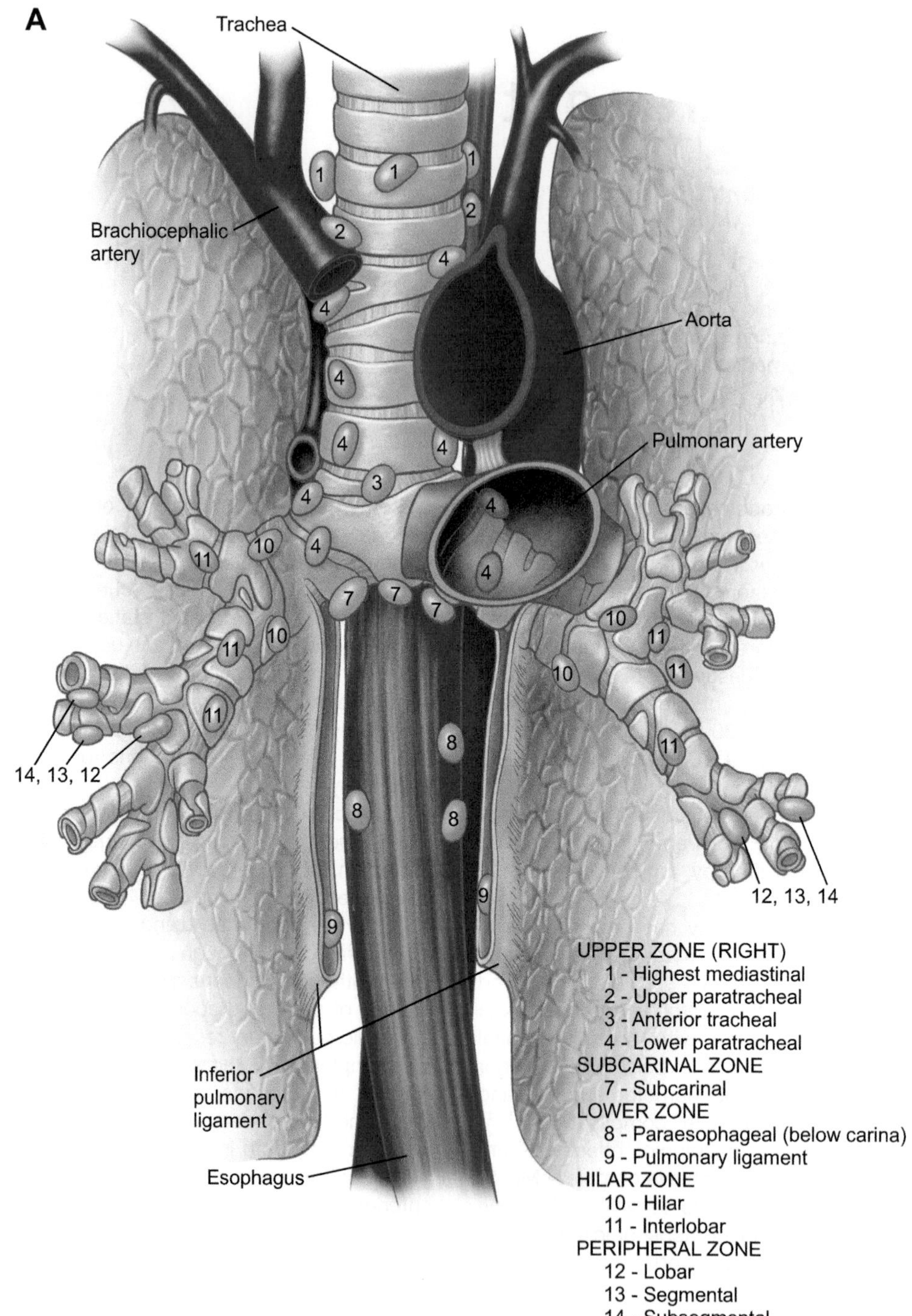

Fig. 1. Mountain-Dresler (MD) lymph node map. The lymph node zones are shown superimposed on the MD-ATS (American Thoracic Society) map. (*Adapted from* Mountain CF, Dresler CM. Regional lymph node classification for lung cancer staging. Chest 1997;111:1718–23; with permission.)

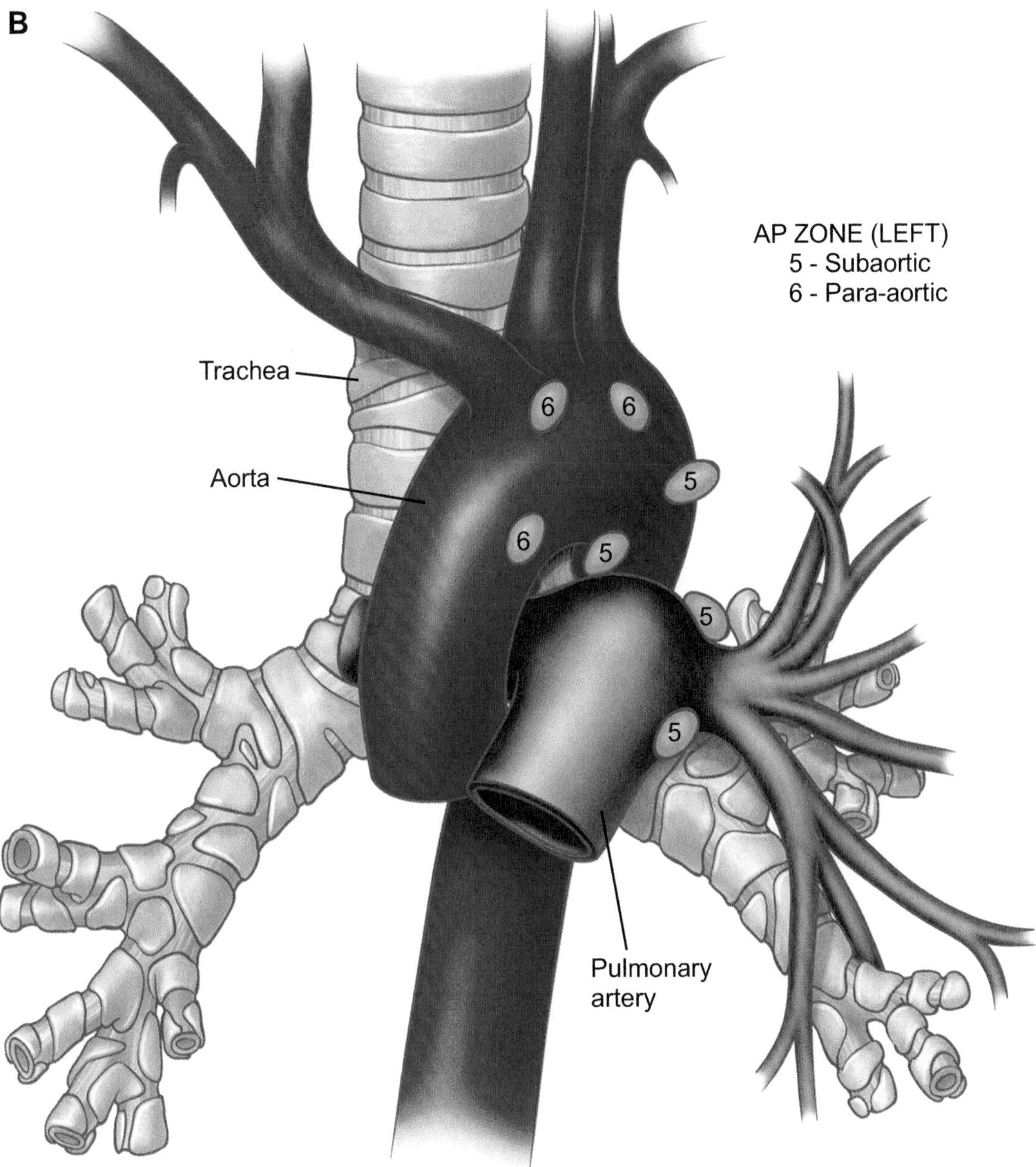

Fig. 1. (*continued*)

be performed using a combination of sharp dissection with clips, blunt dissection, electrocautery, or an alternative energy source. The magnification provided by the use of a videoscope improves the ability to recognize normal structures and identify anomalous conditions, minimizing the risk of complications during nodal dissection.[23]

Anterior paratracheal mediastinal nodal dissection includes resection of all soft tissue (nodal tissue and adipose tissue) between the superior vena cava (anterior border), trachea (posterior border), the pericardium (medial border), the azygos vein (inferior border), and the intersection of the innominate artery and trachea (superior border) (**Fig. 2**). Care should be taken to avoid dissection close to the innominate artery to minimize risk of injury to the right recurrent laryngeal nerve.[23]

Subcarinal lymph node dissection from the right includes the nodal tissue encompassed by the right and left main bronchi, esophagus, and pericardium (**Fig. 3**). Visualization of the thoracic duct is possible in many cases owing to the thoracoscopic camera angles and image magnification,

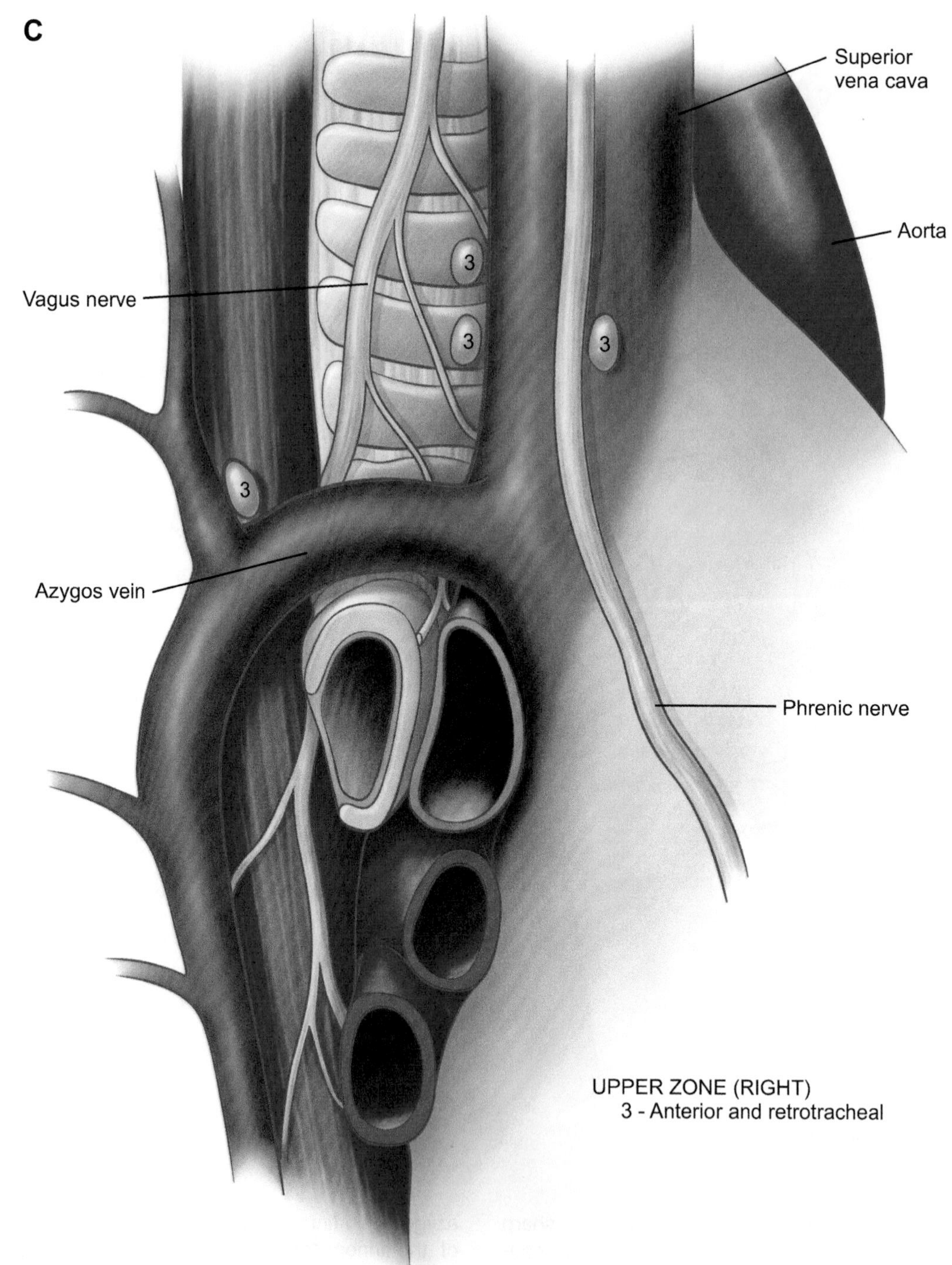

Fig. 1. (*continued*)

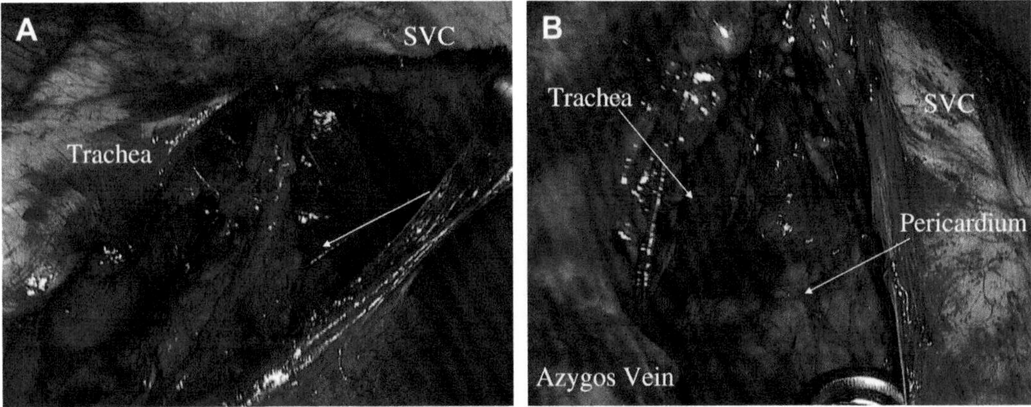

Fig. 2. (*A*) Right anterior paratracheal mediastinal nodal dissection. (*B*) Completed paratracheal mediastinal nodal dissection.

minimizing the risk of postoperative chylothorax[22] (**Fig. 4**). Judiciously increasing the tidal volume delivered to the dependent (left) lung may improve the exposure of the subcarinal station, although barotrauma must be avoided.

On the left, dissection of the lymph nodes in the aortopulmonary window (level 5) and para-aortic station (level 6) is enhanced by video-assisted approach with magnification, allowing thorough and precise nodal dissection with avoidance of the recurrent laryngeal nerve (**Fig. 5**). Thoracoscopic dissection of the subcarinal station from the left side is more difficult than from the right side because the open approach is used. Nevertheless, complete nodal dissection is achieved with adequate retraction and visualization.

Lymphadenectomy of the subcarinal station (or other stations) during mediastinoscopy is an alternative strategy to achieve complete MLND when thoracoscopic lobectomy is performed on the left side.[24–26] Kuzdzal and colleagues[24,25] have demonstrated the feasibility of transcervical extended mediastinal lymphadenectomy (TEMLA) to achieve lymph node dissection. Compared with mediastinoscopy, the sensitivity and the negative predictive value of TEMLA in detecting mediastinal metastases are significantly better. Although TEMLA has not been compared with open or thoracoscopic MLND, it does seem that this technique represents a reasonable strategy to achieve lymphadenectomy. Video-assisted mediastinal lymphadenectomy has been demonstrated to be successful as well, with improved optics and visualization using a camera with magnification.[26]

COMMENT

The ideal strategy of assessment of mediastinal lymph nodes is a topic of debate, which may be settled by a recently completed clinical trial.[5] Purported advantages of complete MLND (as compared with systematic sampling) include

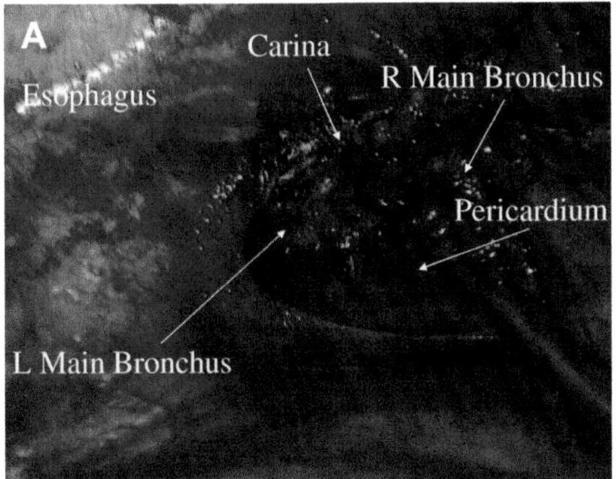

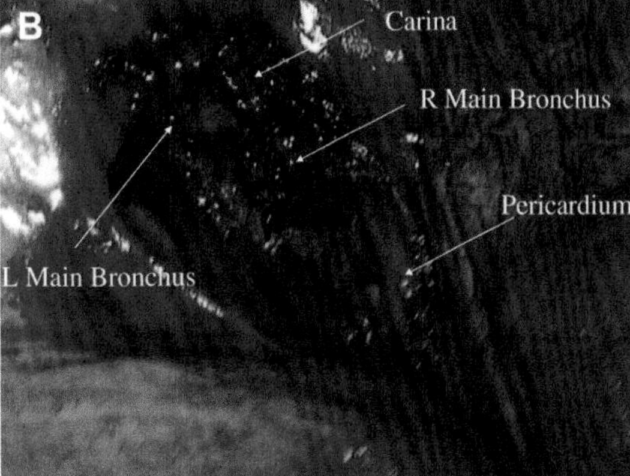

Fig. 3. (*A*) Subcarinal lymph node dissection. (*B*) Completed subcarinal lymph node dissection.

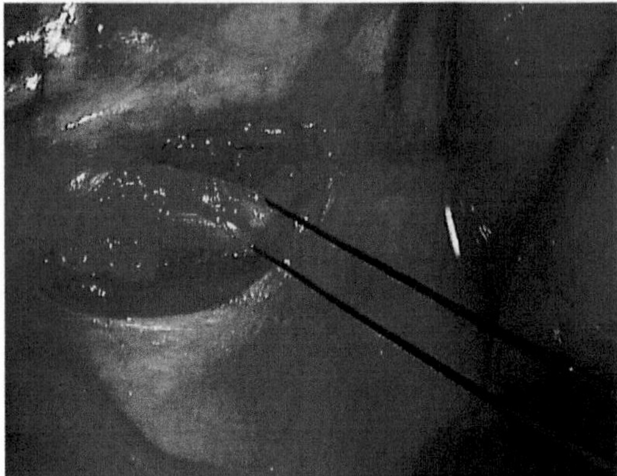

Fig. 4. Thoracic duct.

superior staging as well as improvement in local control and survival.[3,4] There is evidence to support the concept that complete MLND is performed just as effectively using the thoracoscopic approach.

Several studies have been performed, comparing thoracoscopic dissection with conventional lymph node dissection.[27–29] In one study, Kondo and colleagues[29] performed complete MLND during thoracoscopic lobectomy followed by thoracotomy. In this study, 27to 48 lymph nodes were resected thoracoscopically, and subsequent thoracotomy yielded minimal extra lymph node tissue: mean 1.3 and median zero lymph nodes. In the randomized study by Sugi and colleagues,[30] there was no difference in the number of hilar or mediastinal lymph nodes resected using the open or thoracoscopic approaches. Watanabe and colleagues[31] demonstrated similar lymph node resection rates for the open and thoracoscopic approaches in a lobe-specific study.

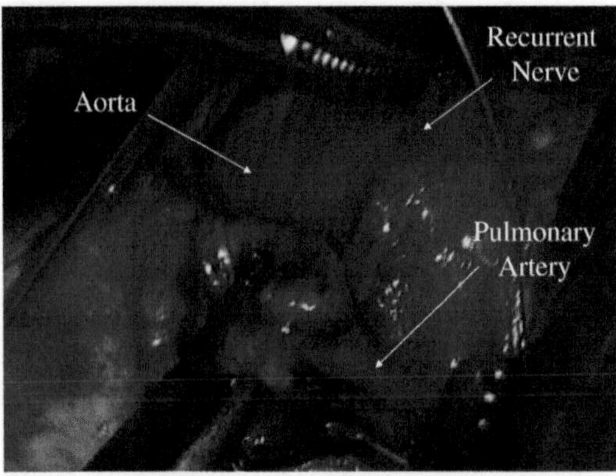

Fig. 5. Aortopulmonary window and para-aortic lymph node stations.

SUMMARY

Mediastinal lymphadenectomy is a crucial element of staging in patients with resectable NSCLC. Thoracoscopic pulmonary resection, accepted as a viable option for patients with clinical stage I and stage II disease, must include effective resection of mediastinal lymph nodes. During thoracoscopic lobectomy, MLND at all stations may be performed safely and effectively, with oncologic results comparable with those of open procedures. In addition, there are many advantages compared with the open procedure, including improved quality of life, fewer complications, and better compliance with adjuvant chemotherapy. The optics of modern video equipment may further improve the efficacy of mediastinal lymphadenectomy, with superior clarity and magnification.

REFERENCES

1. Ettinger DS, Akerly W, Bepler G, et al. National Comprehensive Cancer Network (NCCN). Non-small cell lung cancer clinical practice guidelines in oncology. J Natl Compr Canc Netw 2008;6:228–69.
2. Whitson BA, Groth SS, Maddaus MA. Surgical assessment and intraoperative management of mediastinal lymph nodes in non-small cell lung cancer. Ann Thorac Surg 2007;84:1059–65.
3. Passlick B, Kubuschock B, Sienel W, et al. Mediastinal lymphadenectomy in non-small cell lung cancer effectiveness in patients with or without nodal micrometastases—results of a preliminary study. Eur J Cardiothorac Surg 2002;21:520–6.
4. Keller SM, Adak S, Wagner H, et al. Mediastinal lymph node dissection improves survival in patients with stages II and IIIa non-small cell lung cancer. Eastern Cooperative Oncology Group. Ann Thorac Surg 2000;70:358–65.
5. Allen MS, Darling GE, Pechet TT, et al. Morbidity and mortality of major pulmonary resections in patients with early-stage lung cancer: initial results of the randomized, prospective ACOSOG Z0030 trial. Ann Thorac Surg 2006;81:1013–9.
6. Arriagada R, Bergman B, Dunant A, et al. Cisplatin-based adjuvant chemotherapy in patients with completely resected non-small-cell lung cancer. N Engl J Med 2004;350:351–60.
7. Winton TL, Livingston R, Johnson D, et al. Vinorelbine plus cisplatin vs. observation in resected non–small cell lung cancer. N Engl J Med 2005;352:2589–97.
8. Onaitis MW, Petersen PR, Balderson SS, et al. Thoracoscopic lobectomy is a safe and versatile procedure: experience with 500 consecutive patients. Ann Surg 2006;244:420–5.

9. McKenna RJ, Houck W, Fuller CB. Video-assisted thoracic surgery lobectomy: experience with 1,100 Cases. Ann Thorac Surg 2006;81:421–6.
10. Swanson SJ, Herndon JE, D'Amico TA, et al. Video-assisted thoracic surgery (VATS) lobectomy–report of CALGB 39802: a prospective, multi-institutional feasibility study. J Clin Oncol 2007;25:4993–7.
11. Demmy TL, Curtis JJ. Minimally invasive lobectomy directed toward frail and high-risk patients: a case control study. Ann Thorac Surg 1999;68:194–200.
12. Nagahiro I, Andou A, Aoe M, et al. Pulmonary function, postoperative pain, and serum cytokine level after lobectomy: a comparison of VATS and conventional procedure. Ann Thorac Surg 2001;72:362–5.
13. Petersen RP, Pham D, Burfeind WR, et al. Thoracoscopic lobectomy facilitates the delivery of chemotherapy after resection for lung cancer. Ann Thorac Surg 2007;83:1245–9.
14. Nicastri DG, Wisnivesky JP, Litle VR, et al. Thoracoscopic lobectomy: report on safety, discharge independence, pain, and chemotherapy tolerance. J Thorac Cardiovasc Surg 2008;135:642–7.
15. Park BJ, Zhang H, Rusch VW, et al. Video-assisted thoracic surgery does not reduce the incidence of postoperative atrial fibrillation after pulmonary lobectomy. J Thorac Cardiovasc Surg 2007;133: 775–9.
16. Cattaneo SM, Park BJ, Wilton AS, et al. Use of video-assisted thoracic surgery for lobectomy in the elderly results in fewer complications. Ann Thorac Surg 2008;85:231–6.
17. Villamizar NR, Darrabie MD, Burfeind WR, et al. Thoracoscopic lobectomy is associated with lower morbidity compared to thoracotomy. J Thorac Cardiovasc Surg 2009;138(2):419–25.
18. D'Amico TA. Long-term outcomes after thoracoscopic lobectomy. Thorac Surg Clin 2008;18(3): 259–62.
19. Whitson BA, Andrade RS, Boettcher A, et al. Video-assisted thoracoscopic surgery is more favorable than thoracotomy for resection of clinical stage I non-small cell lung cancer. Ann Thorac Surg 2007; 83:1965–70.
20. Mountain CF, Dresler CM. Regional lymph node classification for lung cancer staging. Chest 1997; 111:1718–23.
21. Rusch VW, Crowley J, Giroux DJ, et al. The IASLC lung cancer staging project: proposals for the revision of the N descriptors in the forthcoming seventh edition of the TNM classification for lung cancer. J Thorac Oncol 2007;2:603–12.
22. Burfeind WR, D'Amico TA. Thoracoscopic lobectomy. J Thorac Cardiovasc Surg 2004;9:98–114
23. D'Amico TA. Complications of mediastinal surgery. In: Little AG, editor. Complications in cardiothoracic surgery. Elmsford (NY): Blackwell; 2004.
24. Kuzdzal J, Zielinski M, Papla B, et al. Transcervical extended mediastinal lymphadenectomy—the new operative technique and early results in lung cancer staging. Eur J Cardiothorac Surg 2005;27:384–90.
25. Kuzdzal J, Zielinski M, Papla B, et al. The transcervical extended mediastinal lymphadenectomy versus cervical mediastinoscopy in non-small cell lung cancer staging. Eur J Cardiothorac Surg 2007;31: 88–94.
26. Leschber G, Holinka G, Linder A. Video-assisted mediastinoscopic lymphadenectomy (VAMLA)—a method for systematic mediastinal lymph node dissection. Eur J Cardiothorac Surg 2003;24: 192–5.
27. Naruke T, Tsuchiya R, Kando H, et al. Lymph node sampling in lung cancer: how should it be done? Eur J Cardiothorac Surg 1999;16:S17–24.
28. Asamura H, Nakayama H, Kondo H, et al. Lymph node involvement, recurrence, and prognosis in resected small, peripheral non-small cell lung carcinomas: are these carcinomas candidates for video-assisted lobectomy? J Thorac Cardiovasc Surg 1996;111:1125–34.
29. Kondo T, Sagawa M, Tanita T, et al. A prospective trial of video-assisted lobectomy for cancer of the right lung. J Thorac Cardiovasc Surg 1998;116: 651–2.
30. Sugi K, Kaneda Y, Esato K. Video-assisted thoracoscopic lobectomy achieves a satisfactory long-term prognosis in patients with clinical stage IA lung cancer. World J Surg 2000;24:27–31.
31. Watanabe A, Koyanagi T, Ohsawa H, et al. Systematic node dissection by VATS is not inferior to that through an open thoracotomy: a comparative clinicopathologic retrospective study. Surgery 2005; 138:510–7.

Transcervical Extended Mediastinal Lymphadenectomy

Marcin Zieliński, MD, PhD

KEYWORDS

• Lung cancer • Surgery • Mediastinum • Staging

Mediastinal staging plays a central role in the treatment of non–small cell lung cancer (NSCLC).[1,2] Most investigators agree that patients with stage I-II disease should be offered radical surgery; however, some patients with stage IIIA and a select group of patients with stage IIIB disease are probably best managed with neoadjuvant therapy and subsequent operative treatment. Therapeutic impact of mediastinal lymphadenectomy on late survival rate is possible but not proved.[3–6] In recent years, a new imaging technique, positron emission tomography (PET) with CT, and endoscopic techniques, including endobronchial ultrasonography with transbronchial fine-needle biopsy (EBUS/TBNA) and endoesophageal ultrasonography and fine-needle aspiration (EUS/FNA), have been developed.[7–9] Invasive techniques, however, remain a cornerstone of preoperative mediastinal staging.[2] The methods of preoperative invasive staging of the mediastinum include classic cervical mediastinoscopy or video-mediastinoscopy, videothoracoscopy, anterior mediastinotomy, video-assisted mediastinal lymphadenectomy (VAMLA), and transcervical extended mediastinal lymphadenectomy (TEMLA), introduced by the author in 2004.[10–14] This report presents the author experience with use of TEMLA in staging and treatment of NSCLC.

MATERIAL AND METHODS

TEMLA was performed on patients with proved NSCLC who were candidates for pulmonary resection, regardless of the state of the mediastinal nodes on CT or PET/CT, after negative result of EBUS/TBNA or EUS. The aim of TEMLA was to maximally and accurately stage and possibly improve late results of treatment of NSCLC. All mediastinal nodal stations (according to the Mountain-Dresler map), except for the pulmonary ligament nodes (station 9), were removed during procedure.[15]

SURGICAL TECHNIQUE

The operation starts with a 58-cm collar incision in the neck. The platysma muscle is divided and the anterior jugular veins are exposed, suture ligated, and divided. Visualization and protection of the laryngeal recurrent nerves bilaterally is a priority. The technique of visualization of the laryngeal recurrent nerves is described elsewhere.[16] In brief, to reach the nerve below the level of the thyroid gland, divide the deep cervical fascial layers covering the carotid arteries until the clean wall of the artery is reached. Traction is applied on the carotid artery in the lateral direction and on the trachea in the opposite direction. This maneuver stretches the tissue between these structures containing the laryngeal recurrent nerves. With use of a blunt dissection with a peanut sponge, the laryngeal recurrent nerves are visualized safely and almost instantly. The rule is not to dissect the nerve circumferentially and to leave the deepest layer of the fascial tissue covering the nerve. These maneuvers protect the nerve from injury. The right recurrent nerve runs from the division of the innominate artery to the larynx. The left laryngeal recurrent nerve lies in the groove between the trachea and the esophagus. Such position of both nerves is almost always constant; the author and colleagues have never seen any anatomic variability of the position of the laryngeal recurrent nerve in more than 1200 operations with

Department of Thoracic Surgery, Pulmonary Hospital, Ul. Gładkie 1 34 500 Zakopane, Poland
E-mail address: marcinz@mp.pl

Thorac Surg Clin 20 (2010) 215–223
doi:10.1016/j.thorsurg.2010.02.007
1547-4127/10/$ – see front matter

the laryngeal recurrent nerve dissection (including TEMLA, transcervical-subxiphoid–video-assisted thoracoscopic maximal thymectomies, resection of the various mediastinal lesions, and esophageal resections).

After visualization of both laryngeal recurrent nerves, the sternal manubrium is elevated with a sharp 3-teeth hook connected to the Rochard frame (Aesculap-Chifa Company) to widen the access to the mediastinum.

The highest mediastinal nodes (station 1) are dissected first. These nodes are located above the upper margin of the left innominate vein and belong to the anterior lymphatic flow from the chest. The fatty tissue containing these nodes is dissected from the right carotid artery and the right innominate veins (laterally, on the right side), from the left carotid artery (laterally, on the left side); then, it is dissected from the trachea (posteriorly) and from the left innominate vein (inferiorly). The piece of tissue containing the station 1 nodes is resected en bloc along with the upper poles of the thymus gland.

To enter the right paratracheal space containing stations 2R and 4R, it is necessary to dissect along the right vagus nerve, which lies between the right carotid artery and the right jugular vein. The dissection proceeds along the nerve, below the division of the innominate artery. The origin of the right laryngeal recurrent nerve is clearly visible and protected from injury. Dissection proceeds toward the tracheal bifurcation. The whole fatty tissue containing the 2R and 4R nodes lying between the right innominate vein and the right mediastinal pleura (laterally), the ascending aorta and trachea (medially), the back wall of the superior vena cava (anteriorly), the esophagus and the thoracic spine (posteriorly), and the right main bronchus, and the azygos vein and the right pulmonary artery (inferiorly) is removed. Any

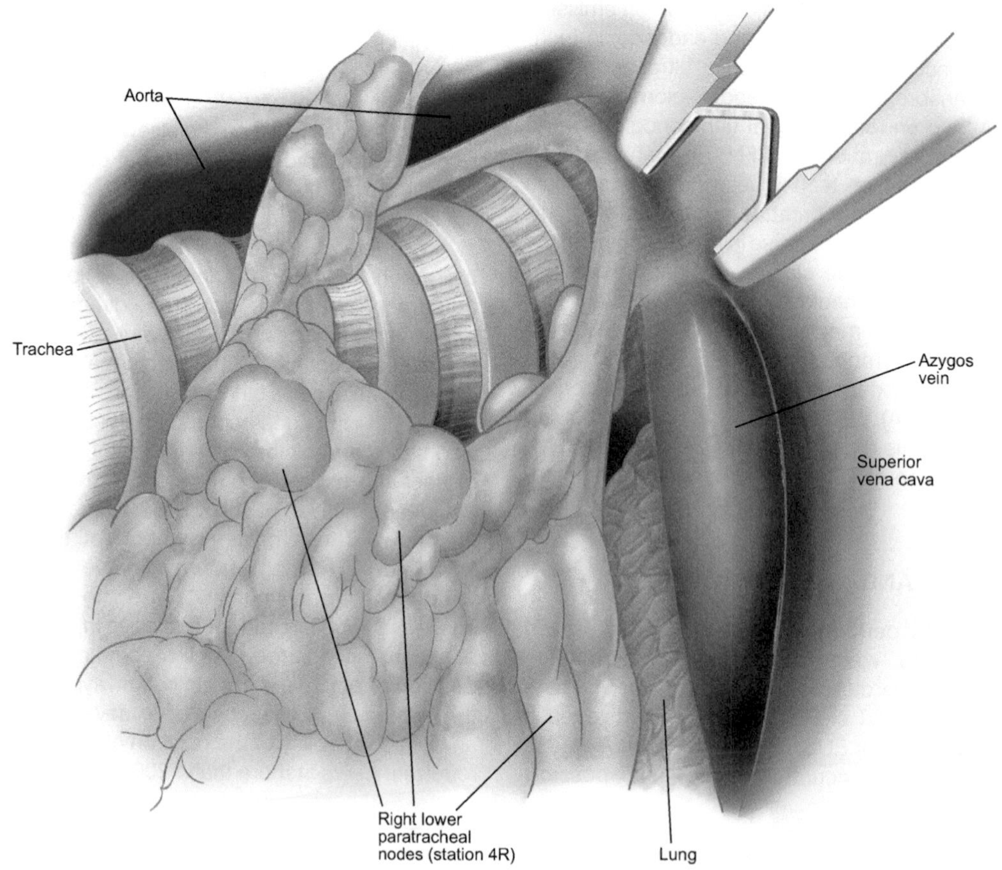

Fig. 1. Any vessels in this area are managed with vascular clips or cautery.

vessels in this area are managed with vascular clips or cautery (**Fig. 1**).

The next step is the dissection of the left paratracheal space: retracting the trachea to the right side and the left common carotid artery to the left and upwards enables excellent visualization of the whole left paratracheal space to the level of one-third of the left main bronchus.

The dissection proceeds along the left laryngeal recurrent nerve below the level of the tracheal bifurcation. The nerve is dissected from the left wall of the trachea and the left main bronchus with a peanut sponge; lateral connections of the nerve are preserved to maintain the blood supply to the nerve. Division of the fascial layer covering the nerve is usually necessary to visualize the nerve (**Fig. 2**). In most patients, the left upper paratracheal nodes (station 2L) are located medially and in front of the nerve, whereas the lower paratracheal nodes (station 4L) almost always lie behind the nerve. Carefully preserving the left laryngeal recurrent nerve, the lymph nodes 2L and 4L are dissected.

To enter the subcarinal nodes, it is necessary to divide the firm fascial layer covering the station 7 nodes anteriorly. Dissection proceeds along the medial walls of both main bronchi for the distance of 4 to 5 cm. The package containing the station 7 and 8 nodes is dissected from the pulmonary artery and the pericardium covering the left atrium (anteriorly) and the esophagus (posteriorly) and removed en bloc (**Fig. 3**).

For removal of the subcarinal and periesophageal nodes (stations 7 and 8), the mediastinoscope is used; the author and colleagues prefer the operative Wolf video-mediastinoscope (Richard Wolf GmbH, Knittlingen, Germany), equipped with moving blades, which are useful in retracting the pulmonary artery from the carina during dissection of node station 7 and the left atrium from the esophagus during dissection of node station 8, to a level 5 to 8 cm below the carina. The mediastinoscope is used for retracting of these structures

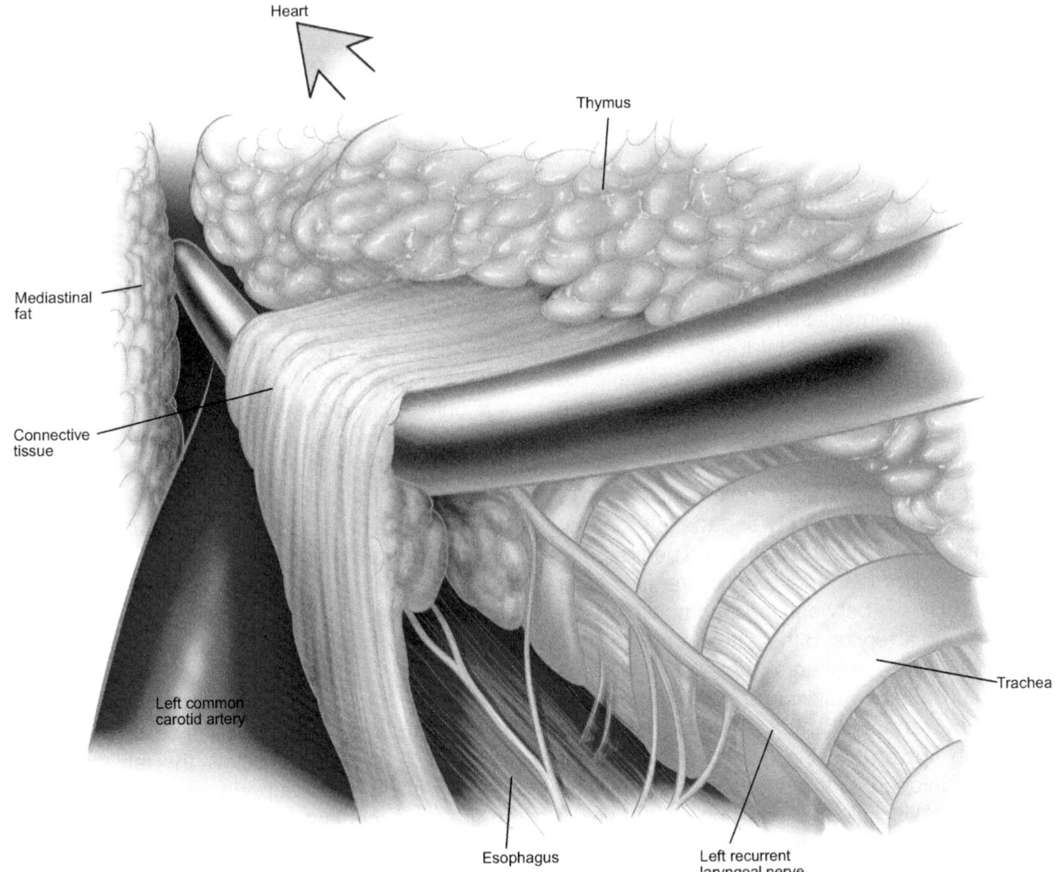

Fig. 2. Division of the fascial layer covering the nerve is usually necessary to visualize the nerve.

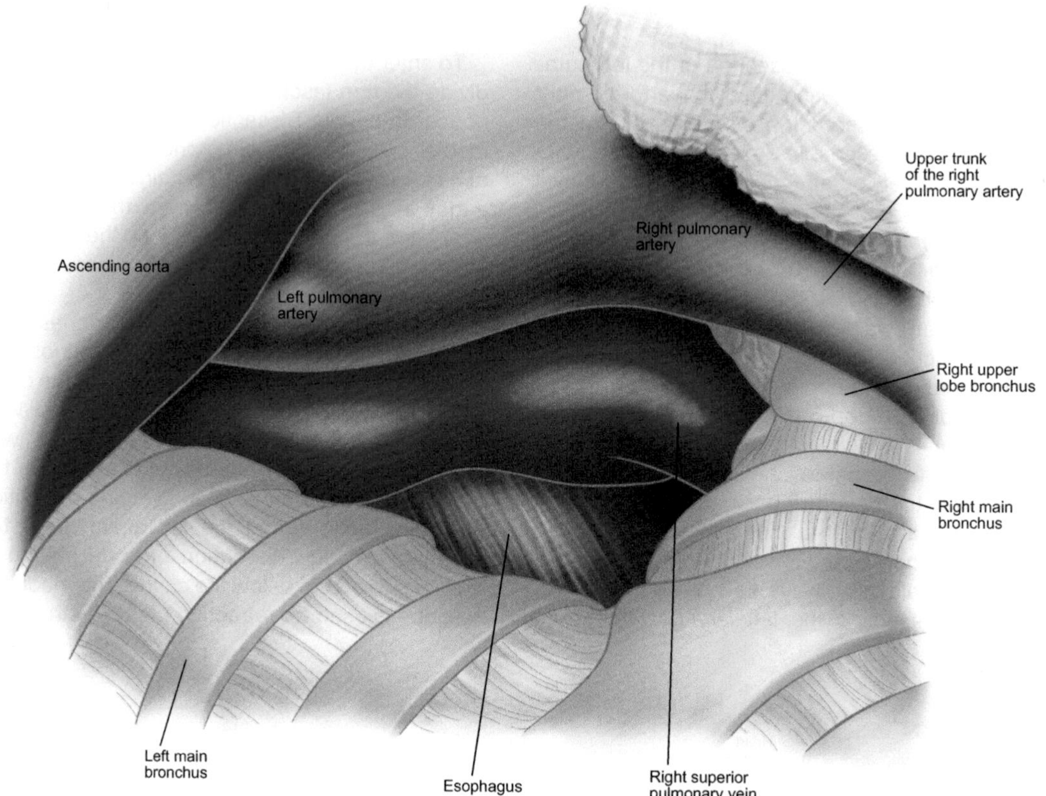

Fig. 3. The package containing station 7 and 8 nodes is dissected from the pulmonary artery and the pericardium covering the left atrium (anteriorly) and the esophagus (posteriorly) and removed en bloc.

and visualization only—the removal of lymph nodes is performed using a standard dissector for open surgery, introduced through the right paratracheal space along the mediastinoscope. In some patients, the mediastinoscope is also helpful in removal of the most distal lower paratracheal nodes (station 4L) (**Fig. 4**). In these patients, removal of the lower paratracheal nodes (station 4L) is postponed until the subcarinal and the periesophageal nodes are removed.

The entrance to the aorto-pulmonary window and station 6 nodes lies between the left innominate vein and the left carotid artery. The first step to reach this area is the division of the firm layer of the fascial tissue between the innominate artery, the left carotid artery, and the left innominate vein. The fascial layer obscures the view of these vessels and after its division the left innominate vein can be retracted anteriorly. After retracting of the vein upwards using a long retractor, the plane is developed at the anterior surface of the aortic arch. With blunt dissection with use of a peanut sponge the fatty tissue containing the station 6 nodes is dissected of the ascending aorta until the left pulmonary artery is reached. The left vagus nerve is a landmark of dissection. The nodes located in above the convexity of the aortic arch and lying in front of the vagus nerve, crossing the aortic arch, the Botallo ligament, are the para--aortic nodes (station 6). The nodes located below the aortic arch and behind the Botallo ligament are the pulmonary window nodes (station 5). The left pulmonary artery, left phrenic nerve, and left superior pulmonary vein are clearly visible after completion of dissection (**Fig. 5**). In a case of opening of the mediastinal pleura, there is no need for drainage of the mediastinum. Insertion of the piece of fibrin sponge and hyperinflation of the lungs during closure of the wound are all that is necessary in such patients. The same rule is valid if the mediastinal pleura are opened on the right side.

Stations 3A (prevascular nodes) and 3P (retrotracheal nodes) are removed in selected patients. Station 3A nodes lies below the left innominate vein, in front of the superior vena cava, medially to the right mediastinal pleura and laterally to the ascending aorta. These nodes are dissected after removal of station1 nodes. The left innominate vein and the superior vena cava are retracted

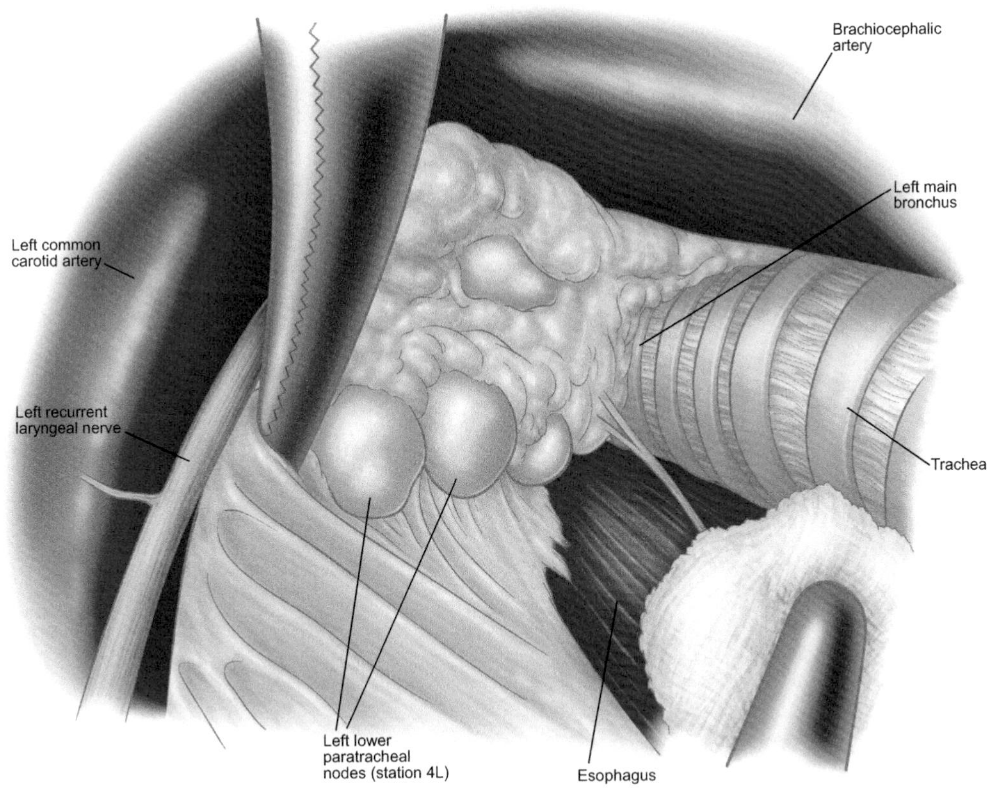

Fig. 4. In some patients, the mediastinoscope is also helpful in removal of the most distal lower paratracheal nodes (station 4L).

posteriorly with a peanut sponge and the fatty tissue containing the 3A nodes is dissected from the structures (discussed previously). In the author and colleagues' experience, these nodes are rarely the site of metastasis, which are found only in case of right-sided tumors.

The retrotracheal nodes (station 3P) are located behind the bifurcation of the trachea. This area is approached in same fashion as the right paratracheal nodes. The tracheal bifurcation is retracted anteriorly, which enables visualization of the nodes lying in front of the esophagus. The nodes are easily removed; however, the author and colleagues never found any metastatic nodes in this station and most often there were no visible nodes in this location at all. During TEMLA, all mediastinal lymph nodal stations and the surrounding fatty tissue are removed with the exception of the pulmonary ligament, station 9 nodes.

The author and colleagues try to follow the rule of performance of lymphadenectomy in en bloc fashion, with resection of the whole package of the lymphatic tissue without separation of the individual nodes. It is possible to remove all the nodes of station 1 in one piece, also containing the upper pole soft the thymus. Afterwards, stations 2R and 4R are removed in one piece, as with stations 7 and 8 and stations 5 and 6. The nodes of stations 2L and 4L are removed separately because they almost never occur in one piece of tissue.

Generally, most part of TEMLA is an open procedure, with the exception of dissection of the subcarinal (station 7), the periesophageal (station 8) nodes, and the left lower paratracheal (station 4L) nodes, which are dissected in the mediastinoscopy-assisted fashion with aid of Wolf 2-blade mediastinoscope. The para-aortic, station 6, and aorto-pulmonary window, station 5 nodes are sometimes dissected with aid of a videothoracoscope introduced to the mediastinum through the operative wound.

Bilateral supraclavicular lymphadenectomy and even deep cervical lymph node dissection is possible during TEMLA through the same incision, although the author and colleagues do not recommend these additions in routine use for NSCLC.

Currently, the indications for TEMLA in NSCLC in the author and colleagues' department include preoperative staging of potentially operable

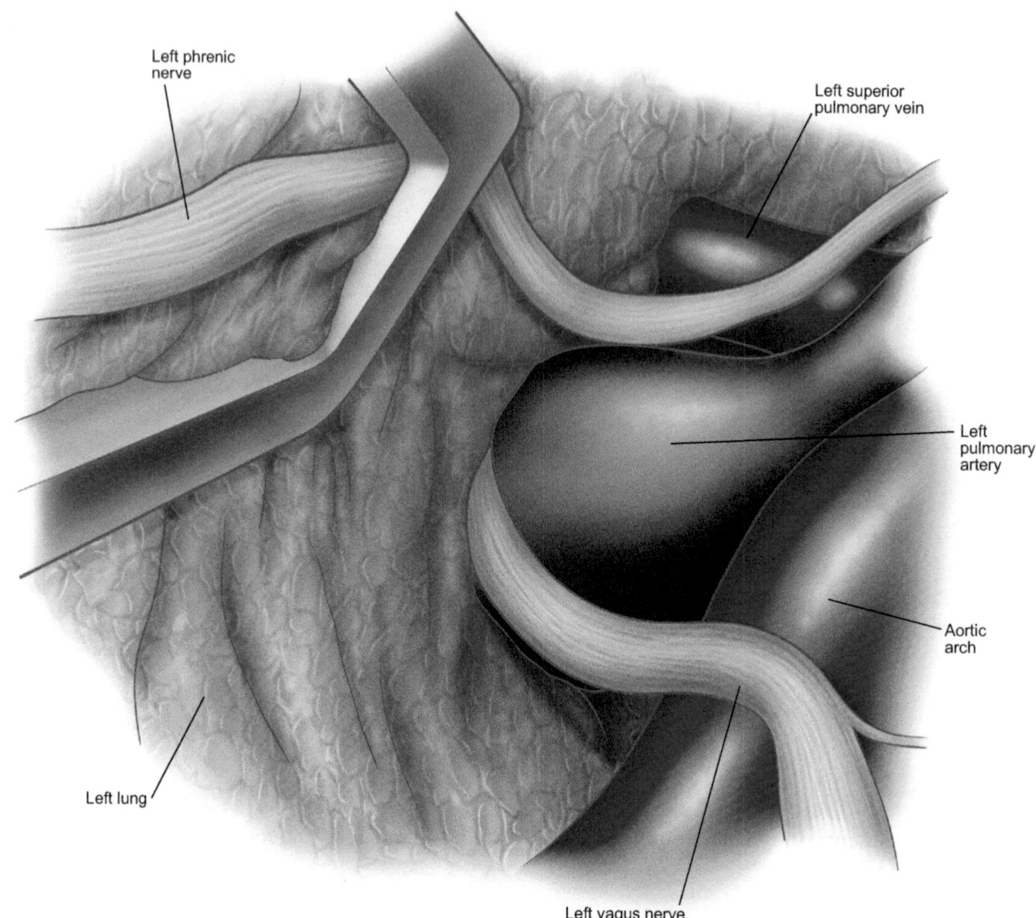

Fig. 5. Left pulmonary artery, the left phrenic nerve and the left superior pulmonary vein are clearly visible after completion of dissection.

patients, regardless of the mediastinal nodal status on CT or PET/CT. In all patients, TEMLA is preceded by previous combined EBUS/EUS examination. In cases of positive result of EBUS/EUS, patients are referred to neoadjuvant chemotherapy.

The results of TEMLA were estimated in regard to the diagnostic yield, prevalence of N2-3 metastatic involvement of the mediastinal nodes, and nodal stations, and the number of patients who underwent thoracotomy with pulmonary resection after negative TEMLA were calculated.

RESULTS

There were 587 patients, 480 men and 107 women ages 41 to 79 (mean age 60.8), studied from January 1, 2004, to January 31, 2009. There were 431 squamous cell carcinomas, 114 adenocarcinomas, 20 large cell carcinomas, and 22 other carcinomas. Time of operation was 80 to 330 minutes (mean 161 minutes). In the last 100 patients, mean time of operation was 112.3 minutes. There were no intraoperative injuries of the vitally important structures, including major vessels, tracheobronchial tree, or the esophagus. There were 5 postoperative deaths unrelated to the procedure (mortality 0.9%). Complications of TEMLA occurred in 40 of 587 of patients (6.8%) with temporary laryngeal nerve palsy in 16 of 587 patients (2.7%) and permanent nerve palsy in 2 of 587 patients (0.3%). Pneumothorax necessitating pleural drainage occurred in 1 of 587 patients (0.2%) and pleural effusion in 11 of 587 patients (1.9%). Asymptomatic widening of the mediastinum was noted in approximately 40% of patients. It necessitated no treatment, subsided after several days, and was not regarded a postoperative complication. The complications of TEMLA are shown in **Table 1**.

Table 1
Complications of 587 TEMLA procedures

Complication	N (%)
Pleural effusion (conservative treatment)	12 (2.0)
Laryngeal recurrent nerve palsy—overall	16 (2.7)
Temporary left laryngeal recurrent nerve palsy	2 (0.3)
Temporary right laryngeal recurrent nerve palsy	1 (0.2)
Temporary bilateral laryngeal recurrent nerve palsy	2 (0.3)
Permanent laryngeal recurrent nerve palsy	2 (0.3)
Pneumothorax (necessitating chest drainage)	1 (0.2)
Pneumothorax (conservative treatment without chest drainage)	3 (0.5)
Respiratory insufficiency (ventilator)	5 (0.9)
Postoperative psychosis	2 (0.3)
Perforation of the duodenal ulcer	1 (0.3)
Cerebral ischemia	1 (0.3)
Subarachnoid hemorrhage	1 (0.3)
Cardiovascular insufficiency	1 (0.3)
Overall morbidity	43 (7.3)
Death[a]	5 (0.9)

[a] Causes of death: exsanguinating respiratory hemorrhage on remote day after procedure (2 patients), intracranial hemorrhage (1 patient), myocardial infarct (1 patient), unknown (1 patient).

The number of dissected nodes during TEMLA was 15 to 85 (mean 38.9). Metastatic N2 nodes were found in 128 of 587 patients (21.8%) and N3 nodes were found in 25 of 587 patients (4.3%). Metastatic nodes were most prevalent in station 7, station 4R, station 2R, station 5, and station 4L. Subsequent thoracotomy was performed in 368 of 434 patients (84.8%) after negative result of TEMLA. There were 88 pneumonectomies, 31 sleeve lobectomies, 231 lobectomies/bilobectomies, 3 sublobar resections, and 15 explorations (4.1%) (**Table 2**). During thoracotomy, omitted N2 was found in 7 of 368 (1.9%) patients and omitted normal mediastinal nodes were found in 49 of 368 patients (13.3%). Omitted N2 nodes were found in station 5 (2 patients), station 4L (1 patient), station 7 (1 patient), station 4R (1 patient), station 8 (1 patient), and station 9 (1 patient). Postoperative mortality after pulmonary resection in all patients operated on for NSCLC in the author and colleagues' institution (in some of them TEMLA was not performed) in the period from January 1, 2004, to January 30, 2009, was 1.6% (11/680). The mortality was 4.3% (5/115) in 2004 and 1.1% (6/565) in the years 2005–2009. In the period 2002–2003, before introduction of TEMLA, the postoperative mortality in the author and colleagues' department was 3.5%. There was a 25% decrease in the number of pulmonary resections for NSCLC in the years 2004–2005 in comparison to the period 2002–2003.

Table 2
Types of pulmonary resections in 368 patients operated on after negative result of TEMLA

Type of Pulmonary Resection	Number of Patients
Pneumonectomy	88
Sleeve lobectomy	31
Lobectomy/bilobectomy	231
Sublobar resection	3
Exploratory thoracotomy	15

Sensitivity of TEMLA in discovery of N2-3 nodes was 95.6%, specificity was 100%, accuracy was 98.8%, negative predictive value (NPV) was 98.4%, and positive predictive value (PPV) was 100% (**Table 3**). In the last 100 patients, all these parameters were 100%.

COMMENT

The main advantage of TEMLA for staging of NSCLC is the possibility of removing almost all mediastinal lymph nodes with the surrounding fatty tissue. A mean number of 38.9 nodes per

Table 3
Diagnostic yield of TEMLA for NSCLC

Diagnostic Parameter	Value (%)
Sensitivity	95.9
Specificity	100
NPV	98.4
PPV	100
Accuracy	98.8

procedure was removed (from 15 to 85 nodes/procedure). Such complete removal of the mediastinal nodes increases the reliability of staging. No other invasive staging technique enables such complete assessment of the mediastinal nodes. For comparison, a mean number of 8.7 to 20.7 nodes was removed during VAMLA.[10,11] During mediastinoscopy, normally, 1 to 2 lymph nodes from each of 5 stations accessible in this procedure (stations 2R,4R, 2L, 4L, and 7) were biopsied and a mean number of 1 to 2 nodes was biopsied during EBUS and EUS procedures.[8,9,17] In 7 patients who underwent TEMLA, omitted N2 nodes were found during subsequent thoracotomy. The reasons for omitting of these nodes were dependent on the learning curve; in the last 100 TEMLA procedures, there were no false-negative results and all diagnostic parameters of TEMLA were 100% for this large subgroup.

In our recently presented prospective randomized trial, diagnostic accuracy of TEMLA proved statistically better than in standard mediastinoscopy (sensitivity 100% versus 37.5%; NPV 100% versus 66.7%; $P<.05$).[18] The impairment of pulmonary function after TEMLA and standard mediastinoscopy reflecting invasiveness of both surgical procedures were not statistically different.[19] Also, the morbidity of TEMLA in the whole group was relatively low. Most of the complications were minor and subsided during the follow-up period and there were no life-threatening intraoperative complications. Two of 5 postoperative deaths can be attributed to the progression of cancer (fatal hemorrhage secondary to the fistula between the pulmonary artery and the bronchial tree) and 2 other were independent events (myocardial infarct and intracerebral hemorrhage). In 1 patient, the cause of death was unknown; a postmortem was not obtained. These data showed that invasiveness of TEMLA was limited. Despite moderate invasiveness, TEMLA is a time-consuming procedure; however, it was well tolerated by the patients. Current mean operative time has been substantially reduced, however, from 160 to 112 minutes, due to the growing experience of the surgeons of the team.

Due to liberal inclusion criteria to TEMLA, there were several patients who did not undergo subsequent thoracotomy after negative result of TEMLA (operability 84.8%). Results of 368 patients who underwent thoracotomy indicate that previous TEMLA was not an obstacle to perform safely all kinds of pulmonary resections, including sleeve lobectomies and pneumonectomies.

Diagnostic yield of TEMLA for NSCLC was high and if the results of the last 100 patients were analyzed, all the diagnostic parameters were 100%. False-negative results of TEMLA were noted mostly in the author and colleagues' early experience and were due to the learning curve. The only nodal station inaccessible during TEMLA is station 9.

Possible higher postoperative mortality and morbidity of pulmonary resections after prior TEMLA due to the inflammation and scarring of the mediastinal tissue was a concern initially, after introduction of TEMLA. The postoperative mortality in 2004, the first year when TEMLA was used, however, was 4.3%, and in the years 2005 to 2009, the postoperative mortality decreased to 1.1%. In the period 2002 to 2003, before introduction of TEMLA, the postoperative mortality in the author and colleagues' department was 3.5%. These data indicate that introduction of TEMLA is not associated with increased risk of postoperative mortality but, conversely, it leads to decrease the mortality, probably due to better selection of patients for pulmonary resection. Due to more accurate preoperative staging, there was a 25% decrease of the number of pulmonary resections for NSCLC after introduction of TEMLA.

In addition to the staging of NSCLC, TEMLA might have a therapeutic impact. The author and colleagues' preliminary late results are encouraging. Survival rates of patients who underwent radical R0 resection after negative TEMLA are probably better than the previous results of survival for patients who were operated on before introduction of TEMLA. Additionally, locoregional nodal recurrence occurred in only 5 patients whereas all other recurrences were the intrabronchial ones or occurred in distal organs (predominantly in the brain, the bones, and the liver). It is, however, too early to ultimately estimate probable therapeutic impact of TEMLA in the treatment of NSCLC.

The advantage of TEMLA in regard to the patients sent to neoadjuvant therapy is no need for invasive restaging of the mediastinal nodes, which is otherwise impossible. In such patients, only the imaging or endoscopic studies are possible.

Other uses of the technique of TEMLA include resection of the mediastinal tumors, resection of the metastatic nodes to the mediastinum, and transcervical right upper lobectomy.[20]

In the author's opinion, a promising use of TEMLA is esophageal resection with 3-field lymphadenectomy (combined with laparotomy, which was done in 5 patients, or with laparoscopy, which was done in 1 patient). The last technique is probably the least invasive technique of the esophageal resection that has been reported.

SUMMARY

Operative technique of a new surgical method, TEMLA, is described in detail. TEMLA enables almost complete en bloc removal of the mediastinal nodes in semiopen fashion. Sensitivity and NPV of TEMLA for staging were 95.6% and 98.4%, respectively, and for restaging, 95.7% and 98.4%, respectively. Other uses of TEMLA include resection of the mediastinal tumors and resection of the metastatic nodes to the mediastinum, esophagectomy with 3-field dissection (combined with laparoscopy or laparotomy), closure of postpneumonectomy fistula, and right upper pulmonary lobectomy.

REFERENCES

1. Lardinois D, De Leyn P, Van Schil P, et al. ESTS guidelines for intraoperative lymph node staging in non-small cell lung cancer. Eur J Cardiothorac Surg 2006;30:787–92.
2. De Leyn P, Lardinois D, Van Schil PE, et al. ESTS guidelines for preoperative lymph node staging for non-small cell lung cancer. Eur J Cardiothorac Surg 2007;32:1–8.
3. Wright G, Manser R, Byrnes G, et al. Campbell: surgery for non-small cell lung cancer: systematic review and meta-analysis of randomized controlled trials. Thorax 2006;61:597–603.
4. Passlick B, Kubuschock B, Sienel W, et al. Mediastinal lymphadenectomy in non-small cell lung cancer: effectiveness in patients with or without nodal micrometastases—results of a preliminary study. Eur J Cardiothorac Surg 2002;21:520–6.
5. Wu Y, Huang Z, Wang S, et al. A randomized trial of systematic nodal dissection in resectable NSCLC. Lung Cancer 2002;36:1–6.
6. Lardinois D, Suter H, Hakki H, et al. Morbidity, survival, and site of recurrence after mediastinal lymph-node dissection versus systematic sampling after complete resection for non-small cell lung cancer. Ann Thorac Surg 2005;80:268–74.
7. Cerfolio R, Buddhiwardhani O, Bryant A, et al. The accuracy of integrated PET-CT compared to dedicated PET alone for the staging of patients with non-small cell lung cancer. Ann Thorac Surg 2004;78:1017–23.
8. Herth F, Ernst A, Eberhardt R, et al. Endobronchial ultrasound-guided transbronchial needle aspiration of lymph nodes in the radiologically normal mediastinum. Eur Respir J 2006;28:910–4.
9. Annema J, Hoeksstra O, Smit E, et al. Toward a minimally invasive staging strategy in NSCLC: analysis of PET positive lesions by EUS-FNA. Lung Cancer 2004;44:53–60.
10. Hurtgen M, Friedel G, Toomes H, et al. Radical video-assisted mediastinoscopic lymphadenectomy (VAMLA)—technique and first results. Eur J Cardiothorac Surg 2002;21:348–51.
11. Leschber G, Holinka G, Linder A. Video-assisted mediastinoscopic lymphadenectomy (VAMLA)—a method for systematic mediastinal lymphnode dissection. Eur J Cardiothorac Surg 2003;24:192–5.
12. Kuzdzal J, Zielinski M, Papla B, et al. Transcervical extended mediastinal lymphadenectomy—the new operative technique and early results in lung cancer staging. Eur J Cardiothorac Surg 2005;27:384.
13. Zielinski M, Kuzdzal J, Nabialek T, et al. Transcervical extended mediastinal lymphadenectomy. Multimedia Manual of Cardiothoracic Surgery. MMCTS (October 9, 2006). DOI: 10.1510/mmcts.2005.001693.
14. Zieliński M. Transcervical extended mediastinal lymphadenectomy: results of staging in two hundred fifty-six patients with non-small cell lung cancer. J Thorac Oncol 2007;2:370–2.
15. Mountain CF, Dresler CM. Regional lymph node classification for lung cancer staging. Chest 1997;111:1718.
16. Zieliński M, Kużdżał J, Szlubowski A, et al. A safe and reliable technique for visualization of the laryngeal recurrent nerves in the neck. Am J Surg 2005;189:200–2.
17. Venissac N, Alifano M, Mouroux J. Video-assisted mediastinoscopy: experience from 240 consecutive cases. Ann Thorac Surg 2003;76:208–12.
18. Kuzdzal J, Zielinski M, Papla B, et al. The Transcervical Extended Mediastinal Lymphadenectomy (TEMLA) versus cervical mediastinoscopy in NSCLC staging. Eur J Cardiothorac Surg 2007;31:88–94.
19. Kuzdzal J, Zielinski M, Papla B, et al. Effect of bilateral mediastinal lymphadenectomy on pulmonary function. Eur J Cardiothorac Surg 2007;31:161–6.
20. Zieliński M, Pankowski J, Hauer L, et al. The right upper lobe pulmonary resection performed through the transcervical approach. Eur J Cardiothorac Surg 2007;32:766–9.

Awake Video-Assisted Thoracoscopic Biopsy in Complex Anterior Mediastinal Masses

Eugenio Pompeo, MD*, Federico Tacconi, MD, Tommaso C. Mineo, MD

KEYWORDS

• VATS • Thoracic surgery • Awake anesthesia
• Epidural anesthesia • Local anesthesia
• Mediastinum • Mass • Biopsy

Rapidly evolving anterior mediastinal masses can develop from a wide spectrum of pathologic conditions, most of which are malignant in nature and require prompt diagnosis for immediate initiation of the appropriate treatment.

In many instances, these lesions remain silent until when they enlarge enough to cause symptoms induced by compression of the airways and/or the upper venous system. Associated intrathoracic conditions such as pleural and pericardial effusions can also contribute to severity of symptoms leading to a complex clinical picture (**Figs. 1** and **2**).

Several nonsurgical and surgical methods have been used to manage these complex anterior mediastinal masses.[1] Video-assisted thoracoscopic surgery (VATS) is often preferred because of its limited invasiveness and optimal versatility that allows wide biopsy samples to be obtained and coexisting intrathoracic conditions needing surgical management to be treated.[2–5] On the other hand, VATS has been mostly performed through general anesthesia and one-lung ventilation, which can induce several adverse effects in these patients, eventually leading to prolonged postoperative ventilatory support and a morbidity rate as high as 20%.[6–12]

Having gained experience with awake VATS that we now routinely use to perform several thoracic surgery procedures,[13–16] we have decided to extend the indication to patients with complex anterior mediastinal masses.

This article describes and discuss the indications, surgical technique, and results of this novel and minimally invasive surgical option.

INDICATIONS

The presence of an undetermined mass in the anterior mediastinum associated with other intrathoracic conditions requiring surgical management should be considered as elective indications for the awake VATS approach (**Table 1**). For this purpose, we have arbitrarily defined as complex anterior mediastinal masses those fulfilling 2 or more of the criteria summarized in **Table 2**.

Contraindications for the thoracoscopic approach include imaging-based suspicion of dense pleural adhesions, especially when corroborated by a clinical history of previous pleural-pulmonary infections or previous thoracic surgery procedures on the side targeted for the operation that should prompt a preference for anterior mediastinotomy. On the other hand, the presence of severe anxiety or other psychiatric conditions potentially jeopardizing the patient's full cooperation must be excluded before planning an awake VATS biopsy.

Department of Thoracic Surgery, Fondazione Policlinico Tor Vergata, Tor Vergata University, Viale Oxford, 81, Rome 00133, Italy
* Corresponding author.
E-mail address: pompeo@med.uniroma2.it

Thorac Surg Clin 20 (2010) 225–233
doi:10.1016/j.thorsurg.2010.01.003
1547-4127/10/$ – see front matter

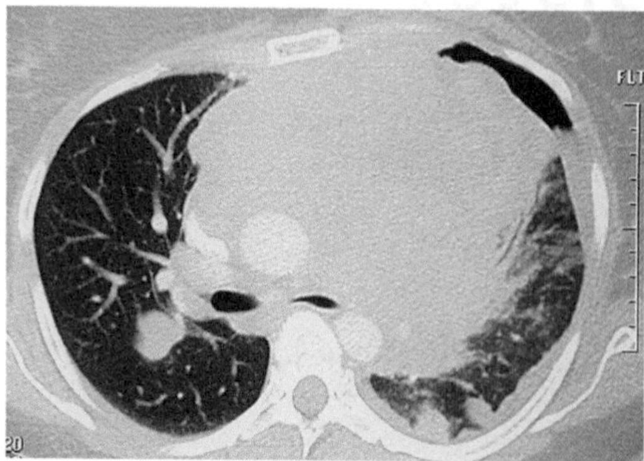

Fig. 1. Computed tomography (CT) image showing a bulky mediastinal mass compressing the airways associated with pleural effusion, lung nodules, and pneumothorax consequent to nondiagnostic agobiopsy.

Table 1 Indications for awake VATS biopsy
Complex anterior mediastinal mass
Absence of peripheral lymphadenopathy or skin metastases
Full acceptance of the awake procedure
No anxiety or other psychic disorders
No bleeding disorders
No history of previous surgery on the chest side involved
No history of pleural-pulmonary infections on the side involved

PREOPERATIVE WORKUP

Preoperative workup is not different from that of patients scheduled for VATS under general anesthesia. A careful assessment of all superficial node stations amenable to simpler surgical biopsy is mandatory before proceeding to awake VATS biopsy.

When the procedure is not performed on an emergency-based regimen, echocardiography is useful to assess the contractile function of the heart, spirometry performed in a sitting position as well as in supine and lateral decubitus positions permits estimation of fixed airway compression.[17] Radiologic workup includes chest roentgenograms and integrated whole-body computed tomography (CT) plus positron emission tomography; these are mandatory for accurate clinical staging of the disease (**Figs. 3** and **4**). Fiber-optic bronchoscopy is usually avoided in these patients, but it is routinely performed if signs of bronchial or pulmonary involvement exist, provided there is no

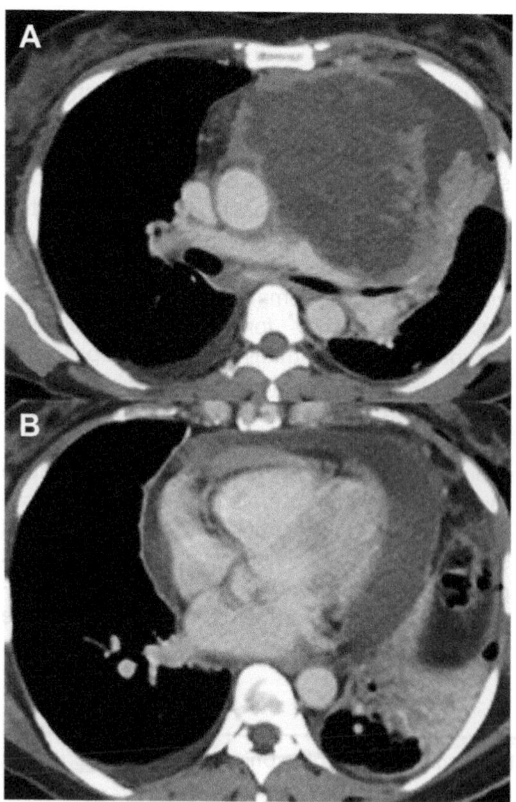

Fig. 2. CT images showing a nonhomogeneous mediastinal mass with large necrotic areas (*A*) associated with pericardial effusion (*B*).

Table 2 Definition of complex anterior mediastinal mass
Bulky mediastinal mass with MTR $\geq$0.35
An MTR <0.35 with at least 1 of the following conditions:
1. Compression of trachea or main stem bronchi
2. Superior vena cava syndrome
3. Radiologic evidence of pleural-pericardial effusion or solid implants
4. Pneumothorax
5. Lung nodules, opacities, or recent-onset fibrosis requiring diagnosis
6. Compression of major vessels other than superior vena cava
7. Arrhythmias
8. Left ventricular ejection fraction <50%

Abbreviation: MTR, mediastinal-thoracic ratio at axial CT images.

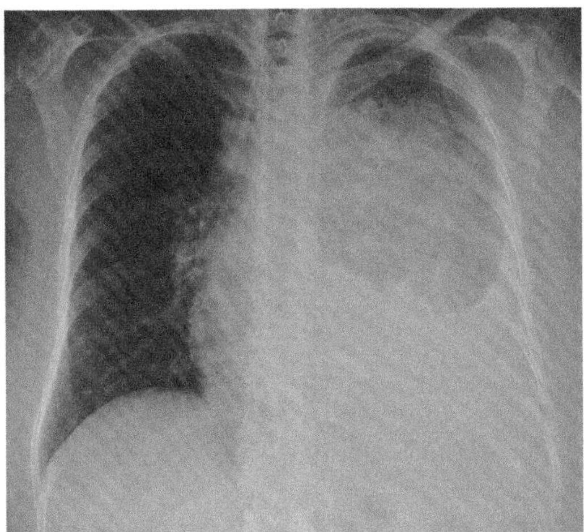

Fig. 3. Chest roentgenogram of a patient with complex mediastinal mass mimicking massive pleural effusion.

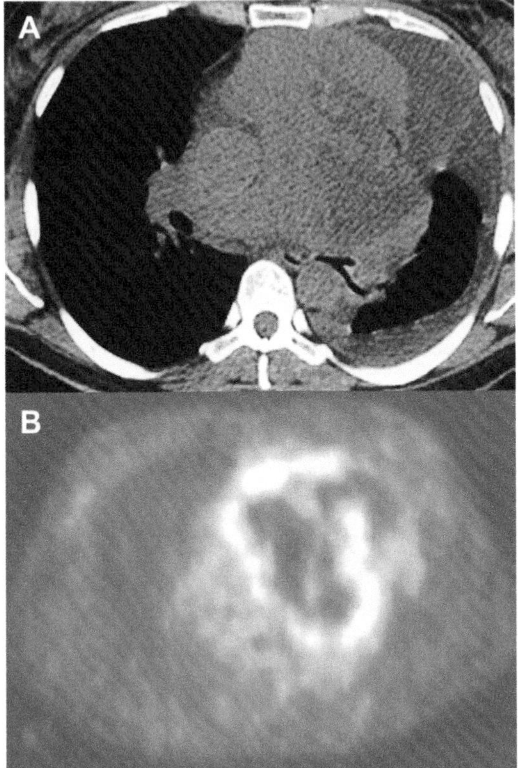

Fig. 4. CT image showing a bulky mediastinal mass compressing both airways and left lung (*A*) integrated by positron emission tomography assay (*B*), which provides additional information regarding focal increased metabolic activity of some areas of the mass that are better suited for awake VATS biopsy.

unstable cardiopathy or severe impairment in respiratory function.

Preoperative administration of steroids is avoided whenever possible because they can lead to artifacts in the biopsy samples. Fluid intake is slightly restricted and low-dose diuretics are used to limit the risk of airway edema. Aerosolized and oral bronchodilators are also given to limit bronchial reactivity. Cough sedatives are usually withdrawn although they can be useful to avoid sleep disturbance in cases of nocturnal coughing.

ANESTHESIA

In the operating room, venous and radial artery catheters are inserted. Premedication is usually not necessary unless selective minimal sedation with midazolam is considered worthwhile. The technique of thoracic analgesia entails an epidural catheter placed at the T4 to T5 level via a loss-of-resistance technique. Warm-cold and pin-prick discrimination tests can be used to assess the degree of thoracic analgesia. Alternatively, sole intercostal block can be performed by local injection of a 50% mixture of lidocaine 2% and ropivacaine 7.5% at the site chosen for insertion of the trocar.

Perioperatively, fluids are given at a minimum rate to ensure adequate urinary output. If necessary, oxygen is administered via a Venturi mask to keep arterial oxygen saturation more than 90%. Before induction of the surgical pneumothorax, the patient must be warned that this maneuver can render spontaneous ventilation less comfortable although oxygen saturation is maintained at a satisfactory level. In rare instances, panic attacks triggered by anxiety or mild dyspnea can develop although they can be mostly controlled without conversion to general anesthesia by simply increasing sedation with subhypnotic boluses of propofol (0.5–1 mg/kg). Should conversion to general anesthesia become necessary, orotracheal intubation is usually done without changing the patient's position. In such instances, videolaringoscopy and a fiber-optic bronchoscopy can be useful to aid faster and easier intubation with the patient lying in lateral decubitus position.

The beneficial effects of thoracic epidural anesthesia include increased myocardial blood flow and reduced myocardial oxygen consumption,[18] which may be particularly useful in patients with impaired cardiorespiratory function. However, in some instances, including the presence of superior vena cava obstruction or the need for anticoagulant therapy at admission, intercostal blockade by local anesthesia might be preferred to epidural anesthesia because of the potential increased risk of spinal hematoma related to the use of epidural anesthesia. Placement of a thoracic epidural catheter may be difficult in patients with congenital or acquired spinal deformities in whom intercostal blockade should also be chosen.

SURGICAL TECHNIQUE

The side for the VATS approach is chosen based on the main bulge of the mass and the associated intrathoracic conditions needing surgical management. As for every type of awake VATS procedure, 1 chest tube with its water-sealed chamber is kept ready on the nurse's table to allow immediate interruption of the procedure whenever necessary.

Care is also taken to place the patient in a comfortable position and to prepare and drape the operating field so that the patient's face is free thus facilitating spontaneous breathing and the patient's cooperation with the surgical staff. We consider it important that the medical and nursing personnel create a friendly and empathic environment in the operating room. Some patients feel reassured if they can follow their vital parameters and even the operation itself on the monitors,[19] although others do not. In addition, low-volume classical music is played in the operating room because it has been shown to reduce anxiety and the need for pharmacologic sedation during awake surgical procedures.[20]

The patient is placed in semilateral, 30-degree, off-center, decubitus position with mild trunk elevation and the arm adducted (**Fig. 5**). In most instances, the entire procedure can be performed through a single port with surgical access resembling that used for simple insertion of a thoracic drain. One 20-mm flexible trocar is inserted in the sixth or seventh intercostal space, on the anterior axillary line. A 30-degree 10-mm camera is used to facilitate oblique vision of the anterior mediastinum and coaxial surgical maneuvering (**Fig. 6**). A supplemental 7-mm flexible trocar can sometimes be inserted to aid division of pleural adhesions or to create a pericardial window in the presence of major pericardial effusion. Instrumental retraction of the lung is not necessary to reach the anterior mediastinum because the surgical pneumothorax usually creates enough space in the pleural cavity; because of the semilateral position, the lung tends to fall posteriorly by gravity.

The mediastinal pleura is incised and multiple biopsies are then taken under direct vision in the most representative target sites, with spoon-shaped forceps. Usually this maneuver does not elicit pain even in patients without epidural analgesia. A few milliliters of 2% lidocaine can be

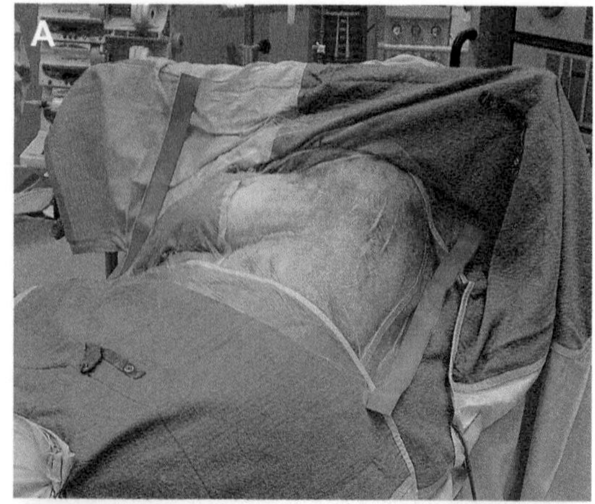

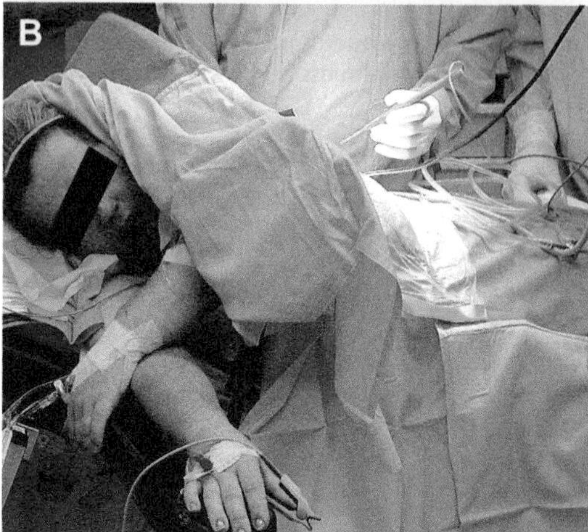

Fig. 5. Patient positioning: dorsal view (*A*) and ventral perioperative view (*B*).

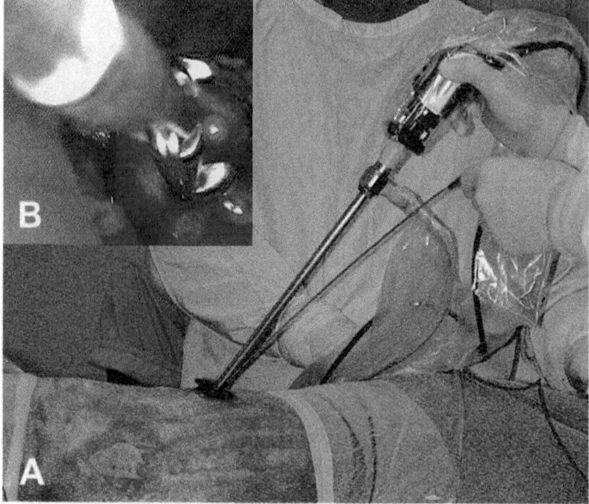

Fig. 6. Intraoperative view of the single-trocar access with coaxial camera and biopsy forceps insertion (*A*) and biopsy (*B*).

released over the mediastinal pleura via a plastic catheter whenever needed. To avoid electrocautery artifacts, coagulation must be avoided during the procedure (**Fig. 7**). Next, hemostasis is revised and oxidized cellulose is placed on the biopsy area. Additional measures such as pleural talc poudrage or sampling, pericardial fenestration, and lung wedge resection can be easily performed according to standard techniques whenever required.

At the end of the operation a double-lumen chest tube is placed through a water seal and the patient is asked to cough repeatedly while the trocar port(s) are occluded, to restore intrapleural negative pressure and aid lung re-expansion (**Fig. 8**).

In patients operated via thoracic epidural analgesia, the epidural catheter is left in place for 24 hours. When sole intercostal blocks are used, a small-sized catheter is inserted beneath the parietal pleura under direct thoracoscopic vision along the intercostal space through which the chest tube has been passed. Subsequently, a double-way elastomeric device is connected to the extrapleural catheter and the second lumen of the chest tube to release ropivacaine 0.2% at the apex of the pleural cavity as well as along the neurovascular intercostal bundle for continuous analgesia.[21]

Postoperative care follows a fast track policy and involves a brief stay in the recovery room and rapid transfer to the ward with overnight stay and subsequent discharge. Once in the ward, oral fluid intake and mobilization of the patient is allowed immediately. Discharge is usually planned for 24 hours after the procedure although recently, some patients have been operated on a day-surgery regimen.

COMMENT

The awake VATS approach for patients with complex anterior mediastinum masses represents

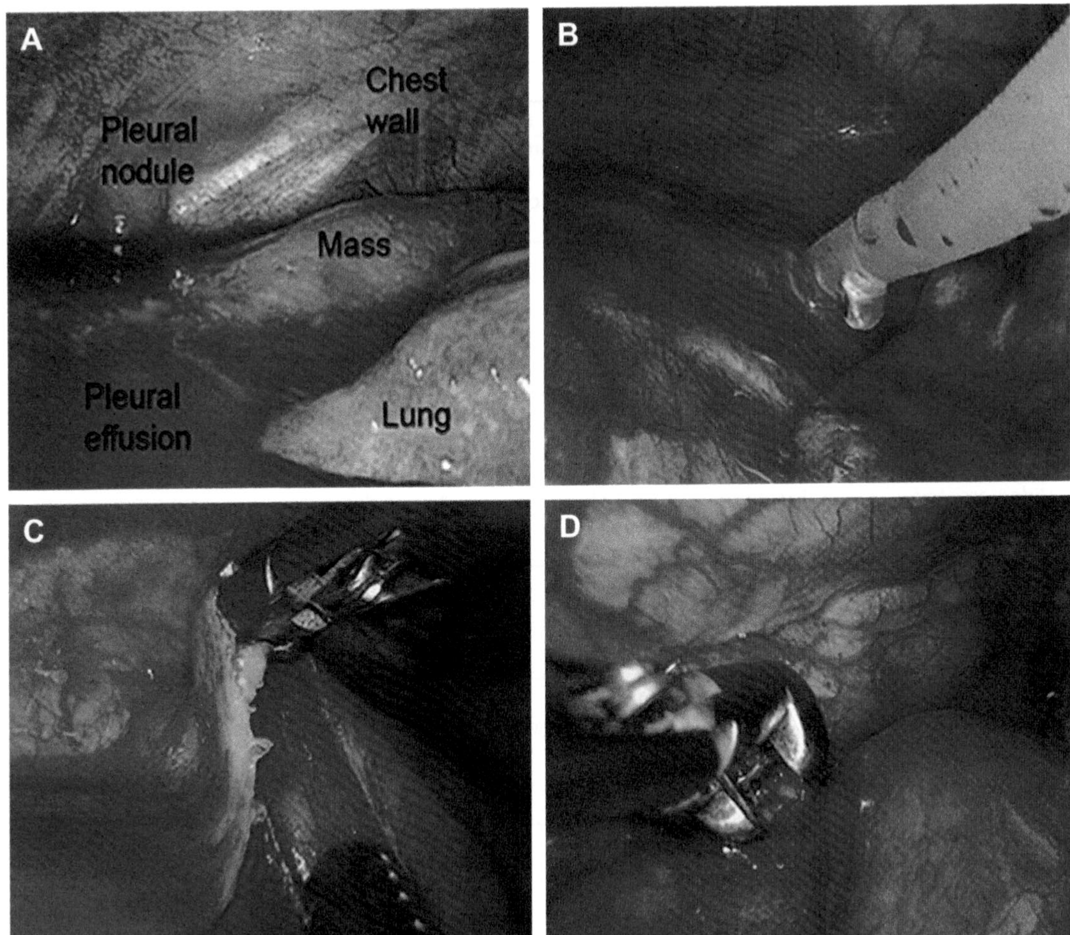

Fig. 7. Thoracoscopic view following creation of the surgical pneumothorax (*A*); topical anesthesia onto the mediastinal pleura through a plastic catheter (*B*); noncoagulating opening of the mediastinal pleura to avoid biopsy artifacts (*C*) and multiple biopsy of the mass (*D*).

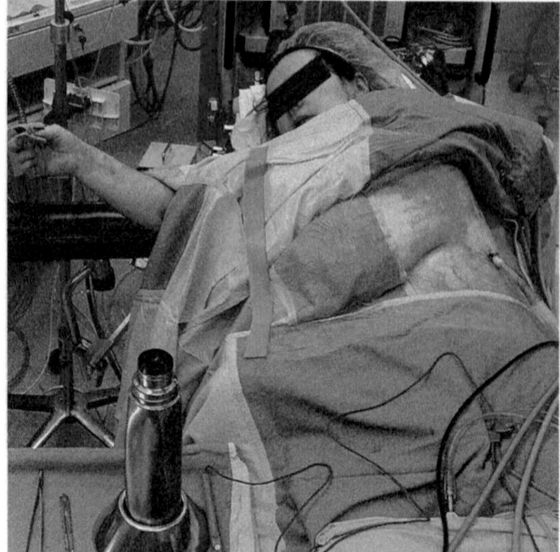

Fig. 8. Immediately after the procedure the patient can comfortably ventilate and be mobilized without additional oxygen.

a further step within our policy of minimizing invasiveness of surgery and anesthetics.[13–16]

In our experience, awake VATS is feasible and safe in all patients with complex mediastinal masses and results in a diagnostic yield of 100%; it is associated with no perioperative cardiopulmonary adverse events and negligible morbidity (**Table 3**).

Our current results contrast with those reported so far for surgical biopsy performed using general anesthesia, which can be associated with difficult weaning, prolonged mechanical ventilation, and a morbidity rate as high as 20%.[6–9] The adverse effects of general anesthesia are not to be underestimated and include barotrauma, volutrauma, atelectrauma, and biotrauma. These adverse effects are particularly dangerous in patients with bulky mediastinal masses that cause compression of the airways and the upper venous system. The reasons for this are probably multifactorial; lung volumes are reduced by 500 to 1000 mL as a result of the loss of diaphragm and abdominal muscle relaxation[6,9]; smooth muscle relaxation may favor

Table 3
Surgical and nonsurgical diagnostic methods for anterior mediastinal masses

Procedure	Diagnostic Yield	Complication Rate[a]	Advantages	Limits
Surgical methods				
Extended mediastinoscopy[22–24]	Excellent (>95%)	~3%	Minimally invasive	Risk for vascular injury Supine position needed
Anterior mediastinotomy[25–28]	Good (85%–96%)	7%–16%	Minimally invasive Local anesthesia possible	Limited access Supine position needed
Video-assisted thoracoscopy[2–5,29,30]	Excellent (93%–100%)	2%–4%	Minimally invasive Multisite sampling	One-lung ventilation needed
Awake video-assisted thoracoscopy	Excellent (100%)	–	Minimally invasive Multisite sampling Avoidance of general anesthesia	Lack of large clinical evaluation
Nonsurgical Methods				
CT-guided FNA/CB[25,26,31–35]	Satisfactory (71%–91%)	5%–11%	Short procedure, minimal discomfort	Less accurate for lymphomas and germ-cell tumors
Ultrasound-guided needle biopsy[36,37]	Satisfactory (79%–89%)	~3%	Minimal discomfort Cost-saving	Difficult procedure with advanced emphysema (inadequate window)

Abbreviations: CB, core biopsy; FNA, fine-needle aspiration cytology.
[a] Postoperative morbidity rate includes major and minor surgery-related complications.

compression of the tracheobronchial tree exerted by the mass.[6] The absence of spontaneous ventilation reduces the negative pleural pressure gradient, which contributes to airways' patency under normal conditions.[6–9] Furthermore, it has been postulated that, in cases of preexisting central airway obstruction, mechanical ventilation may enhance poststenotic turbulence of the inhaled gases, which may critically reduce alveolar ventilation.[6,8,9] Great vessels including the superior vena cava and the main pulmonary artery can also be compressed by the mass reducing the right ventricular preload and decreasing pulmonary perfusion.[8,10] These adverse effects are exaggerated by the supine position, which increases compression of the mediastinal structures by gravity.

From these findings, local anesthesia with spontaneous ventilation has been advocated as the safest type of anesthesia to be used in surgical management of patients with bulky mediastinal masses although so far, this type of approach has been anecdotally reported. In the 1970s, Ward[38] reported on the use of mediastinoscopy under local anesthesia as a minimally invasive diagnostic tool. The author emphasized the easy feasibility of this procedure and some peculiar advantages, including reduced bleeding compared with open biopsy performed under general anesthesia. However, standard mediastinoscopy is not suitable for biopsy of anterior mediastinal masses. In 1977, Arom and colleagues[39] proposed inserting a mediastinoscope through a subxiphoid incision to allow exploration and biopsy of anterior mediastinal compartments. Subsequently, Sibert and colleagues[40] reported on a patient with a bulky mediastinal mass and superior vena cava obstruction who was managed via anterior thoracotomy with awake intubation and spontaneous ventilation. In 2002, Rendina and colleagues[41] reported on the use of an optical mediastinoscope inserted through a parasternal incision under local anesthesia in patients with anterior mediastinal lesions. With this procedure, the investigators reached a 100% diagnostic yield with no mortality and limited (4.3%) morbidity. More recently, awake VATS has been reported for management of pericardial effusion[42,43] and even thymectomy.[44,45]

Theoretic concerns regarding this approach include the risk of ventilatory impairment induced by the surgical pneumothorax, loss of airway patency, and compression of the dependent lung by the mediastinal mass. However, we have been encouraged by the highly satisfactory results observed with other thoracic surgery procedures[13–16] including our awake nonresectional lung volume reduction surgery technique[16] and awake VATS biopsy performed in patients with diffuse lung disease. We immediately noticed that arterial oxygenation was easily maintained within highly satisfactory ranges and no patient required ventilatory support.

Anterior mediastinotomy is one of the most commonly used surgical alternatives to our new approach.[25,26] However, we believe that the limited visualization, less than ideal scarring, the potential delay in starting salvage radiotherapy because of the anterior location of the skin incision and the need for additional access for insertion of a thoracic drain or even additional VATS management of other associated intrathoracic conditions, constitute clear disadvantages of anterior mediastinotomy compared with the awake VATS approach.

The pros and cons of awake VATS management in patients with complex mediastinal masses must be balanced against the choice of nonsurgical methods that include CT-guided fine-needle aspiration or core biopsy. These methods have become increasingly popular, although there is a certain discordance on the actual diagnostic accuracy of these techniques. Agid and colleagues[46] have reported a diagnostic yield of only 82.5% in a large retrospective review of patients with mediastinal lymphomas undergoing CT-guided biopsy. Furthermore, in a prospective study by Fang and colleagues[25] comparing anterior mediastinotomy with CT-guided biopsy for bulky mediastinal masses, the latter resulted in a diagnostic yield of 41.7%. A similar conclusion has been made by Watanabe and colleagues.[26] Gossot and colleagues[31] reported a 75% failure rate with CT-guided needle biopsy in restaging residual lymphomas after antiblastic treatment.

Besides the possibility of failures, one has to keep in mind that imaging-guided biopsy is not completely risk free. Pneumothorax and bleeding are reported to occur at a low but constant rate after the procedure although iatrogenic pneumothorax resulting from percutaneous needle biopsy is usually regarded as a minor complication.

We believe that, in patients with anterior mediastinal masses, the advantages of awake VATS over the other methods include safety, wide visual control of mediastinal sampling, and accurate assessment of the disease extension with an excellent diagnostic yield. Because most anterior mediastinal masses are lymphoproliferative disorders, pathologists appreciate the possibility of analyzing multiple biopsy specimens from different sites of the mass to allow precise histologic characterization because of the possible coexistence of Hodgkin and non-Hodgkin features in the same lesion. In addition, awake VATS offers the possibility of performing pleural-pulmonary biopsies and draining concomitant pleural-pericardial effusions through a single access that is identical to that used to insert a simple thoracic drain. Immediate management of pericardial effusion is not to be underestimated because this condition has been found to be predictive of life-threatening complications and even to significantly affect survival[47] in patients with bulky mediastinal masses.[8]

Using a transpleural route avoids any potential delay for salvage radiation therapy because the skin incision is located far from fields targeted for mediastinal irradiation. Lateral decubitus and avoidance of muscle relaxation may contribute to reduce compression of the airways by the mass during surgery.[48]

SUMMARY

In our hands, awake VATS was well tolerated by patients and is a safe and reliable approach for surgical management of complex anterior mediastinal masses. Using this approach we achieved a 100% diagnostic yield with no adverse cardiopulmonary events and negligible morbidity. Although further investigation is needed, this approach should be included in the thoracic surgeon armamentarium within the framework of minimally invasive options as a new tool that seems suited for all patients with anterior mediastinal masses, and particularly when these are associated with other intrathoracic conditions requiring surgical management. Anterior mediastinal masses can develop from a wide spectrum of pathologic conditions, most of which are malignant in nature and require prompt diagnosis for immediate initiation of the appropriate treatment. Clinical pictures can be variable and complicated by associated intrathoracic conditions requiring surgical management such as pleural and pericardial effusions or nodules (complex anterior mediastinal masses).

We have employed a single-trocar VATS approach using thoracic epidural or sole local anesthesia in awake patients. Advantages of awake VATS biopsy include avoidance of all potential adverse effects related to the use of general anesthesia, wide visual control of mediastinal sampling, and accurate assessment of the disease extent with the possibility of obtaining multiple biopsy specimens from different sites of the mass. In addition, adequate surgical management of associated intrathoracic conditions is possible through a single skin incision that resembles that used to insert a simple thoracic drain.

This novel and less invasive surgical option might thus be included within the framework of most reliable methods currently available to manage patients with undetermined anterior mediastinal masses.

REFERENCES

1. Date H. Diagnostic strategies for mediastinal tumors and cysts. Thorac Surg Clin 2009;19:29–35.
2. Sugarbaker DJ. Thoracoscopy in the management of anterior mediastinal masses. Ann Thorac Surg 1993;56:653–6.
3. Roviaro G, Varoli F, Nucca O, et al. Videothoracoscopic approach to primary mediastinal pathology. Chest 2000;117:1179–83.
4. Yim AP. Video-assisted thoracoscopic management of anterior mediastinal masses. Preliminary experience and results. Surg Endosc 1995;9:1184–8.
5. Cirino LM, Milanez de Campos JR, Fernandez A, et al. Diagnosis and treatment of mediastinal tumors by thoracoscopy. Chest 2000;117:1787–92.
6. Goh MH, Liu XY, Goh YS. Anterior mediastinal masses: an anaesthetic challenge. Anaesthesia 1999;54:670–4.
7. Azizkhan RG, Dudgeon DL, Buck JR, et al. Life-threatening airway obstruction as complication to the management of mediastinal masses in children. J Pediatr Surg 1985;20:816–22.
8. Bechard P, Létourneau L, Lacasse Y, et al. Perioperative cardiorespiratory complications in adults with mediastinal mass. Anesthesiology 2004;100:826–34.
9. Erdos G, Kunde M, Tzanova I, et al. Anasthesiologisches Management bei mediastinale Raumforderung [Anaesthesiological management of mediastinal tumors]. Anaesthesist 2005;54:1215–28 [in German].
10. Power CK, Buggy D, Keogh J. Acute superior vena caval syndrome with airway obstruction following elective mediastinoscopy. Anaesthesia 2007;52:989–97.
11. Pullerits J, Holzman R. Anaesthesia for patients with mediastinal masses. Can J Anaesth 1989;36:681–8.
12. Prakash UB, Abel MD, Hubmayr RD. Mediastinal mass and tracheal obstruction under general anesthesia. Mayo Clin Proc 1988;63:1004–11.
13. Pompeo E, Tacconi F, Mineo D, et al. The role of awake video-assisted thoracoscopic surgery in spontaneous pneumothorax. J Thorac Cardiovasc Surg 2007;133:786–90.
14. Pompeo E, Mineo D, Rogliani P, et al. Feasibility and results of awake thoracoscopic resection of solitary pulmonary nodules. Ann Thorac Surg 2004;78: 1761–8.
15. Pompeo E, Mineo TC. Awake pulmonary metastasectomy. J Thorac Cardiovasc Surg 2007;133:960–6.
16. Mineo TC, Pompeo E, Mineo D, et al. Awake nonresectional lung volume reduction surgery. Ann Surg 2006;243:131–6.
17. Meysman M, Vincken W. Effects of body posture on dynamic lung functions in young non-obese Indian subjects. Chest 1998;114:1042–7.

18. Mineo TC. Epidural anesthesia in awake thoracic surgery. Eur J Cardiothorac Surg 2007;32:13–9.
19. Bayar A, Tuncay I, Atasoy N, et al. The effect of watching live arthroscopic views on postoperative anxiety of patients. Knee Surg Sports Traumatol Arthrosc 2008;16:982–7.
20. Lepage C, Drolet P, Girard M, et al. Music decreases sedative requirements during spinal anesthesia. Anesth Analg 2001;93:912–6.
21. Forcella D, Pompeo E, Coniglione F, et al. A new technique for continuous intercostal-intrapleural analgesia in videothoracoscopic surgery. J Thorac Cardiovasc Surg 2009;127:e48–9.
22. Lopez L, Varela A, Freixinet J, et al. Extended cervical mediastinoscopy: prospective study of fifty cases. Ann Thorac Surg 1994;57:555–7.
23. Metir M, Sayar A, Turna A, et al. Extended cervical mediastinoscopy in the diagnosis of anterior mediastinal masses. Ann Thorac Surg 2002;73:250–2.
24. Freixinet Gilart J, Garcia PG, de Castro FR, et al. Extended cervical mediastinoscopy in the staging of bronchogenic carcinoma. Ann Thorac Surg 2000;70:1641–3.
25. Fang W, Xu M, Chen G, et al. Minimally invasive approaches for histological diagnosis of anterior mediastinal masses. Chin Med J 2007;120:675–9.
26. Watanabe M, Takagi K, Aoki T, et al. A comparison of biopsy through a parasternal anterior mediastinotomy under local anesthesia and percutaneous needle biopsy for malignant anterior mediastinal tumors. Surg Today 1998;28:1022–6.
27. Steiger Z, Chaundhry S, Wilson RF. The use of anterior mediastinotomy to assess intrathoracic lesions. Am Surg 1981;47:251–3.
28. Martigne C, Velly JF, Clerc P, et al. Value and current role of anterior mediastinotomy in the diagnosis of mediastinal diseases. Apropos of a series of 100 cases. Ann Chir 1989;43:171–3.
29. Solaini L, Bagioni P, Campanini A, et al. Diagnostic role of videothoracoscopy in mediastinal diseases. Eur J Cardiothorac Surg 1998;13:491–3.
30. Landrenau RJ, Hazelrigg SR, Mack MJ, et al. Thoracoscopic mediastinal lymph node sampling: useful for mediastinal lymph node stations inaccessible by cervical mediastinoscopy. J Thorac Cardiovasc Surg 1993;106:554–8.
31. Gossot D, Girard P, de Kerviler E, et al. Thoracoscopy or CT-guided biopsy for residual intrathoracic masses after treatment of lymphoma. Chest 2001; 120:289–94.
32. Desai F, Shah M, Patel S, et al. Fine needle aspiration cytology of anterior mediastinal masses. Indian J Pathol Microbiol 2008;51:88–90.
33. Priola AM, Priola SM, Cataldi A, et al. CT-guided percutaneous transthoracic biopsy in the diagnosis of mediastinal masses: evaluation of 73 procedures. Radiol Med 2008;113:3–15.
34. Gupta S, Wallace MJ, Morello FA Jr, et al. CT-guided percutaneous needle biopsy of intrathoracic lesions by using the transsternal approach: experience in 37 patients. Radiology 2002;222:57–62.
35. Greif J, Staroselsky AN, Gernjac M, et al. Percutaneous core needle biopsy in the diagnosis of mediastinal tumors. Lung Cancer 1999;25:169–73.
36. Hsu WH, Chiang CD, Hsu JY, et al. Ultrasonically guided needle biopsy of anterior mediastinal masses: comparison of carcinomatous and non-carcinomatou masses. J Clin Ultrasound 1995;23: 349–56.
37. Yu CJ, Yang PC, Chang DB, et al. Evaluation of ultrasonically guided biopsies of mediastinal masses. Chest 1991;100:399–405.
38. Ward P. Mediastinoscopy under local anesthesia. A valuable diagnostic technique. Calif Med 1970; 112:15–22.
39. Arom KV, Franz JL, Grover FL, et al. Subxiphoid anterior mediastinal exploration. Ann Thorac Surg 1977;24:289–90.
40. Sibert KS, Biondi JW, Hirsch NP. Spontaneous respiration during thoracotomy in a patient with mediastinal mass. Anesth Analg 1987;66:904–7.
41. Rendina EA, Venuta F, De Giacomo T, et al. Biopsy of anterior mediastinal masses under local anesthesia. Ann Thorac Surg 2002;74:1720–2.
42. Katlic MR. Video-assisted thoracic surgery utilizing local anesthesia and sedation. Eur J Cardiothorac Surg 2006;30:529–32.
43. De Bellis P, Delfino R, Robbiano F, et al. High epidural thoracic anesthesia for pericardial surgery. Minerva Anestesiol 2005;71:595–9.
44. Al-Abdullatief M, Wahood A, Al-Shirawi N, et al. Awake anaesthesia for major thoracic surgical procedures: an observational study. Eur J Cardiothorac Surg 2007;32:346–50.
45. Matsumoto I, Oda M, Watanabe G. Awake endoscopic thymectomy via an infrasternal approach using sternal lifting. Thorac Cardiovasc Surg 2008; 56:311–3.
46. Agid R, Sklair-Levy M, Bloom AI, et al. CT-guided biopsy with cutting-edge needle for the diagnosis of malignant lymphoma: experience of 267 biopsies. Clin Radiol 2003;58:143–7.
47. Neragi-Miandoab S, Linden PA, Ducko CT, et al. VATS pericardiotomy for patients with known malignancy and pericardial effusion: survival and prognosis of positive cytology and metastatic involvement of the pericardium: a case control study. Int J Surg 2008;6:110–4.
48. Cho Y, Suzuki T, Yokoi M, et al. Lateral position prevents respiratory occlusion during surgical procedure under general anesthesia in the patient of huge anterior mediastinal lymphoblastic lymphoma. Jpn J Thorac Cardiovasc Surg 2004; 52:476–9.

Extended Transcervical Video-Assisted Thymectomy

Christopher B. Komanapalli, MD[a],
James I. Cohen, MD, PhD[b], Mithran S. Sukumar, MD[c,*]

KEYWORDS

- Transcervical thymectomy • Transsternal technique
- Video-assisted thoracoscopic thymectomy
- Myasthenia gravis

Transcervical thymectomy (TCT) was first performed by Sauerbruch in 1912 for myasthenia gravis (MG).[1] Blalock and colleagues[2] published a series of transsternal thymectomies in 1941 for both thymoma and myasthenia that led to the widespread use of this technique. However, it was not until the 1960s that Crile[3] repopularized thymectomy via the transcervical route.

In 1973, Masaoka and colleagues[4] established the "extended thymectomy"—the en bloc resection of all anterior mediastinal adipose tissue along with the thymus via median sternotomy. Adipose tissue from around the upper poles of the thymus, the brachiocephalic veins, and the pericardium are all meticulously removed. The extent of the dissection is from the diaphragm inferiorly, the thyroid superiorly, and the phrenic nerves laterally.

In 1988, Jaretzki and colleagues[5] coined the term "maximal" thymectomy, which consisted of a cervical incision to completely dissect the gland in the neck and a sternotomy via which all anterior mediastinal and hilar adipose tissue was removed between the phrenic nerves. They reported an improved remission rate for myasthenia and this became the standard against which other techniques are measured.[6] In the same year, Cooper and colleagues[7] reported a modified technique of TCT employing the use of a custom sternal retractor which allowed improved visualization of the mediastinum by anterior retraction of the sternum. Subsequently, series employing this technique have reported comparable rates of remission to that of maximal thymectomy.[8]

Thoracoscopy has been added to the techniques by which thymectomy can be accomplished with a left or right chest approach; and series have reported a short-term remission equivalent to the previous techniques.[9] In 2002, Keshavjee[10] described the addition of thoracoscopy to the transcervical route, which improved illumination and visualization of the mediastinum facilitating transcervical thymectomy. Most recently, robotics has been added to the techniques available to perform a thymectomy.[11] Maximal thymectomy utilizing a combined transcervical, subxiphoid, and thoracoscopic approach has also been recently described.[12]

This article describes the transcervical approach with thoracoscopic visualization allowing the performance of an extended thymectomy,

[a] Department of Surgery, Oregon Health & Sciences University, Portland Veterans Affairs Medical Center, L223A, 3181 SW Sam Jackson Park Road, Portland, OR 97239, USA
[b] Department of Surgery, Portland Veterans Affairs Medical Center, Oregon Health & Sciences University, 3710 SW US Veterans Hospital Road, Portland, OR 97239, USA
[c] Division of Cardiothoracic Surgery, Department of Surgery, Portland VA Medical Center, Oregon Health & Sciences University, L353, 3181 SW Sam Jackson Park Road, Portland, OR 97239, USA
* Corresponding author.
E-mail address: sukumarm@ohsu.edu

Thorac Surg Clin 20 (2010) 235–243
doi:10.1016/j.thorsurg.2010.02.004
1547-4127/10/$ – see front matter. Published by Elsevier Inc.

thereby incorporating the minimally invasive nature of the transcervical method with the extensive anterior mediastinal dissection.

PATIENT SELECTION

The transcervical video-assisted extended approach is well suited for patients undergoing thymectomy for MG, thymic cysts, thymoma less than 2 cm, and a mediastinal parathyroid adenoma within the thymus.[8] Thin, young women patients may be best suited for this approach as they have a more pliable thoracic cage and less muscular chest wall compared to men, allowing a larger working space within the mediastinum.

Obesity is a relative contraindication to this approach as the anterior mediastinal exposure is limited by body shape and fat, and the ability of the Rultract Skyhook (Rultract Inc, Corporate Headquarters, Cleveland, OH, USA) sternal retractor to provide adequate exposure in these patients.

Patients who have had median sternotomy or prior radiation to the anterior mediastinum are not suitable for this approach owing to adhesions that are present that prevent expansion of the anterior mediastinal space after placement of the sternal retractor, which is a requirement to perform the operation safely.

PREOPERATIVE PREPARATION

Investigations

All patients are imaged with CT scan and have pulmonary functions checked. Those with myasthenia are optimized medically by a neurologist prior to surgery.

Anesthesia

General anesthesia via a double lumen endotracheal tube is used as single-lung ventilation facilitates exposure during the mediastinal dissection.

Positioning

The patient is positioned supine with an inflatable pressure bag placed horizontally or vertically behind the shoulders to extend the neck and to allow for improved exposure of the anterior mediastinum later in the procedure. A large bore (16 G) intravenous line is placed in a peripheral vein and a radial arterial line is also placed. The endotracheal tube is positioned to the left of the mouth and the head of the patient can be turned to the left to further improve access to the mediastinum. The entire neck and anterior chest are prepped and draped so that access to the sternum is easily available should conversion to sternotomy be required.

The surgeon wears a headlight to help with illumination of the mediastinum and loops to improve visualization when performing the cervical dissection as well as parts of the mediastinal dissection, which are performed under direct vision. A thirty-degree thoracoscope is used to provide illumination and visualization within the lower anterior mediastinum and the pleural cavity. Insertion of the scope through the cervical incision is done carefully to avoid smearing of the lens and it is maintained at the right end of the cervical incision while dissecting the left mediastinum, and vice versa when dissecting the right. The surgeon is positioned at the head of the bed so a direct view of the mediastinum from superior to inferior is obtained. The assistant stands to the right or left of the surgeon, depending on the position of the thoracoscope. The video monitor is best positioned at the foot of the bed so that the surgeon and assistant have the same view of the mediastinum.

Surgical Technique

The steps of the operation are summarized below:

1. A transverse curved 5 cm cervical incision is made 2 cm above the sternal notch between the sternocleidomastoid muscles. Subplatysmal skin flaps are raised superiorly to thyroid cartilage and inferiorly to the sternal notch. The strap muscles are dissected in the midline and down to the sternal notch. In patients with a short or thick neck, inferior division and superior reflection of the sternothyroid muscles improves the exposure in the neck and into the upper mediastinum. The upper poles of the thymus are identified on the posterior aspect of the strap muscles where they have the appearance of encapsulated fat and can be bluntly dissected with a Kittner dissector from the surrounding tissue. The thyrothymic ligament at the superior extent of the poles are ligated and divided between 2-0 silk ligatures, which are left long on the thymic end. This allows for traction on the gland, which facilitates the dissection into the superior mediastinum.
2. The plane just posterior to the sternum is developed bluntly with a finger and the Rultract retractor is placed and the skyhook used to elevate the sternum.[13] The inflatable pressure bag posterior to the shoulder and spine is deflated allowing the anterior mediastinum to further expand as the rest of the mediastinum falls away from the sternum.
3. The thymus is then dissected into the superior mediastinum using blunt, sharp, and

cautery dissection interchangeably. The thoracoscope is useful to provide illumination of the wound at this time and often helps with visualization due to the magnified view it provides (**Fig. 1**). The thymic veins are encountered posterior to the gland draining into the anteroinferior aspect of the innominate vein. These are isolated and ligated using 2-0 silk ligatures. Clips are not used as the repeated passage of instruments through this area during the operation may cause them to dislodge. Extension of the gland behind the innominate vein can be dissected at this time. The gland should be completely dissected from the left innominate vein, right innominate vein, and the upper aspect of the superior vena cava at this time, leaving attachments only at the upper lateral margins of the gland that can be dissected when the pleura have been opened and the phrenic nerves can be visualized.

4. The substernal plane is then created bluntly using tonsil sponges on a curved ring clamp. This dissection extends from the sternal notch

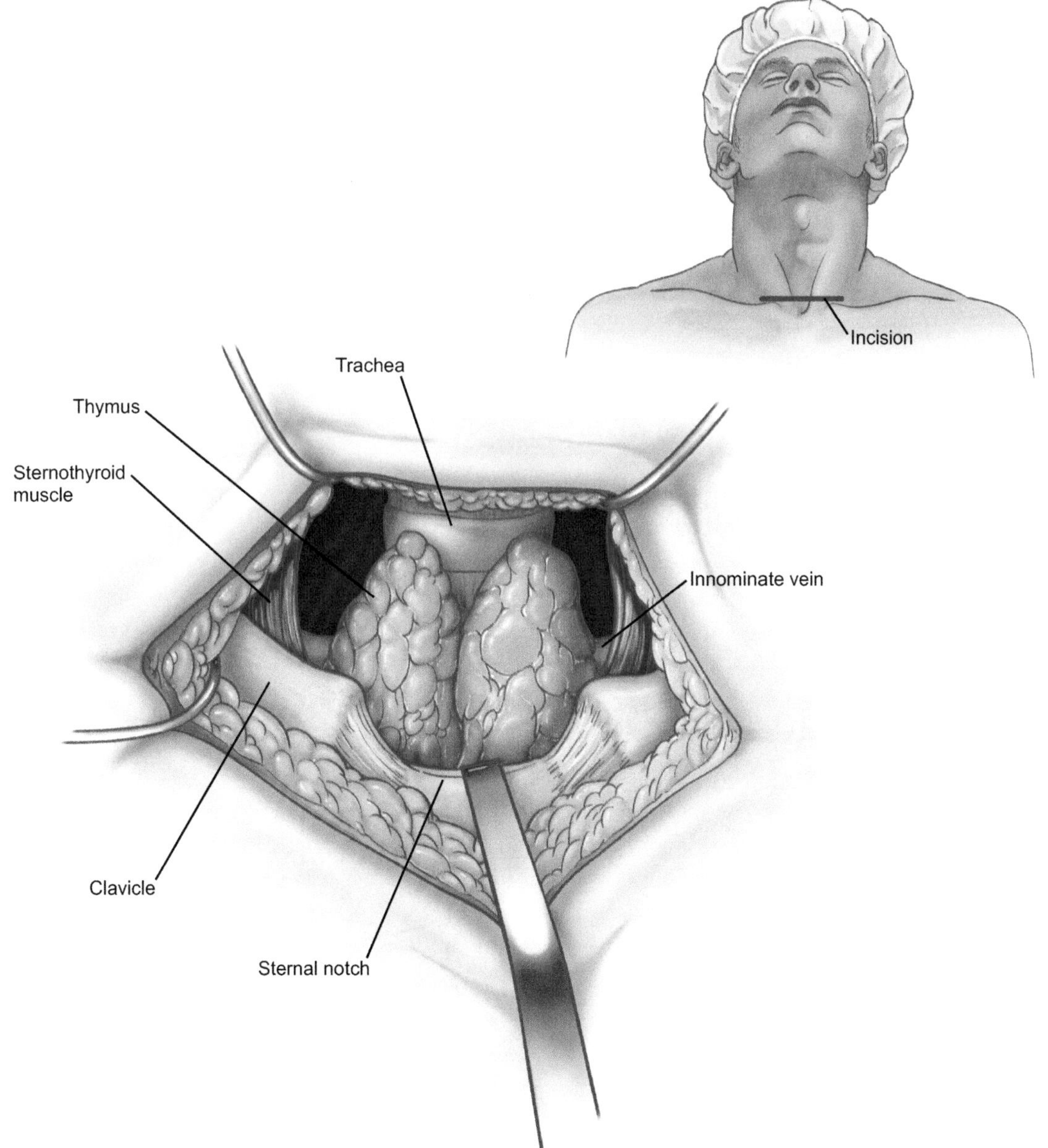

Fig. 1. Open neck showing superior aspect of thymus and innominate vein.

to the domes of the diaphragm and laterally to the pleural reflections. This can be done blindly, under direct vision, or with the thoracoscope, which is introduced through either end of the neck wound.

5. The left lung is deflated and the mediastinal pleura widely opened or resected from the diaphragm to below the sternal notch. The thoracoscope provides excellent illumination and improved visualization at this stage allowing the phrenic nerve to be clearly seen. Collapsing the left lung aids in the ease of performing a complete anterior mediastinal dissection and allowing the phrenic nerve to be kept in view at all times. Use of a Yankauer suction cup keeps the field free of smoke and it can be used to place tension on the pleural edge as the pleura is opened and to bluntly dissect the lateral margin of the thymus. Rolling the operating room table to the contralateral side of the mediastinal dissection improves visualization and makes this part of the mediastinum more accessible.
6. After the left phrenic nerve is identified, the pleural opening is continued superiorly ensuring that the nerve or the mammary vessels are not damaged as the dissection proceeds superiorly (**Fig. 2**).
7. The thymus is grasped with a thoracoscopic ring clamp, retracted to the right and—starting just below the aorto-pulmonary window—dissected medial to the nerve using a combination of sharp (thoracoscopic scissors) and blunt techniques (Kittner or tonsil sponge) continuing distally to the left inferior pole. Vessels that are encountered can be clipped using a 5 mm endoclip applier and divided. Once the left margin of the gland has been dissected, this is continued medially, separating it from the anterior surface of the pericardium sharply or bluntly.

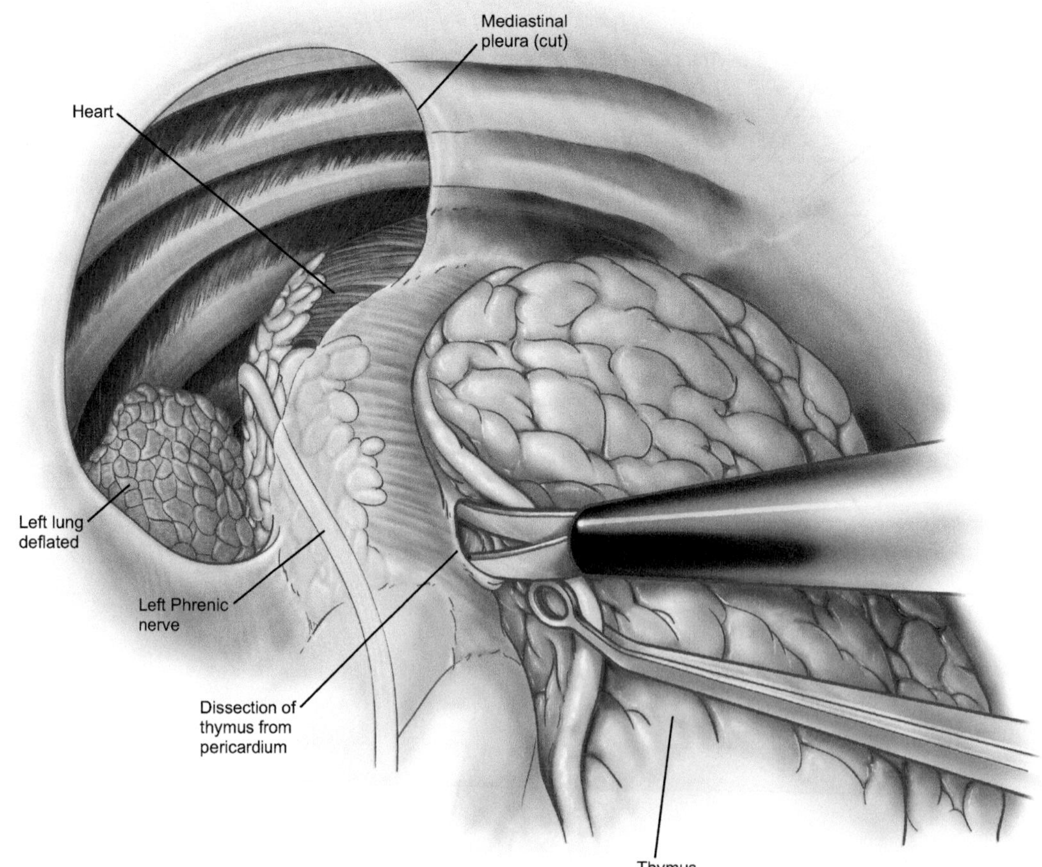

Fig. 2. Looking down into the mediastinum with the pleural cavities open.

The use of cautery on the pericardium should be minimized as this reduces the chance of pericarditis and pericardial effusion postoperatively. The diaphragmatic dissection of the mediastinal fat and gland is done in a similar fashion. This dissection is continued as far right of the midline as possible. The left lung is then re-expanded.

8. The right pleura is then opened after collapsing the right lung. This opening is started inferiorly and continued superiorly, taking care to protect or divide the internal mammary vein at the upper extent of the opening if this facilitates further exposure. The phrenic nerve running over the anterior hilum is visualized and avoided as the right margin of the gland is dissected, after retracting it to the left, by grasping it with a thoracoscopic ring clamp, starting superiorly or inferiorly. Particular care is paid to the position of the phrenic nerve when dissecting the superior aspect of the gland. The dissection is continued medially until all except the upper part of the gland is attached to the anterior surface of the pericardium. Dissection of the lateral right upper part of the gland that had previously been dissected from the innominate vein and the superior vena cava is now completed staying just medial to the phrenic nerve.
9. The gland is grasped in the midline at the level of the innominate vein and retracted anteriorly and to the left and the posterior aspect of the gland dissected sharply to the anteroposterior window. Once this is complete, the left upper margin of the gland is dissected anteriorly from the phrenic nerve just medial from the anteroposterior window. With this, the gland is freed from the mediastinum and is removed through the cervical incision.
10. Any remaining anterior mediastinal and pericardial fat can now be removed. At the conclusion of the operation, the entire anterior mediastinum should be clear of thymic tissue and fat (**Fig. 3**).
11. A no. 19 Blake drain is placed via the neck into the anterior mediastinum and pleural cavities and the lung reinflated. The neck incision is then closed in layers.

At any time during the procedure, if exposure is not adequate to perform the extended thymectomy then a sternotomy or thoracoscopy can be performed to aid in the dissection and completion of thymectomy. This is a matter of surgical judgment and the surgeon must always ensure that the intended operation is not compromised due to a desire to use a minimally invasive technique.

Postoperative Management

Patients are extubated in the operating room and are transferred to a monitored surrounding depending on their underlying disease process. Patients can resume a diet and ambulate as tolerated immediately. Pain is managed with intravenous patient controlled aneasthesia (for the first 24 hours), oral anti-inflammatories, and then with oral narcotics. The drain is removed once drainage is less than 200 cc in 24 hours and patients are able to discharge on postoperative day 1 or 2.

RESULTS

Transsternal Technique

Transsternal-extended thymectomy has traditionally been the standard technique for complete excision of the thymus in patients with MG with or without thymoma and all other techniques are measured against this benchmark.[2,4]

In 1996, Masaoka and colleagues[4] described their 20-year consecutive series of 375 patients with MG who underwent either extended thymectomy (286 patients without thymoma) or extended thymectomy with total resection of thymoma (89 patients). Preoperatively, patients were classified by the following classes: I, ocular symptoms only; IIa, mild generalized MG; IIb, severe generalized MG; and III, acute fulminating MG. Patients were seen up to 20-years postoperatively with their functional status categorized as: group A, asymptomatic without medications; group B, increased functional status with less medication; group C, no change; group D, more medication or worsening symptoms; and group E, death due to MG. There were no operative deaths; however, 29 patients died perioperatively: 14 (4.9%) in the nonthymoma group and 15 (16.9%) in the thymoma group. Eleven of these patients died from complications of MG (5, nonthymoma and 6, thymoma). There was no discussion about hospital length of stay or complication-morbidity rates. Remission rates in nonthymoma patients (patients who were asymptomatic without disease per total number of patients at that follow-up point): 36.9% at 3 years and 45.8% at 5 years, with a 20-year remission rate of 50%. This same group's clinical palliation rate (asymptomatic patients and patients improved on less medication per total patients at the follow up point) was 91.6% at 3 years and 92.2% at 5 years with a 20-year palliation rate of 91.7%. Patients with a thymoma had significantly worse remission rates of 32.4% at 3 years and 23% at 5 years with a 20-year remission rate of 37.5%. Similarly, palliation rates were significantly diminished compared to the nonthymoma group

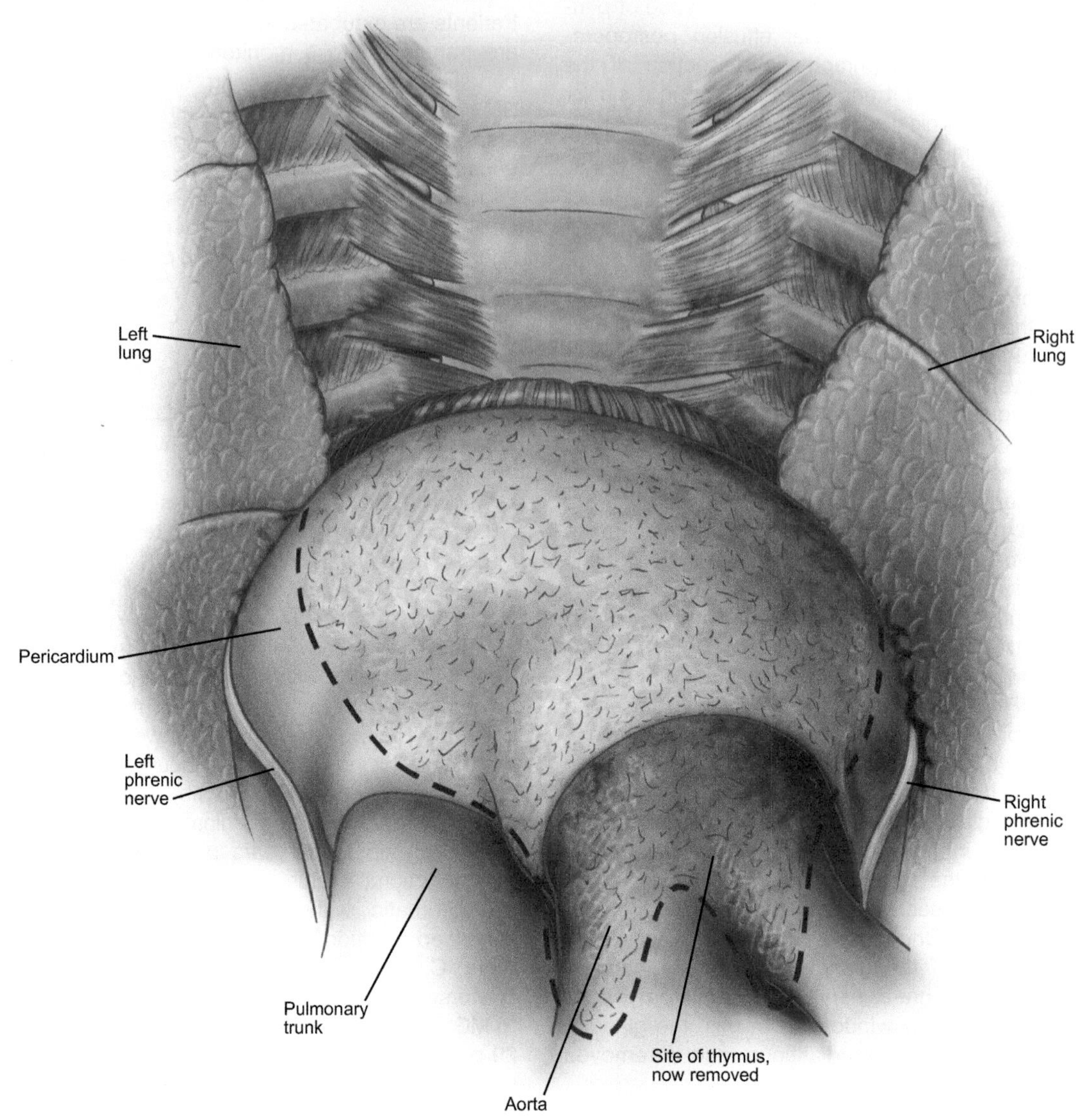

Fig. 3. Mediastinum after the thymus has been removed.

with 3- and 5-year palliation rates of 76.5% and 85.2% with a 20-year rate of 87.5% ($P<.05$). Subgroup analysis of functional status revealed that there was no difference between groups in the nonthymoma group, whereas patients with thymoma and minimal symptoms had the best remission rate with declining remission rates in more symptomatic patients. They concluded that a transsternal approach provides excellent remission rates in patients with nonthymoma MG; and, in thymomatous MG patients with short duration and minimal symptoms, thymectomy offers improvement in functional status.

Video-assisted Thoracoscopic Thymectomy

Subsequently, video-assisted thoracoscopic thymectomy has been shown to be an acceptable alternative approach. Mack and colleagues,[9] in 2009, described their series of 95 patients who underwent either transsternal (47) or video-assisted thoracic surgery (VATS) (48) for MG. The groups were not significantly different in terms of gender, preoperative duration of symptoms, and operative times. Mean age was slightly older in the VATS group (34.4 years, transsternal vs 39.8 years, VATS). There were more patients in MG functional class III in the transsternal group;

however, there were more patients in the MGFA class IV group in the VATS group. Their transsternal approach is similar to the technique described by Masaoka and colleagues,[4] but with a limited skin incision. The VATS approach involves single-lung ventilation; four right-sided ports are placed. Dissection is initiated anterior to the phrenic nerve, and all anterior mediastinal tissue is dissected off the sternal table anteriorly and the pericardium posteriorly. The tissues are swept cephalad. Tissues surrounding the innominate veins are dissected and the thymic vein doubly clipped and ligated. Then, carbon dioxide insufflation is used to facilitate exposure of the upper poles of the thymus. Lastly, the thymus is dissected from the left phrenic nerve bluntly. The specimen is removed through an Endocatch bag (Covidien, North Haven, CT, USA) and the chest desufflated. No chest tubes are placed. Patients are extubated in the operating room. Postoperative care is performed in the general ward and patients are discharged the next day.

They determined several important outcome-related differences between the two groups. There was a statistically significant difference in hospital length of stay (LOS) of 4.6 days in the transsternal compared to 1.9 days in the VATS group ($P<.001$). There were four deaths in the series, unrelated to MG. In their analysis, they were able to determine that patients undergoing VATS had a complete stable remission (CSR) rate of 34.9% compared to 15.8% in the transsternal group. Pharmacologic remission (other than anticholinesterase inhibitors) in 7.9% of transsternal compared to 4.7% in the VATS group. They concluded that VATS offers reduction in hospital LOS, and similar remission rates.

Transcervical Approach

For a time, the TCT was sparingly performed by thoracic surgeons because of the popularity of the transsternal extended and maximal thymectomy based on their results and, possibly, the familiarity of the sternotomy among cardiothoracic surgeons.

There are now numerous series demonstrating the efficacy of the TCT in myasthenic patients with improvement in functional status and CSR similar to those of sternotomy with significantly less morbidity.[7,8,14–16]

While the transcervical approach was reintroduced in the 1960s for resection of the thymus, one of the first series was reported in 1994 by DeFilippi and colleagues[14] in a retrospective analysis of 53 patients who had MG without thymoma. The patients had a mean age of 27.5 and a mean duration of symptoms of 2 years. Their Osserman classification was as follows: Class I, 13%; Class IIA, 53%; Class IIB, 28%; Class III, 6%. Average hospital LOS was 3 days and there were no deaths in their series. Eighty-one percent were asymptomatic and 43% were in complete remission at 5-years follow-up postoperatively. There was no difference in Osserman classification, thymic histology, or patient age in respect to overall outcome. The investigators concluded that this was an effective technique for patients with non-thymoma MG.

The transcervical technique was further improved with the advent of the robust Cooper thymectomy retractor (Pilling Co, Fort Washington, PA, USA). Calhoun and colleagues[15] described their series of 100 patients who underwent TCT with the use of the Cooper retractor. In their series, 61% were women with a mean age of 38 years. The mean duration of symptoms was 1.7 years. Average hospital LOS was 1.2 days, 85% were discharged on the first postoperative day and 96% by postoperative day 2. There were eight complications in this series: one patient developed seizures, another developed myasthenic crisis, and one developed deep vein thrombosis that was treated with systemic anticoagulation. Five patients were found to have apical pneumothorax postoperatively; two of which underwent aspiration with prompt resolution. Eighty-five percent of patients had clinical improvement of at least one Osserman grade. Thirty-five percent were in remission (symptom and medication free) and 71% had no generalized symptoms at 5-years follow-up time. Fourteen percent had no change in Osserman grade and one patient had deteriorated one Osserman grade. The investigators reported that, since patients are often on chronic prednisone empirically postoperatively to prevent re-emergence of symptoms, their remission rate would otherwise be 46%, comparable to the outcomes of Masaoka and colleagues.[4] Calhoun and colleagues[15] concluded that TCT offers a low morbidity and zero mortality rate compared to as high as 33% morbidity rate with "maximal" thymectomy (reported by Jaretzki and colleagues[6] using a combined transsternal and cervicomediastinal approach).

Calhoun and colleagues[15] also reported that, given that the operative times, hospital LOS, and morbidity rates were all less than more radical approaches, that the cost difference would be significant. Lastly, they reported that the rapid return to work and a favorable cosmetic result offers improved patient satisfaction.

In the largest series to date, reported in 2006 by Shrager and colleagues,[16] 164 patients with MG underwent an attempted TCT. Thirteen required further extension of the procedure (VATS, partial or full sternotomy), leaving 151 patients undergoing TCT. The mean age was 42.5 years and 60.3% were women. Mean preoperative Osserman class was 2.3; of which 21.2% were class I, 39.1% class II, 27.6% class III, and 12.2% class IV. Preoperative duration of symptoms was greater than 2 years in 31.4% of patients. The average LOS was 1.10 days, and there were no perioperative deaths. Eleven patients (7.3%) experienced complications, which were described as seroma, pleural effusion, pneumothorax, wound infection, myasthenia flare, pneumonia, or vocal cord paralysis.

Their crude CSR rate was 43% and 45% at 3 and 6 years, respectively, in patients who are asymptomatic or on minimal immunosuppression therapy. Patients who were asymptomatic without any medication comprised 33% and 35% of patients at 3 and 6 years, respectively. They noted that none of their patients who had an initial complete remission relapsed. A univariate analysis determined that Osserman class was associated with postoperative remission rate such that a lower Osserman grade was associated with higher crude CSR. Multivariate analysis further showed the preoperative Osserman class was associated with postoperative CSR. They concluded that extended transsternal or maximal thymectomy offer similar CSR rates to transcervical approaches and that the small difference that is offered by more radical dissection is tempered by significant increases in morbidity.

COMMENT

Based on a recent series, the transcervical route is now proven equivalent to the transsternal route for thymectomy in selected patients.[16]

The combination of the transcervical route and the technique of extended thymectomy are now possible and theoretically allow for the benefits of both procedures to be combined. The use of a cervical incision, single-lung ventilation, a special retracting system, the thoracoscope, and widely opening the pleura allows complete resection of the thymus and anterior mediastinal fat (extended thymectomy), yet avoids the morbidity associated with a sternotomy. The technique described in this article differs from TCT in that single-lung ventilation is always used and the pleura is widely opened on both sides.

The transcervical approach to thymectomy with video-assistance is a safe, reliable technique to perform a complete thymectomy with a low morbidity and hospital stay and equivalent remission rates in MG.[16]

The authors' preliminary experience appears to follow that of the TCT series so far published, but confirmation of this will have to determined in the future.

To date there are no published series or trials involving transcervical video-assisted extended thymectomy. Whether this procedure results in increased morbidity over routine transcervical thymectomy or improvement in the remission rate for myasthenia is unknown and will have to await further study.

SUMMARY

The technique of transcervical video-assisted extended thymectomy allows for complete removal of the thymus and anterior mediastinal fat and avoids the morbidity of a sternotomy.

REFERENCES

1. Schumacher E, Roth J. Thymektomie bei cenum Fall von Morbus Basedowii mit myasthenia. Mit a. d. Grezgeb d. Med Chir 1912;25:746 [in German].
2. Blalock A, McGehee H, Ford F. The treatment of myasthenia gravis by removal of the thymus gland. J Am Med Assoc 1941;117:1529.
3. Crile G Jr. Thymectomy through the neck. Surgery 1966;59(2):213–5.
4. Masaoka A, Yamakawa Y, Niwa H, et al. Extended thymectomy for myasthenia gravis patients: a 20-year review. Ann Thorac Surg 1996;62(3):853–9.
5. Jaretzki A 3rd, Wolff M. "Maximal" thymectomy for myasthenia gravis. Surgical anatomy and operative technique. J Thorac Cardiovasc Surg 1988;96(5):711–6.
6. Jaretzki A 3rd, Penn AS, Younger DS, et al. "Maximal" thymectomy for myasthenia gravis. Results. J Thorac Cardiovasc Surg 1988;95(5):747–57.
7. Cooper JD, Al-Jilaihawa AN, Pearson FG, et al. An improved technique to facilitate transcervical thymectomy for myasthenia gravis. Ann Thorac Surg 1988;45(3):242–7.
8. Shrager JB, Deeb ME, Mick R, et al. Transcervical thymectomy for myasthenia gravis achieves results comparable to thymectomy by sternotomy. Ann Thorac Surg 2002;74(2):320–6 [discussion: 326–7].
9. Mack MJ, Landreneau RJ, Yim AP, et al. Results of video-assisted thymectomy in patients with myasthenia gravis. J Thorac Cardiovasc Surg 1996;112(5):1352–9 [discussion: 1359–60].
10. Keshavjee R. Videothoracoscopic transcervical thymectomy. In: Pearson FG, editor. Thoracic surgery. Churchill Livingstone; 2002. p. 1769–73.
11. Rea F, Marulli G, Bortolotti L, et al. Experience with the "da Vinci" robotic system for thymectomy in

patients with myasthenia gravis: report of 33 cases. Ann Thorac Surg 2006;81(2):455–9.
12. Zielinski M, Kuzdzał J, Szlubowski A, et al. Transcervical-subxiphoid-videothoracoscopic "maximal" thymectomy–operative technique and early results [review]. Ann Thorac Surg 2004;78(2):404–9 [discussion: 409–10].
13. Komanapalli CB, Person TD, Schipper P, et al. An alternative retractor for transcervical thymectomy. J Thorac Cardiovasc Surg 2005;130(1):221–2.
14. DeFilippi VJ, Richman DP, Ferguson MK. Transcervical thymectomy for myasthenia gravis. Ann Thorac Surg 1994;57(1):194–7.
15. Calhoun RF, Ritter JH, Guthrie TJ, et al. Results of transcervical thymectomy for myasthenia gravis in 100 consecutive patients. Ann Surg 1999;230(4):555–9 [discussion: 559–61].
16. Shrager JB, Nathan D, Brinster CJ, et al. Outcomes after 151 extended transcervical thymectomies for myasthenia gravis. Ann Thorac Surg 2006;82(5):1863–9.

Extended Transsternal Thymectomy

Vincent C. Daniel, MD, Cameron D. Wright, MD*

KEYWORDS

• Thymectomy • Myasthenia • Thymoma • Surgery

The 2 primary indications for thymectomy are the treatments of patients with thymoma and patients with myasthenia gravis. Several different methods have been described to remove the thymus gland, including transcervical-transsternal "maximal" thymectomy, extended transsternal thymectomy, classic transsternal thymectomy, (extended) transcervical thymectomy, and video-assisted thoracoscopic (VATS) thymectomy. The purpose of this article is to focus on the technical aspects of performing an extended transsternal thymectomy and the published results of extended transsternal thymectomy as compared with other techniques available.

Several early reports linked the thymus to myasthenia gravis, including those by Oppenheim in 1889[1,2] and Weigert in 1901,[3] who noted that at autopsy, patients with myasthenia gravis also had a high proportion of thymic tumors present. After this, there were several isolated reports of thymic tumors being removed from patients with myasthenia gravis, with subsequent improvement in their myasthenic symptoms.[4,5] However, it was Alfred Blalock at the Johns Hopkins Hospital who popularized the procedure of thymectomy in patients with myasthenia gravis. He performed transsternal thymectomy on a series of patients with nonthymomatous myasthenia gravis and noted that there was an improvement in their symptoms, thus initiating the modern experience of performing thymectomy on patients with significant myasthenia gravis symptoms despite medical therapy.[6,7]

The development of the thymus gland begins around the sixth week of gestation, at which time an epithelial outpouching develops from the third branchial pouch and begins to descend caudally. This outpouching of tissue, in addition to giving rise to the inferior parathyroid glands, further differentiates and moves to the midline to ultimately give rise to primordial thymic tissue.[8] Around the tenth week of gestation, migration of lymphocytes occurs from the fetal liver and yolk sac to populate the primordial thymus. At birth, the thymus gland weighs approximately 15 g, and it continues to enlarge in size until puberty, reaching its maximum weight of approximately 35 g. Subsequently, the gland progressively involutes and regresses throughout the remainder of life. The primary role of the thymus includes the development of immunocompetent T cells, differentiation of T-cell subsets, and the development of immunologic self tolerance. Genetic mutations in thymus-specific genes, as seen for example in DiGeorge syndrome, result in impaired immunologic function.

At birth, the thymus resides as a bilobed structure in the anterior superior mediastinum, usually between the thyroid superiorly and resting on the pericardium inferiorly (**Fig. 1**). The blood supply of thymic tissue is provided by the internal mammary arteries and the inferior thyroid artery. Venous drainage is provided either directly into the innominate vein or through thyroid venous tributaries. The size and shape of the adult thymus is variable with involution and fatty replacement as aging occurs.

Patients with myasthenia gravis referred for thymectomy require a careful preoperative neuromuscular evaluation before undergoing surgery. Approximately 30% of patients with thymoma also have myasthenia gravis.[9,10] Preoperative planning is critical in patients with myasthenia gravis in order to avoid postoperative complications such as

Division of Thoracic Surgery, Massachusetts General Hospital, Blake 1570, 55 Fruit Street, Boston, MA 02114, USA
* Corresponding author.
E-mail address: cdwright@partners.org

Thorac Surg Clin 20 (2010) 245–252
doi:10.1016/j.thorsurg.2010.02.005

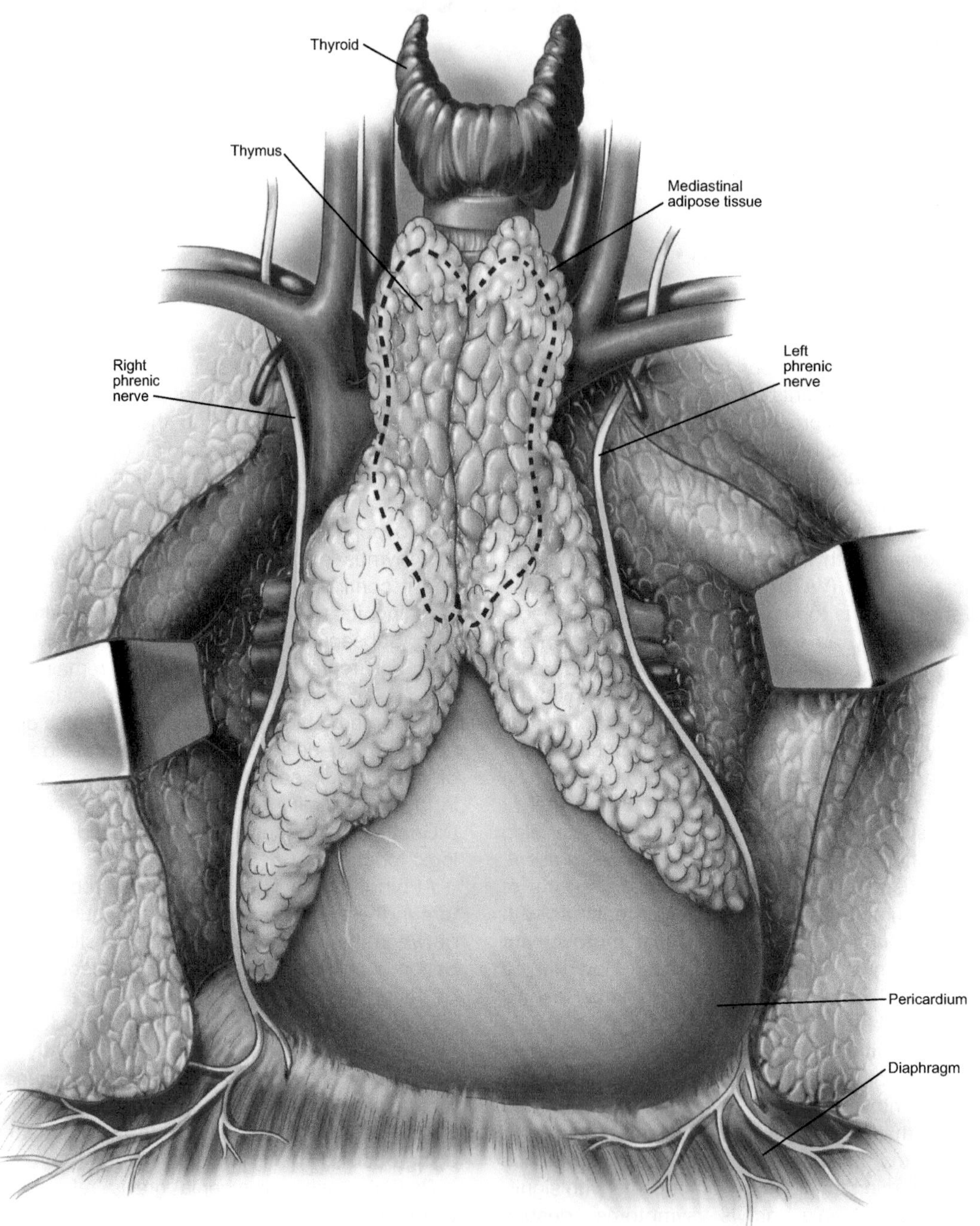

Fig. 1. The relationship of the thymus to the mediastinal and cervical structures. The thymus is quite variable, and can be fused or has separate lobes. The lower poles can extend down for a variable distance toward the diaphragm.

aspiration, postoperative respiratory failure, or myasthenic crisis. Patients with myasthenia gravis should receive a computed tomography scan because 10% to 15% will also have a thymoma present.[9,11] Most patients take pyridostigmine (Mestinon), which should be continued up to the time of surgery. Patients may also take prednisone or other immunosuppressive medications, and these should also be continued up until surgery. Spirometry preoperatively may help identify those patients who are at increased risk of having problems postoperatively. Patients with a vital capacity less than 2.9 L, forced expiratory force less than 40 to 50 cm H_2O, previous respiratory insufficiency secondary to myasthenia gravis, or a history of myasthenia gravis for more than 6 years should be considered as at higher risk for postoperative difficulty.[12–15] Patients with significant bulbar or extrabulbar weakness or those who are identified preoperatively as at high risk for respiratory complications may also benefit from either preoperative plasmapheresis or intravenous immunoglobulin (IVIG) therapy. Plasmapheresis occurs over 3 to 5 sessions performed every other day before surgery. Studies have shown a reproducible benefit to patients who have undergone plasmapheresis treatment.[16–18] IVIG therapy also appears in studies to show a postoperative benefit for patients with myasthenia gravis undergoing thymectomy, but studies comparing IVIG therapy with plasmapheresis are difficult to interpret because there is a bias for patients with the more symptomatic myasthenia gravis to receive plasmapheresis preoperatively.[19] In patients with more modest symptoms, IVIG and plasmapheresis seem to be comparable, with greater ease in treatment noted with IVIG therapy. IVIG treatment is given as a 400-mg/kg/d dose administered over 3 to 5 days.[19]

The goal of thymectomy for either treatment of thymoma or management of myasthenia gravis is the complete removal of all thymic tissue. There is a proven oncologic benefit in thymoma patients in performing a complete resection because essentially all studies demonstrate that a complete resection is the most important prognostic factor.[20,21] In addition, studies appear to demonstrate a higher remission rate and palliation rate with complete removal of all thymic tissue in patients with myasthenia gravis.[22,23] The most effective method of removing all thymic tissue, however, continues to remain controversial. Studies have demonstrated the presence of microscopic deposits of thymic tissue in pericardial fat overlying the heart, in the aortopulmonary window, and behind the innominate vein.[24] Based on this information, some surgeons believe that the presence of any amount of thymic tissue left behind compromises the results of the operation procedure. Whether this assumption is correct continues to be a source of debate.

SURGICAL TECHNIQUE

Extended transsternal thymectomy involves the removal of all thymic tissue in the mediastinum, including the 2 cervical lobes of thymic tissue extending into the neck. It also includes resection of all fatty tissue in the anterosuperior mediastinum between the 2 phrenic nerves from the diaphragm to the bottom of the thyroid gland (**Fig. 2**).

An incision is made in the middle of the sternum from manubrium to xiphoid and the subcutaneous tissue is divided with electrocautery. The sternum is divided, and a retractor is placed after adequate periosteal and bone marrow hemostasis is obtained.

We (the authors of this article) begin our dissection by removing all evidence of thymic tissue and fat from the anterior surface of the pericardium starting at the level of the diaphragm and proceeding cephalad. We routinely enter both pleural spaces early on to locate the phrenic nerves to define the lateral margins of resection and importantly preserve the phrenic nerves. When a thymoma is present, it is also important to examine the entire visceral and parietal pleural surface to confirm the absence of metastatic disease or drop metastasis. The dissection of mediastinal fat and thymic tissue proceeds in an en bloc fashion along the pericardium cephalad, with the lateral extent of resection defined by the right and left phrenic nerves. It is important not to use unipolar cautery too close to the phrenic nerves to avoid injury. Additional caution should be used higher in the mediastinum near the thoracic inlet because the phrenic nerves travel more medially and are prone to injury at this level. There is always a significant amount of fatty tissue around this area, and some judgment is necessary in deciding how much to remove when it is adjacent to the phrenic nerve.

Most times, at this point, it is easier to begin the remainder of the operation at the upper extent of dissection, defined by the cervical lobes of the thymus inferior to the thyroid gland. There is an areolar layer of connective tissue deep to the strap muscles that is readily dissected away from the 2 thymic cervical lobes. We ligate or cauterize each apex of the thymic cervical lobes and then progress caudally, removing all evidence of thymic and adipose tissue down to the level of dissection begun at the pericardium.

Care should be exercised in identifying and ligating thymic veins arising from the innominate vein, of which there are usually 2, but considerable variation exists.

Likewise, the arterial branches from the internal mammary or inferior thyroid arteries should be carefully controlled. At the conclusion of the dissection, the left brachiocephalic vein should be cleaned of overlying adipose tissue, as should the area inferior to the thyroid gland where the cervical lobes reside and the pericardium from the innominate vein to the diaphragm.

A special note should be made for thymectomy in conjunction with resection of thymic tumors invading adjacent structures. Studies have

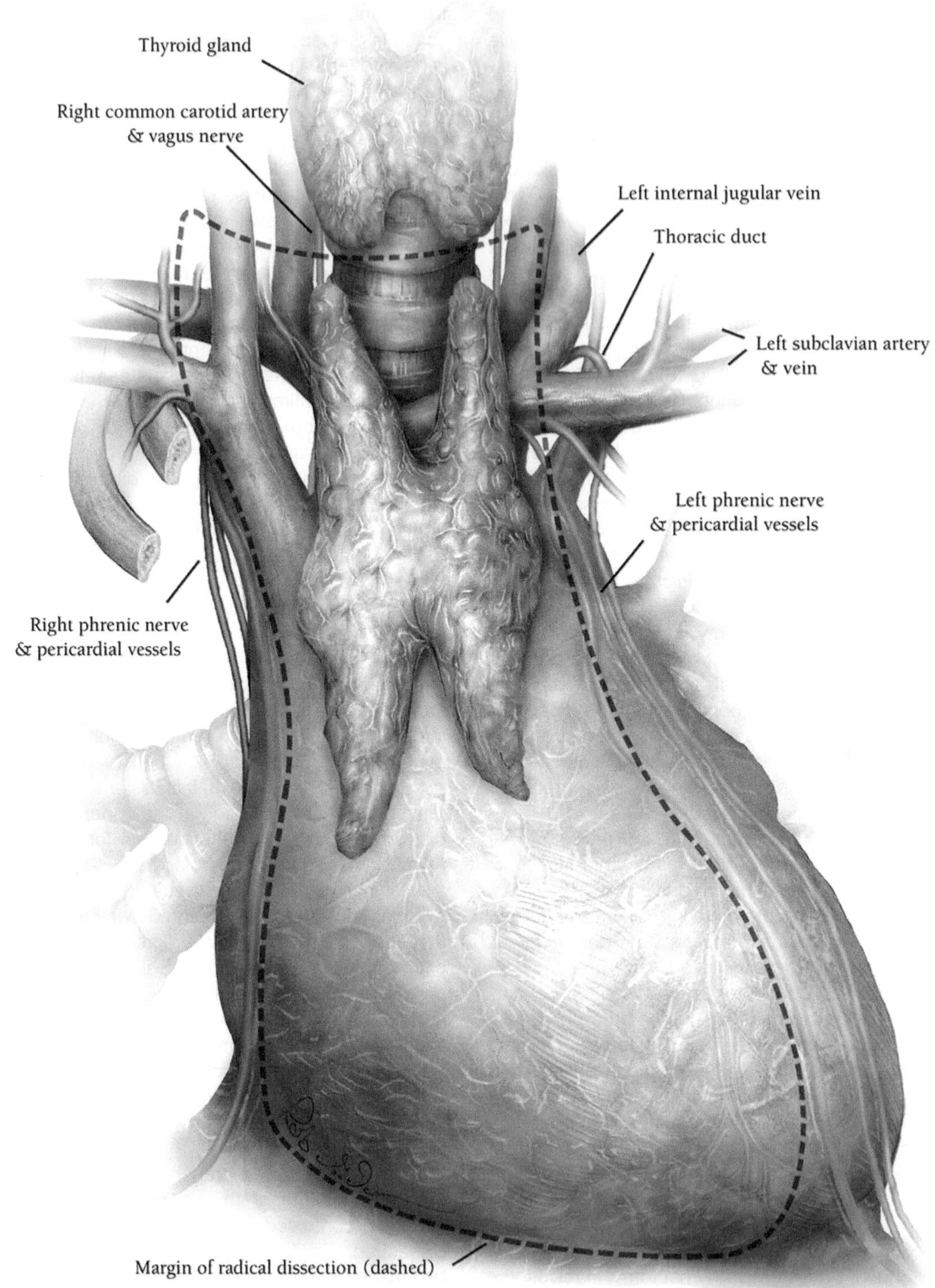

Fig. 2. The extent of resection for an extended transsternal thymectomy. The dotted lines indicate the approximate margins of resection of the mediastinal adipose tissue that encompasses the thymus and presumably thymic rests in the fat. (*Reproduced from* Mason DP. Radical transsternal thymectomy. Operat Tech Thorac Cardiovasc Surg 2005;10(3):231–43; with permission.)

demonstrated that the most important factor in the prevention of thymoma recurrence is to achieve a complete resection.[20,21] Accordingly, there should be no hesitation in resecting adjacent structures involved with tumor. This resection includes lung, pericardium, chest wall, innominate vein or superior vena cava, or a single phrenic nerve, provided both nerves are not involved with tumor. If it is apparent that both phrenic nerves are involved with tumor, the area is debulked as much as possible and clips are placed for future radiation therapy.

On completion of the en bloc resection, mediastinal chest tubes are placed with the tips present in the pleural space. Sternal wires are placed for chest closure, and the periosteal tissue, subcutaneous tissue, and skin are closed. Patient-controlled analgesia is used for pain control for the first 1 or 2 days, then the patient is switched to oral oxycodone. The drainage tubes are usually removed on the second postoperative day. Most patients are discharged on the fourth postoperative day. Serious complications are rare after extended transsternal thymectomy. Death is extremely rare and is usually either due to underlying cardiovascular disease or a myasthenic crisis. Sternal infections are very rare but represent a very serious complication that requires aggressive debridement and reoperation. Atelectasis is common and usually self-limited. Rarely, atelectasis leads to a postoperative pneumonia or an aspiration pneumonia develops. Bleeding requiring reoperation is very rare. Atrial fibrillation is a common complication in older patients, especially if the pericardium is resected. Occasionally the postpericardiotomy syndrome develops after discharge, leading to fever, pleuritic chest pain, and troublesome pleural effusions. This condition is treated with nonsteroidal anti-inflammatory agents.

COMMENT

Convincing evidence has demonstrated that compared with patients with myasthenia gravis undergoing medical therapy alone, those undergoing thymectomy have significantly improved rates of medication-free remission and of being asymptomatic, and have improved disease severity.[25–27] Based on these studies, the Myasthenia Gravis Foundation of America (MGFA) recommends thymectomy as an option to increase the probability of remission or improvement in nonthymomatous myasthenia gravis.[28] However, considerable debate remains as to the best surgical technique of performing thymectomy and the extent of resection needed to produce the best clinical results. To simplify the nomenclature of surgical procedures performed and to standardize future studies comparing various techniques, the MGFA developed a thymectomy classification scheme of the various operative procedures performed for thymic resection (**Table 1**).[29]

In addition, several studies have sought to identify myasthenia gravis patients who would benefit greatest from thymectomy postoperatively. Unfortunately, there are few conclusive studies clearly identifying a patient population most likely to benefit from surgical intervention. Patients undergoing thymectomy for myasthenia gravis with the presence of a thymoma tend to have less favorable remission rates.[30–32] Other factors that have been examined as prognostic indicators of likelihood of remission include age, sex, and severity and duration of illness. Again, no definitive conclusions can be drawn from the available studies. It seems there is greater benefit to thymectomy if symptoms have been present for less than 1 year.[33] Also, younger patients appear to have better response rates and, not surprisingly, decreased morbidity.[34,35] Studies are equivocal, however, on the effect gender plays in thymectomy response rate.[32,36,37] All of these factors remain controversial with regard to their influence on myasthenia gravis remission rates after thymectomy, and should not be used as a basis for determining surgical candidacy.

What also becomes apparent in reviewing published results of thymectomy is the wide variability among studies, making direct comparisons difficult (**Table 2**). Diverse follow-up periods, varying degrees of disease severity, inclusion of thymomatous and nonthymomatous myasthenia gravis, variable definitions of patient response to surgical treatment, and inclusion of multiple surgical techniques within a single study make conclusive

Table 1
Thymectomy classification scheme

T-1	Transcervical thymectomy
A	Basic
B	Extended
T-2	Video-assisted thoracoscopic thymectomy
A	Classic
B	Extended (VATET)
T-3	Transsternal thymectomy
A	Standard
B	Extended
T-4	Transcervical-transsternal thymectomy

Table 2
Recent published outcomes for various thymectomy techniques

Surgery	Author	Year	Institution	Number	Remission Rate	Palliation Rate	Follow-up (Mean)
Extended transsternal	Kattach et al[31]	2006	Oxford	85	17.0%	79%	4.5 y
	Park et al[39]	2006	South Korea	150 (NT + T)	37.0%		7.5 y
	Jaretzki et al[22]	1988	New York	72 (maximal)	46.0%	79%	40 mo
	Masaoka et al[5]	1996	Osaka	286	45.8%		5 y
	Bulkley et al[32]	1997	Baltimore	157 (nT + T)		86%	5 y
Extended transcervical	Calhoun et al[40]	1999	St Louis	100	35.0%	71%	5 y
	DeFilippi et al[41]	1994	Chicago	53	41.0%		
	Shrager et al[42]	2002	Philadelphia	78	40.0%	90%	4.6 y
VATS	Meyer et al[43]	2009	Dallas	95	34.9%		6.1 y
	Tomulescu et al[44]	2006	Bucharest	42	43.0%		5 y
	Mineo et al[45]	2000	Rome	31	36.0%	96%	4 y

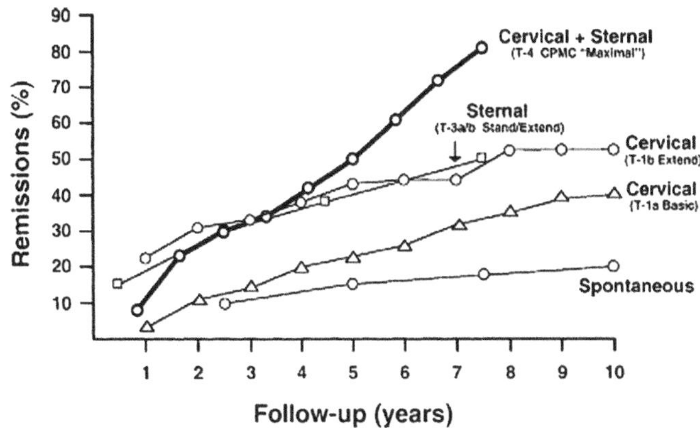

Fig. 3. Life-table analysis of different thymectomy techniques with remission rates over time. Note that the spontaneous remission rate and the remission rate of each thymectomy technique increase with time. These patients are nonrandomized, so great caution must be made in comparing the remission rates among the various techniques. (*Reproduced from* Jaretzki A III. Thymectomy for myasthenia gravis: analysis of controversies – patient management. Neurologist 2003;9:77–92; with permission.)

recommendations difficult. What does seem to be inferred from the available data is that after thymectomy, complete remission (defined as medication and symptom free) results may be expected in 35% to 45% of patients up to 5 years after the procedure, and palliation (defined as symptom free on medication or minimal symptoms on no medication) can be expected in 70% to 90% of patients. Analysis of the data shows a continued clinical improvement associated with passage of time after thymectomy (**Fig. 3**). For this reason, several published reports advocate the use of Kaplan-Meier survival curve analysis as a more accurate method to assess the true rate of remission.[38] With the retrospective data available, however, no major difference can be concluded in the study outcomes provided by the individual methods. More rigorously controlled studies are necessary to make direct comparisons between surgical procedures.

SUMMARY

Thymectomy continues to remain the mainstay in the treatment of thymoma and myasthenia gravis. Extended transsternal thymectomy has historically been the gold standard for thymoma resection and in the treatment of nonthymomatous myasthenia gravis. Techniques more recently reported in the literature such as VATS thymectomy and extended transcervical thymectomy may have similar efficacy in the treatment of nonthymomatous myasthenia gravis. Regardless of the technique used, the purpose of surgery is to remove all thymic tissue possible. The extended transsternal thymectomy can reliably remove the thymus, and most mediastinal adipose tissue with accessory thymic tissue present, with acceptable morbidity and mortality.

REFERENCES

1. Pascuzzi RM. The history of myasthenia gravis. Neurol Clin 1994;12(2):231–42.
2. Oppenheim H. Weiterer Beitrag zur Lehre von der acuten nicht-eitrigen Encephalitis und der Polioencephalomyelitis [Further contribution to the knowledge of acute non-purulent encephalitis and polio encephalitis]. Dtsch Z Nervenheilkund 1899;15:1–27 [in German].
3. Weigert C. Pathologisch-anatomischer Beitrag zur Erb'schen Krankheit (myasthenia gravis) [Pathologic-anatomic contribution to Erb's disease (myasthenia gravis)]. Neurol Zentralbl 1901;20:597–601 [in German].
4. Schumacher R. Thymektomie bei einem Fall von Morbus Basedowi mit Myasthenie [Thymectomy in a case of Basedow disease with myasthenia]. Mitten Grenz Med Chirg 1912;25:746 [in German].
5. Masaoka A, Yamakawa Y, Niwa H, et al. Extended thymectomy for myasthenia gravis patients: a 20 year review. Ann Thorac Surg 1996;62:853–9.
6. Blalock A, Harvey A, Ford F. The treatment of myasthenia gravis by removal of the thymus gland. JAMA 1941;117:1529.
7. Blalock A. Thymectomy in the treatment of myasthenia gravis: report of 20 cases. J Thorac Surg 1944;13:316.
8. Shields TW. The thymus. In: Shields TW, Locicero J III, Ponn RB, et al, editors. 6th edition, In: General thoracic surgery, vol. 2. Philadelphia: Lippincott Williams & Wilkins; 2005. p. 2347–56.
9. Thomas CR, Wright CD, Loehrer PJ. Thymoma: state of the art. J Clin Oncol 1999;17:2280–9.
10. Adams R, Allan FN. Thymectomy in the treatment of myasthenia gravis. Chest 1947;13:436–49.
11. Drachman DB. Myasthenia gravis. N Engl J Med 1994;330:1797–810.
12. Kernstine KH. Preoperative preparation of the patient with myasthenia gravis. Thorac Surg Clin 2005;15:287–95.
13. Younger DS, Braun NMT, Jaretzki A, et al. Myasthenia gravis: determinants for independent

ventilation after transsternal thymectomy. Neurology 1984;34:336–40.
14. Leventhal SR, Orkin FK, Hirsh RA. Prediction of the need for postoperative mechanical ventilation in myasthenia gravis. Anesthesiology 1980;53:26–30.
15. Eisenkraft JB, Papatestas AE, Kahn CH, et al. Predicting the need for postoperative mechanical ventilation in myasthenia gravis. Anesthesiology 1986;65:79–82.
16. Cumming WJK, Hudgson P. The role of plasmapheresis in preparing patients with myasthenia gravis for thymectomy. Muscle Nerve 1986;9:S155–8.
17. d'Empaire G, Hoaglin DC, Perlo VP, et al. Effect of prethymectomy plasma exchange on postoperative respiratory function in myasthenia gravis. J Thorac Cardiovasc Surg 1985;89:592–6.
18. Spence PA, Morin JF, Katz M. Role of plasmapheresis in preparing myasthenic patients for thymectomy: initial results. Can J Surg 1984;27:303–5.
19. Jensen P, Bril VA. Comparison of the effectiveness of intravenous immunoglobulin and plasma exchange as preoperative therapy of myasthenia gravis. J Clin Neuromuscul Dis 2008;9(3):352–5.
20. Mangi AA, Wain JC, Donahue DM, et al. Adjuvant radiation of stage III thymoma: is it necessary? Ann Thorac Surg 2005;79:1834–9.
21. Regnard J-F, Magdeleinat P, Dromer C, et al. Prognostic factors and long-term results after thymoma resection, a series of 307 patients. J Thorac Cardiovasc Surg 1996;112:376–84.
22. Jaretzki A III. Thymectomy for myasthenia gravis: analysis of controversies regarding technique and results. Neurology 1997;48(Suppl 5):S52–63.
23. Jaretzki A, Penn AS, Younger DS, et al. "Maximal" thymectomy for myasthenia gravis: results. J Thorac Cardiovasc Surg 1988;95:747–57.
24. Jaretzki A, Wolff M. "Maximal" thymectomy for myasthenia gravis: surgical anatomy and operative technique. J Thorac Cardiovasc Surg 1988;96:711–6.
25. Buckingham JM, Howard FM Jr, Bernatz PE, et al. The value of thymectomy in myasthenia gravis: a computer-assisted matched study. Ann Surg 1976;184:453.
26. Mantegazza R, Beghi E, Pareyson D, et al. A multicentre follow-up study of 1152 patients with myasthenia gravis in Italy. J Neurol 1990;237:339.
27. Papatestas AE, Genkins G, Kornfeld P, et al. Effects of thymectomy in myasthenia gravis. Ann Surg 1987;206:79.
28. Gronseth GS, Barohn RJ. Practice parameter: thymectomy for autoimmune myasthenia gravis (an evidence-based review): report of the Quality Standards Subcommittee of the American Academy of Neurology. Neurology 2000;55:7–15.
29. Jaretzki A 3rd, Barohn RJ, Ernstoff RM, et al. Myasthenia gravis: recommendations for clinical research standards. Task force of the Medical Scientific Advisory Board of the Myasthenia Gravis Foundation of America. Ann Thorac Surg 2000;70:327.
30. Venuta F, Rendina EA, De Giacomo T, et al. Thymectomy for myasthenia gravis: a 27-year experience. Eur J Cardiothorac Surg 1999;15:621.
31. Kattach H, Anastasiadis K, Cleuziou J, et al. Transsternal thymectomy for myasthenia gravis: surgical outcome. Ann Thorac Surg 2006;81:305–8.
32. Bulkley GB, Bass KN, Stephenson GR, et al. Extended cervicomediastinal thymectomy in the integrated management of myasthenia gravis. Ann Surg 1997;226(3):324–34.
33. Lopez-Cano M, Ponseti-Bosch JM, Espin-Basany E, et al. Clinical and pathologic predictors of outcome in thymoma-associated myasthenia gravis. Ann Thorac Surg 2003;76:1643.
34. Huang CS, Hsu HS, Huang BS, et al. Factors influencing the outcome of transsternal thymectomy for myasthenia gravis. Acta Neurol Scand 2005;112:108.
35. Nieto IP, Robledo JP, Pajuelo MC, et al. Prognostic factors for myasthenia gravis treated by thymectomy: review of 61 cases. Ann Thorac Surg 1999;67:1568.
36. Beghi E, Antozzi C, Batocchi AP, et al. Prognosis of myasthenia gravis: a multicenter follow-up study of 844 patients. J Neurol Sci 1991;106:213.
37. Ozdemir N, Kara M, Dikmen E, et al. Predictors of clinical outcome following extended thymectomy in myasthenia gravis. Eur J Cardiothorac Surg 2003;23:233.
38. Jaretzki A III. Thymectomy for myasthenia gravis: analysis of controversies—patient management. Neurology 2003;9:77–92.
39. Park IK, Choi SS, Lee JG, et al. Complete stable remission after extended transsternal thymectomy in myasthenia gravis. Eur J Cardiothorac Surg 2006;30(3):525–8.
40. Calhoun RF, Ritter JH, Guthrie TJ, et al. Results of transcervical thymectomy for myasthenia gravis in 100 consecutive patients. Ann Surg 1999;230(4):555–61.
41. DeFilippi VJ, Richman DP, Ferguson MK. Transcervical thymectomy for myasthenia gravis. Ann Thorac Surg 1994;57:194.
42. Shrager JB, Deeb ME, Mick R, et al. Transcervical thymectomy for myasthenia gravis achieves results comparable to thymectomy by sternotomy. Ann Thorac Surg 2002;74:320–7.
43. Meyer DM, Herbert MA, Sobhani NC, et al. Comparative clinical outcomes for myasthenia gravis performed by extended transsternal and minimally invasive approaches. Ann Thorac Surg 2009;97:385–91.
44. Tomulescu V, Ion V, Kosa A, et al. Thoracoscopic thymectomy mid term results. Ann Thorac Surg 2006;82:1003–8.
45. Mineo TC, Pompeo E, Lerut TE, et al. Thoracoscopic thymectomy in autoimmune myasthenia: results of left sided approach. Ann Thorac Surg 2000;69:1537–41.

Extended Videothoracoscopic Thymectomy in Nonthymomatous Myasthenia Gravis

Tommaso C. Mineo, MD*, Eugenio Pompeo, MD

KEYWORDS

- Myasthenia gravis • Thymectomy
- Nonthymomatous myasthenia gravis
- Videothoracoscopic thymectomy

Myasthenia gravis (MG) is an uncommon, organ-specific, autoimmune chronic neuromuscular disorder involving the production of autoantibodies directed against the nicotinic acetylcholine receptors (anti-AchRab). It is characterized by weakness and rapid fatigability of voluntary muscles. Ocular muscles are frequently involved rendering ptosis and dyplopia the most common symptoms at onset.

MG was first described by the English physician, Thomas Willis, in a woman with the fatigable weakness of limbs "who temporarily lost her power of speech."[1] The disease was later described in more detail but at that time diagnosis was difficult and it was frequently made only in patients with severe weakness and pneumonia who died within 1 or 2 years of onset. In 1934, Mary Walker[2] showed that physostigmine promptly improved myasthenic symptoms. Since then, anticholinesterase drugs have improved the promptness of diagnosis and facilitated the clinical management of myasthenic patients. A further improvement in clinical course was achieved by use of sulfonomides, antibiotics, and thymectomy.

In 1937, Blalock removed a mediastinal mass from a young woman with MG who improved postoperatively. Later, Blalock's other myasthenic patients improved after surgical removal of the thymus so that thymectomy became an established treatment of MG.[3]

The incidence of MG is 3 to 4 per million per year. The prevalence is about 60 per million, with higher figures in countries where all modern diagnostic and therapeutic measures are available. The distribution of MG is age- and sex-related. The incidence is twice as high in women compared with men. In women, the peak age at onset is in the childbearing years, whereas in men there is no evident peak age. About 15% to 20% of patients with MG experience a myasthenic crisis. Usually, the first crisis occurs within the first 2 years after diagnosis in about 75% of patients. In some patients, MG crisis occurs as the initial presentation of the disease. Patients with MG crisis are typically admitted to an intensive care unit because of acute respiratory failure. In 10% of patients an aspiration pneumonitis is the triggering event. In 30% to 40% of patients no triggering factor is found. Predisposing factors include recent surgery, trauma, thymoma, botulin injections, and the initiation of new medication or change in drugs. As a rule, thymectomy is

Department of Thoracic Surgery, Myasthenia Gravis Unit, Fondazione Policlinico Tor Vergata, Tor Vergata University, Viale Oxford, 81, Rome 00133, Italy
* Corresponding author.
E-mail address: mineo@med.uniroma2.it

Thorac Surg Clin 20 (2010) 253–263
doi:10.1016/j.thorsurg.2010.01.002
1547-4127/10/$ – see front matter

performed early in the course of the disease and is indicated for adults less than 70 years old.[4,5]

For many years, the clinical efficacy of thymectomy has been questioned and so far, its benefits in nonthymomatous MG have not been firmly established. Furthermore, the precise mechanisms of action of thymectomy are unknown although possible explanations include removal of the source of continued antigen stimulation and of the AchRab-recruiting B-lymphocytes as well as immunomodulation. However, thymectomy remains indicated in patients with MG and is widely applied to increase the probability of improvement or remission.

This article presents the evolution of technical and surgical advances achieved within the authors' program of extended endoscopically assisted thymectomy since 1995.[6]

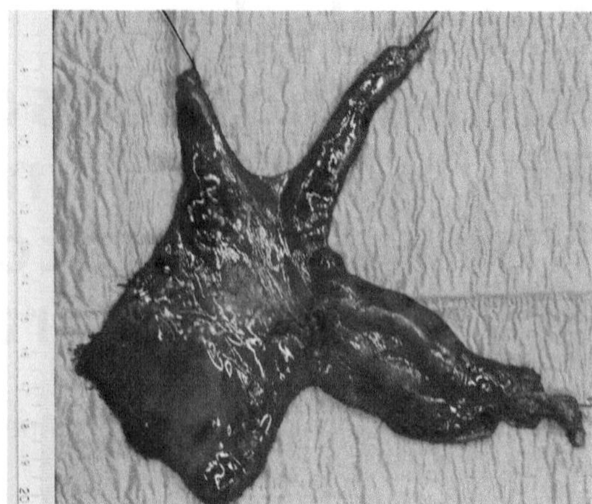

Fig. 1. Thymectomy specimen showing the typical anatomy of the gland in a young adult.

SURGERY

In the adult, the thymus gland is an elongated, lobulated, pinkish-yellow structure comprising fat and thymic tissue. It is situated at the midline in the anterior-superior mediastinum with the superior horns often extending into the lower neck, lying deep to the sternothyroid muscle. Anteriorly, it is related to the sternum, the adjacent parts of the upper 4 costal cartilages, and the sternothyroid and sternohyoid muscles. Posteriorly, the gland is related to the pericardium, the aortic arch and its branches, the left innominate vein, the trachea and, sometimes, the thyroid gland; laterally, with the mediastinal pleura. The thymus is composed of 2 distinct encapsulated elements termed the right and left lobes. The 2 lobes are usually asymmetric; the right lobe is larger than the left, which instead is longer (**Fig. 1**). They do not fuse and are easily separable with smooth dissection. There may be significant variation in its size, shape, or extent. Unencapsulated thymic tissue has also been found variably distributed from the level of the hyoid bone to the diaphragm and behind the phrenic nerves at the level of the hilum. Occasionally, the left or right superior horn passes behind instead of in front the innominate vein as we have observed in a few instances. The thymus has no distinct hilus or single point of entry or exit for vessels. The blood supply is derived from the internal thoracic artery and the inferior thyroid artery. The small arteries enter dorsally through the capsule. As a result of the fusion of smaller veins, a single vein frequently leaves the medial side of each lobe to form a short wide vein, called the great vein of Keynes, which drains into the anteroinferior surface of the left innominate vein. Small additional veins may drain to the inferior superior thyroid vein and the internal thoracic vein.

Preoperative Clinical Evaluation

Twenty years ago we set up an MG unit to optimize the management of myasthenic patients, who are often young women, with neurologic symptoms but no precise diagnosis. The MG unit involves thoracic surgeons, anesthesiologists, neurologists, psychologists, physiotherapists, and nurses working closely together; each patient is evaluated with dedicated care, and therapeutic decisions including timing for surgery are collegially defined. The personal contact between the patient and the MG unit staff provides a more comfortable environment for the patient.

Treatment must be tailored to each myasthenic patient. In particular, each patient must be stabilized before surgery with anticholinesterase drugs and corticosteroids, independently of the surgical approach. If severe weakness and/or bulbar symptoms are present, plasmapheresis may be performed a few days before the operation. Intravenous immunoglobulins are an alternative to plasmapheresis. There is no need to discontinue azathioprine before or after surgery. Whenever feasible, corticosteroids are not used preoperatively and respiratory depressant drugs are carefully avoided.

The final goal of this multimodality management is to reestablish or approximate normal neuromuscular function, minimize adverse effects, and choose the optimal timing for thymectomy.

Selection Criteria

Thymectomy is recommended in patients with nonthymomatous MG as an option to increase the probability of symptomatic improvement or remission. There is a consensus that all adults with generalized symptoms should have thymectomy, particularly if they are younger than 70 years.[4,5] The authors recommend thymectomy for patients with generalized MG and aged between 10 and 70 years, even if they are responding well to anticholinesterase drugs. In our MG unit, surgery is also recommended in patients with isolated ocular disease. We are also convinced that the best clinical response occurs if thymectomy is performed as early as possible in the course of MG.[7,8]

From histopathological findings, anti-AchRab-negative and anti-muscle-specific receptor tyrosine kinase antibody negative (anti-MuSKab) patients have a thymic pattern similar to classic anti-AChRAb-positive MG and should undergo thymectomy. We exclude from thymectomy those patients with antibodies to MuSK in whom a lack of germinative centers and infiltrates of lymphocytes that differentiate the thymus from that of patients with positive anti-AChRAb have been shown.[9]

These general selection criteria are also valid for videothoracoscopic thymectomy.[7,8,10–13] Patients with thymomatous MG are usually operated on through the transsternal approach although there is some evidence that small capsulated thymomas can be safely resected through video-assisted thoracic surgery (VATS).[14] We believe that in any myasthenic patient with preoperative evidence of thymoma, the transsternal approach is preferred for oncologic reasons, mainly to avoid excessive tumor manipulation. Nonetheless, in our experience small encapsulated thymomas incidentally discovered during thoracoscopic thymectomy have been successfully excised by VATS en bloc with the thymic gland (**Fig. 2**).

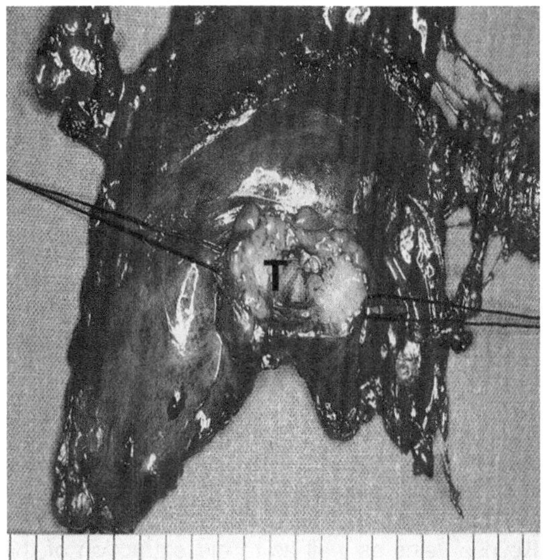

Fig. 2. Thymectomy specimen showing a small incidental thymoma (T).

Other relative contraindications for VATS thymectomy include patient's preference for an open approach, severe obesity, previous long-lasting treatment with oral steroids, and the presence of diffuse bilateral pleural adhesions.

Operative Setup and Position of the Patient

The patient is placed in a 45° off-center position and the table is rotated to place the thorax in a supine position with hyperextension of the head (**Fig. 3**). At the completion of the cervical step of the procedure, the table is rotated back to the initial position to facilitate thoracoscopic access. Thereafter, 3 or 4 flexible trocars are inserted depending on the thymus size and abundance of perithymic fatty tissue (**Fig. 4**).

Fundamental instruments that we commonly use to perform VATS thymectomy include a 30°- angled camera, 10-mm cotton pledgets, 5-mm endoscissors and endograsper, an ultrasonic or radiofrequency coagulator, endoscopic clip appliers, and an endopaddle. We also commonly use standard ring forceps to grasp the thymus during isolation of the innominate and

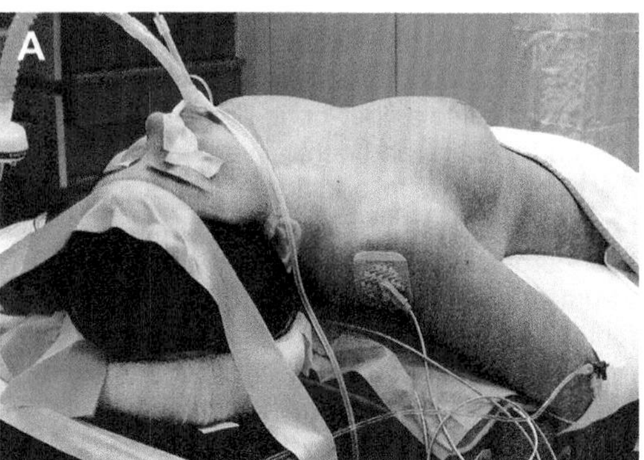

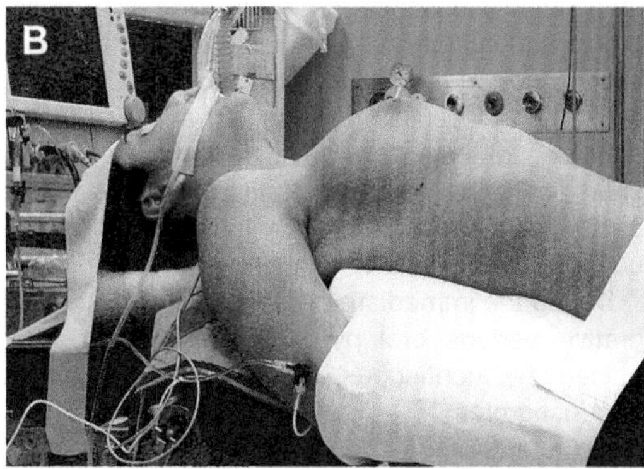

Fig. 3. Patient positioning is changed from a supine position with head hyperextension for the transcervical step (*A*) to a 45° off-center position for optimal videothoracoscopic access (*B*).

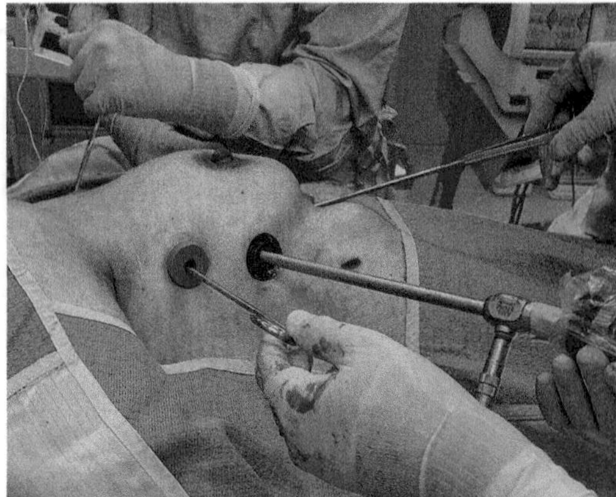

Fig. 4. Typical disposition of trocars for extended thoracoscopic thymectomy.

Keynes veins as well as to aid extraction of the thymus at the completion of the procedure.

Anesthesia and Postoperative Care

When the surgical option is established, assessment of the patient by the anesthesiologist is fundamental and this personal contact continues from the operation until the patient is discharged. The operation is performed under general anesthesia with single-lung ventilation. In rare cases, pretreatment of the tracheobronchial tree with lidocaine 2% can facilitate intubation that can be confirmed using a fiber-optic bronchoscope.

An arterial line and central venous catheter are always inserted. In addition, electrocardiogram, noninvasive blood pressure, pulse oximetry, end-tidal carbon dioxide, airway pressure, ventilatory volume, and fraction of inspired oxygen are routinely monitored.

Anesthesia is induced with propofol (2 mg/kg) and fentanyl (2 mg/kg) and is maintained with isoflurane 1% to 2%, 60% nitrous oxide in oxygen, and a single bolus of morphine. Because myasthenic patients are more susceptible to nondepolarizing neuromuscular relaxants, muscle relaxants are usually not used to avoid potential difficulty at weaning. However, if necessary short-acting nondepolarizing muscle relaxants can be used and monitored by the train of 4 continuous neuromuscular transmission monitoring.[15]

During the immediate preoperative and postoperative periods oral pyridostigmine can be replaced by continuous infusion of intravenous pyridostigmine.

At the end of the operation, we encourage early extubation as well as early physiotherapy and incentive spirometry. Preoperative medication for the control of MG is started as soon as possible. Standard oral analgesics are used as required.

Surgical Technique

Thymectomy demands sufficient familiarity with the anatomy of the neck, the thoracic inlet, and the anterior mediastinum. When planning access to these regions, the skin incision should be made according to Langer lines so that an optimal cosmetic result is obtained. Maximal respect for cosmesis in these areas is requested particularly by young patients and referring physicians.

Initially, we performed VATS thymectomy solely through a left-sided approach.[6,7] More recently, we have changed our strategy and we now selectively choose right or left thoracoscopic access based on the radiologic characteristics of the thymus gland and its vascularization (**Fig. 5**).[8] We now routinely perform an adjuvant cervicotomy as the first surgical step to dissect free the cervical extension of the superior thymic horns and to explore the perithyroid area to maximize removal of the perithymic fatty tissue. The cervicotomy access is also used to lift the sternum during VATS dissection to increase visualization and maneuverability in the anterior-superior mediastina.

The neck and chest are prepared and draped as for a median sternotomy. A minimal transverse collar incision, 4 to 6 cm long, is made at the supraclavicular knotch. The sternohyoid and sternothyroid muscles are retracted laterally and the middle cervical fascia is incised to expose the superior thymic horns that are progressively dissected free by blunt maneuvers up to the thyrothymic ligament. Once these have been completely dissected free, they are ligated and cut (**Fig. 6**A). During this maneuver, the thymus is dissected free down as far as possible usually until the innominate vein is visualized. During thymus dissection great care is taken not to tear the thymic capsula.

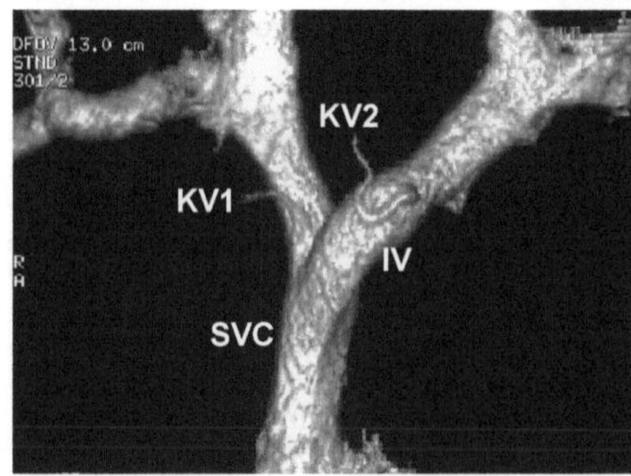

Fig. 5. Three-dimensional computed tomography angiogram showing superior vena cava (SVC), innominate vein (IV) and Keynes' veins (KV1, KV2) suitable for left thoracoscopic access.

After completion of the cervical step of the operation, the patient's position is changed to facilitate VATS and lung collapse is achieved by selective 1-lung ventilation to create conditions for maneuvering of fine instruments. Then, the entire cavity is carefully examined independently of the side chosen for the VATS access, with particular attention to mediastinal organs. First the phrenic nerve must be carefully preserved, then the innominate vein, superior vena cava, aortic arch, and the thymus gland. Pleural adhesions, if present, require adhesiolysis to obtain complete lung collapse, which might be facilitated by sponge-holding compression. A good operating field is mandatory before starting the dissection of the thymus in the cavity.

The mediastinal pleura is incised along the anterior border of the phrenic nerve and all mediastinal tissue including fat is swept away from the nerve (**Fig. 6**B). Subsequently, the inferior horn of the

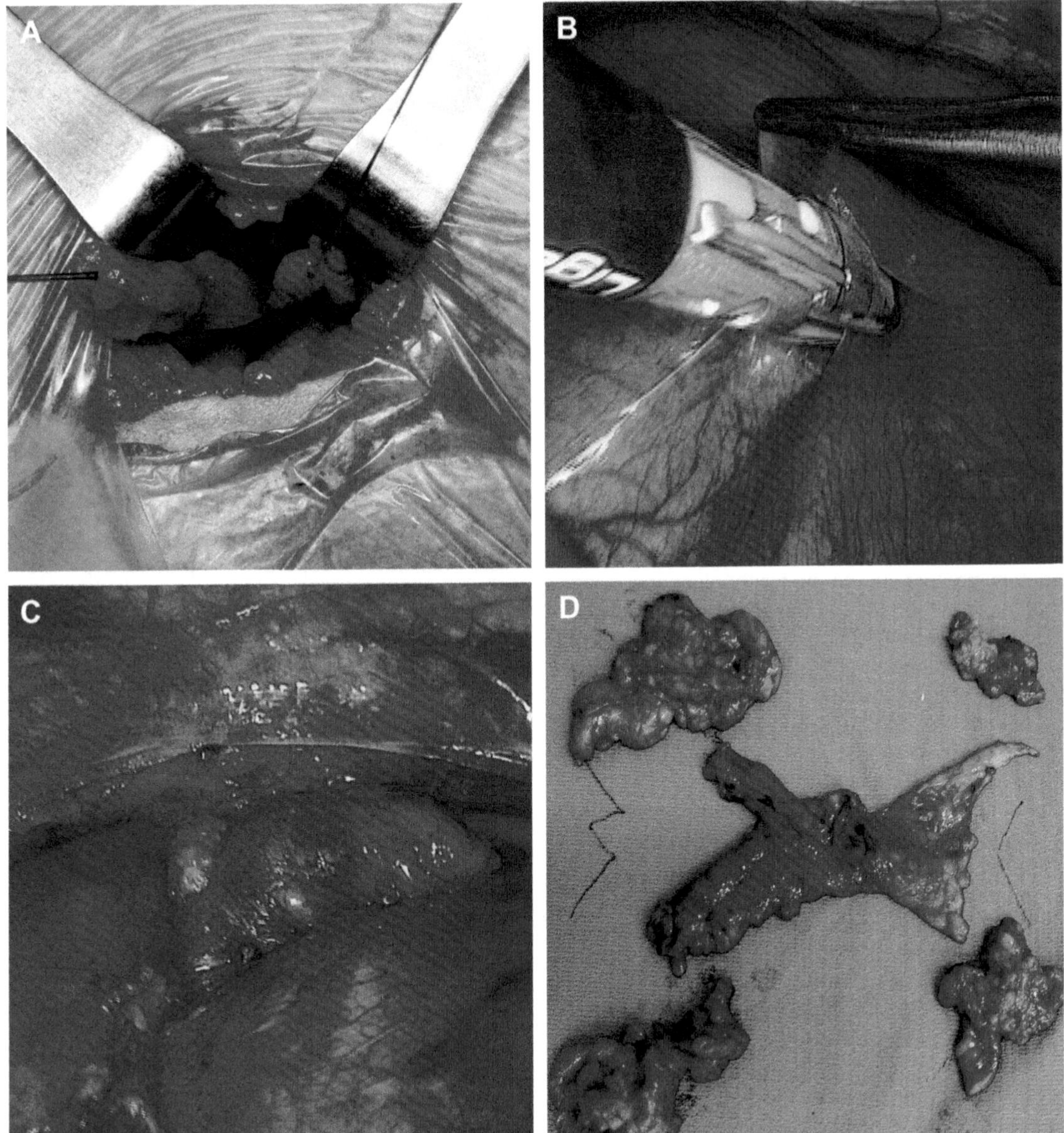

Fig. 6. Intraoperative view showing transcervical dissection of superior thymic horns (*A*); subsequent thoracoscopic incision of the mediastinal pleura by a radiofrequency-based coagulator (*B*); complete mediastinal exenteration with skeletonized innominate vein axis after right thoracoscopic thymectomy (*C*); surgical specimen of extended thoracoscopic thymectomy showing the excised thymic gland with surrounding perithymic fatty, potential sites of unencapsulated ectopic tissue (*D*).

thymus is dissected off the pericardium. The gland is then dissected off the retrosternal area, beginning just below the internal thoracic pedicle, and continuing toward the contralateral mediastinal pleura until this is visualized and the other inferior horn is fully dissected up to the isthmus.

The lower half of the gland is then retracted upward and laterally to aid visualization of the innominate vein. This maneuver is performed more easily from the right because of the visual guide of the superior vena cava and its junction with the innominate axis. By gentle blunt maneuvers and with the aid of 2 pledgets, the innominate vein is widely skeletonized and visualized facilitating identification of the Keynes veins, usually 1 to 3, which are dissected free, clipped, and divided. When radiologic findings indicate a predominantly left-sided origin of the thymic veins, the left-sided approach can be preferred (see **Fig. 5**).

Dissection of the inferior horns of the thymus is facilitated from the left because of the commonly greater development of the left inferior horn; in addition, from the left, removal of adipose tissue in the aortopulmonary window is much easier.

Once the thymic veins are divided, the thymectomy is complete because of the previous transcervical isolation of the superior horns. Thus, the intact gland can be extracted through the cervical incision or the most anterior port of the VATS access where the intercostal space is wider (see **Fig. 6**C). Subsequently, all the mediastinal fat that is present in the pretracheal space, along the internal thoracic pedicles, in the aortopulmonary window as well as in the pericardiophrenic angles, is completely excised to accomplish an anatomically extended thymectomy, which classically entails extracapsular resection with all the fat in anterior mediastinum exenteration, from neck to diaphragm and hilum to hilum (**Fig. 6**D; **Fig. 7**).[16]

Subsequently, hemostasis in the thymic area including the superior vena cava and innominate axis is carefully revised, the chest is drained, and skin incisions are sutured.

In our residency program, teaching thoracoscopic thymectomy follows adequate training with different transsternal access routes to familiarize residents with the anatomy of mediastinal structures and dissection of thymic loggia.

We recommend informing the patient that whenever the surgeon believes thoracoscopic thymectomy is too technically demanding, sternotomy will be performed without hesitation, because this approach ensures the fastest and safest dissection of the thymus in selected instances, such as obese patients with abundant perithymic fatty tissue and patients who have undergone prolonged corticosteroid therapy. Sternotomy should never be considered a failure but rather a tailored and rationale surgical approach to be selectively preferred, when required.

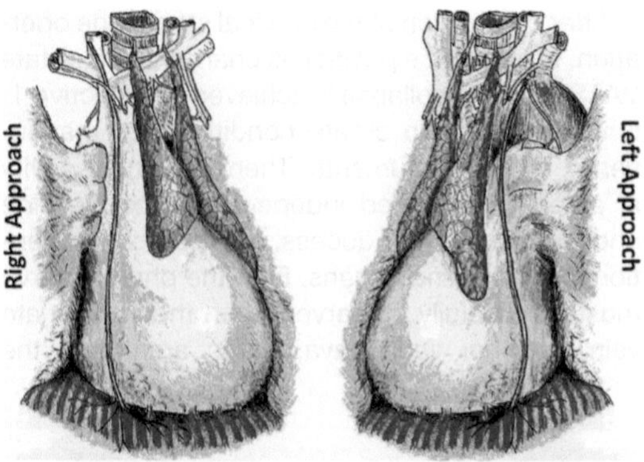

Fig. 7. Anatomic structures visualized by right-sided (*right*) and left-sided (*left*) thoracoscopic access. (*Reprinted from* Mineo TC, Pompeo E, Lerut TE, et al. Thoracoscopic thymectomy in autoimmune myasthenia: results of left-sided approach. Ann Thorac Surg 2000;69:1538; with permission.)

Completion Thymectomy

When clinical myasthenic symptoms and signs after thymectomy are persistent, doubt about a thymic remnant or regrowth is justified. In this case, re-exploration can be considered.[17,18] We believe that the videothoracoscopic approach can facilitate reoperation, particularly when previous transthoracic or transcervical thymectomy has been performed. We have found that a transpleural route facilitates exploration of the anterior-superior mediastina despite the previous dissection. This particular indication must still be considered investigational although in a small series of 9 patients who had undergone transcervical (6 patients) or transsternal (3 patients) thymectomy in other institutions, at reoperation, we found residual thymic tissue in all patients; 7 patients achieved sustained symptomatic improvement postoperatively.[19]

Complications

Major complications of thoracoscopic thymectomy are rare but potentially life-threatening, so we believe that anyone who decides to start a thoracoscopic thymectomy program must be aware of the complications. The main intraoperative risk is vascular injury to the innominate vein, which may occur during isolation of the thymic veins. We experienced 2 bleeding complications requiring conversion to median sternotomy, 1 diffuse and 1 from a left innominate vein lesion in a young female patient. In the latter instance, we found that the adjuvant cervical incision rendered much easier and quicker for an emergency sternotomy.

To limit the risks of vascular injury, we recommend performing delicate blunt dissection of this area to achieve wide and clean visualization of the innominate vein axis that facilitates isolation of Keynes veins.

Ventricular arrhythmias can be triggered by compression of the heart when dissecting the thymus free from the pericardium and, particularly, when using electrocautery. For this reason, we now prefer to use a radiofrequency or ultrasonic coagulator that produces less smoke and does not conduct electricity.[6–8]

Incidental injury to phrenic nerves may occur particularly when dissecting free the lateral aspects of the thymus near the thoracic inlet, where phrenic nerves are lying more medially passing from the cervical region to the anterior-superior mediastina.

Other potential complications include wound infection, hypocalcemia, pneumothorax, contralateral pleural effusion, and intercostals neuralgia. Small opening of the pericardial sac can also occur although this is rare.[10]

RESULTS

Our experience with thymectomy includes transcervical, transsternal, and more recently thoracoscopic thymectomy. Of 43 extended thoracoscopic thymectomies, we have recently reported results of 32 patients with nonthymomatous MG and a follow-up of at least 60 months.[8] There were 21 women and 11 men with a median age of 36 years. Duration of preoperative symptoms averaged 11 months and serum level of anti-AchRab was positive in 22 patients.

According to the clinical Myasthenia Gravis Foundation of America classification,[20] there were 7 patients in class I, 14 patients in class II, 9 patients in class III, and 2 patients in class IV.

Before thymectomy, all patients received anticholinesterase drugs either alone or in combination with corticosteroids (4 patients). Azathioprine was given in 2 patients.

Conversion to median sternotomy is seldom required in thoracoscopic thymectomy, ranging between 0 and 6.7%. Recent series show low morbidity rates and short hospitalization time (**Table 1**).

In our series, 2 obese patients required conversion to median sternotomy because of difficulty in dissecting the thymus and uncontrolled bleeding, respectively. Median operative time was 150 minutes although in the last 10 patients it averaged 110 minutes. All patients were extubated within 24 hours. At pathologic examination, ectopic thymic tissue was found in 18 patients (56%). Ectopic thymic islets with Hassall corpuscles was detected within the anterior mediastinal fat in 10 patients, in the pretracheal fat in 4 patients, and in the aortopulmonary window and cardiophrenic fat in 3 patients each. Two patients had ectopic thymic tissue in 2 distinct locations. There were no operative deaths or major morbidity and the median hospital stay was 4 days.[8]

In another series,[12] VATS thymectomy resulted in less pronounced impairment and faster recovery of pulmonary function than transsternal thymectomy.

We have found that of 32 patients who underwent surgery, 2 had minimal thoracic pain for up to 6 months; none of the patients complained of thoracic pain at 1 year or thereafter.[8]

The long-term clinical results of thoracoscopic thymectomy are still scant although we have observed an 88% rate of improvement and an

Table 1
Surgical results of unilateral thoracoscopic thymectomy

References	Year	Patients	Conversion Rate (%)	Morbidity Rate (%)	Hospital Stay (Days)
Mineo et al[7,a]	2000	31	0	3	5.2
Savcenko et al[21]	2002	36	3	5	1.6
Wright et al[35]	2002	26	4	4	4
Manlulu et al[22]	2005	36	0	11	3
Tomulescu et al[23]	2006	107	0	9	2.3
Toker et al[36]	2008	90	2.2	2.2	2.2
Pompeo et al[8]	2009	32	6.7	0	4.0

[a] Multi-institutional study.

estimated 10-year remission rate of 50%.[8] Other reports[21–25] are in accordance with these findings indicating satisfactory complete remission rates and excellent rates of improvement (**Table 2**).

The cosmetic result is usually rated as excellent by most patients. In our series, 26 (87%) patients rated the cosmetic effect of their operation as excellent (**Fig. 8**).

COMMENT

Since the first successful excision of a thymic lesion in a patient with MG reported by Blalock in 1939,[3] thymectomy in the management of MG was based essentially on empiric observations. Furthermore, because of lack of knowledge of the cause of MG and the function of the thymus gland, for decades indications for thymectomy were developed empirically, mainly from the results achieved by pioneering surgeons. Thus, thymectomy in nonthymomatous MG has been widely performed in an effort to achieve medication-free remission or clinical improvement.[26,27] Gronnseth and Barohn[5] in a meta-analysis of 28 controlled studies showed that after thymectomy, the probability of attaining medication-free remission, pharmacologic remission, or improvement was 2, 1.7 and 1.6 as likely, respectively, although there were differences in demographics and baseline data amongst the series analyzed.

Although thymectomy has not yet been investigated in a prospective, randomized clinical trial in nonthymomatous myasthenic patients, nowadays it represents an integral part of the current management of MG, which also includes anticholinesterase drugs, plasma exchange or specific immunoadsorption procedures, and the use of nonspecific immunosuppressants or immunomodulators. The precise mechanism of action of thymectomy is as yet unknown. At present, there are several controversies related to thymectomy in nonthymomatous MG, including the ideal timing of the operation with respect to onset, course, and patient age, the optimal surgical approach, and whether patients with exclusively ocular disease should undergo thymectomy. However, there is agreement in the belief that it includes removal of the source of continued antigen stimulation, removal of anti-AchRab-recruiting B-lymphocytes, and immunomodulation.[4]

To date, the best surgical approach to the thymus can be a difficult choice. The classic transsternal surgical approach is preferred by advocators of open surgery.[8,27,28] This approach allows total access to the anterior-superior mediastina and also gives adequate exposure of the lower neck to achieve an extended thymectomy. Other

Table 2
Mid- to long-term clinical results of thoracoscopic thymectomy

References	Year	Surgical Approach	Patients (n)	Follow-up (Months)	Improvement Rate (%)	Remission Rate (%)
Savcenko et al[21]	2002	Right-sided	36	53	83	14
Mantegazza et al[24]	2003	Bilateral+cervical incision	159	72	–	54
Manlulu et al[22]	2005	Right-sided	38	69	92	22
Tumulescu et al[23]	2006	Left-sided	107	36	–	59
Bachmann et al[25]	2008	–	22	96	100	48
Pompeo et al[8]	2009	Left- or right-sided+cervical incision	32	119	88	50

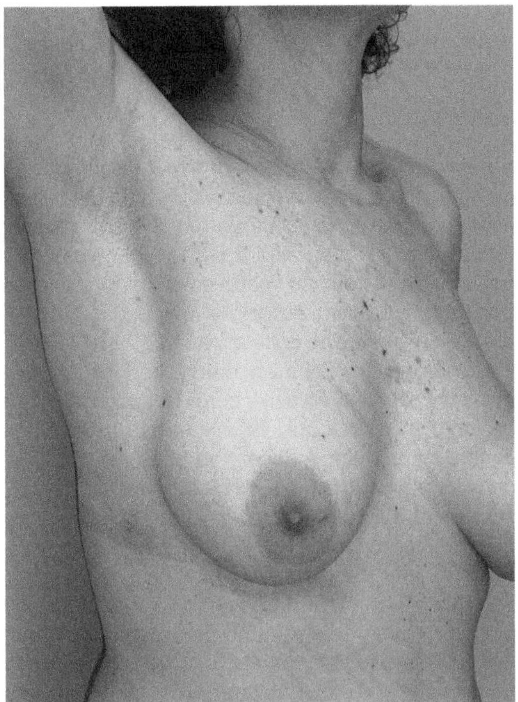

Fig. 8. Excellent cosmetic result following right-sided extended thoracoscopic thymectomy.

open techniques include the combined median sternotomy with transcervical incision, partial sternotomy involving either the upper or lower sternum and transcervical access. However, because many myasthenic patients are young, the surgical decision is influenced by the need to achieve a complete thymectomy and a cosmetically acceptable surgical incision with minor chest trauma.

We believe that VATS thymectomy represents a technological advance and provides a solution to all these requirements.

Thoracoscopic thymectomy is similar to transcervical thymectomy because both are associated with minimal chest wall trauma, low postoperative morbidity, short hospital stay, optimal cosmetic results, and easier acceptance of the procedure by patients and referring neurologists, compared with transsternal thymectomy. However, we agree with the observation of Yim and colleagues[10] that VATS offers additional advantages over the conventional transcervical approach because of the superior visualization and lack of crowding of instruments through a single access site.

This less invasive surgical approach to the thymus has evolved in the last 10 years and several groups have reported satisfactory results with slightly different technical details including the bilateral thoracoscopic approach combined with transcervical incision[29] and robot-assisted thymectomy.[24]

We have periodically revised and slightly modified our surgical approach in an attempt to render it the safest and most effective. Initially, we preferred a left-sided approach, convinced that it offers some advantages because of the commonly greater development of the left inferior thymic horn and the possibility of an easy dissection of the perithymic fatty tissue in the aortopulmonary window, where ectopic thymic tissue is often found. We also initially advocated adjuvant pneumomediastinum (**Fig. 9**) to aid surgical maneuvers within the anterior-superior mediastina.[6]

Yim and colleagues[10] correctly pointed out that from the right side, the landmark of the superior vena cava is easily indentified and acts as a guide to the left innominate vein; yet, they stressed that, because of the wider pleural space, the right-sided approach allows greater maneuverability of instruments and offers an ergonomic advantage for dissection in right-handed surgeons.

Now convinced that each approach has its peculiar advantages, we have started to include a radiological assessment of the vascular anatomy of the thymus to preoperatively visualize the thymic anatomy and vascularity, and selectively choose between a left- or right-sided approach, depending on the peculiar anatomic features of each patient.

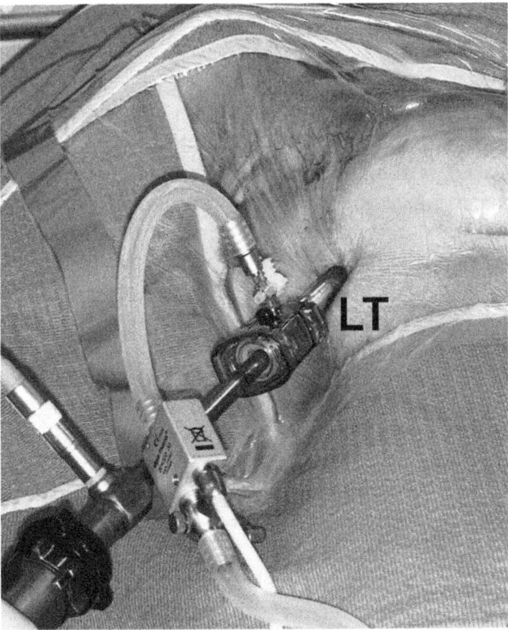

Fig. 9. Adjuvant pneumomediastinum is being induced through a laparoscopic trocar (LT) following thoracoscopic incision of mediastinal pleura to facilitate ungluing of the thymus gland from surrounding structures.

Because of our previous experience with transcervical thymectomy, we have also added an adjuvant cervicotomy to explore the perithyroid area and facilitate isolation of the superior thymic horns.[8] In this way, we have tried to overcome one of the major criticisms of thoracoscopic thymectomy, namely dissection of the lower cervical area through a transthoracic approach.

With a tailored unilateral thoracoscopic approach and adjuvant cervicotomy, we are confident that a classic extended thymectomy can be performed safely. This in the belief that the more complete the removal of thymic tissue, including unencapsulated ectopic thymic tissue, the higher are the chances of achieving control of myasthenic symptoms and signs.

Jaretzki and Wolf[30] observed that 98% of myasthenic patients had anatomic variability in distribution of thymic tissue in the mediastinum; Masaoka and colleagues[31] found that 72% of patients had ectopic thymic tissue within the anterior mediastinal fat; overall, we have found ectopic thymic tissue in 56% of our patients. Nonetheless, so far the role of ectopic thymic tissue remains to be elucidated; there is some evidence that it can be a negative prognostic factor for improvement or remission of symptoms.[32,33]

After thymectomy, prolonged persistence of symptoms and signs refractory to maximized medical treatment can lead to a suspicion of thymic remnants and thus justifies reoperation. In these instances, surgical re-exploration can be facilitated by VATS.[17–19]

Hypothetical concerns have been raised about the risk of chronic thoracic pain after VATS thymectomy because of the transthoracic passage of surgical instrumentation. However, in accordance with previous reports,[10,11] none of our patients complained of chronic thoracic pain in a recent analysis of long-term follow-up data.[8]

Intermediate follow-up data of recent VATS thymectomy series show satisfactory results with complete remission rates between 14%[21] and 59%.[23] In our experience 88% of the patients improved and the estimated 10-year remission rate was 50%.[8] Moreover, in accordance with other reports,[22,23,34] our data suggest that short duration of symptoms and absence of oropharyngeal involvement can be predictors of response to thymectomy.[8]

In conclusion, we believe that VATS thymectomy, including recent technical refinements such as addition of an adjuvant cervical incision, might now be considered a reliable alternative to the most aggressive open approaches aimed at achieving a classic anatomically extended thymectomy. The satisfactory long-term results achieved by this surgical approach corroborate our belief, although more definitive data from future prospective randomized studies are warranted.

SUMMARY

So far, the clinical efficacy of thymectomy on the course of nonthymomatous MG is still difficult to assess. However, thymectomy remains an important step within the integrated treatment of myasthenic patients. Symptomatic improvement or remission is frequently achieved especially in younger thymectomized women with generalized MG.

Nowadays, the operation can be performed using open or minimally invasive surgical access. Video-assisted thoracoscopic thymectomy has become a safe alternative to open approaches. Minimal chest wall trauma, low postoperative morbidity, short hospital stay, improved cosmesis and easy patient acceptance, are the most important advantages of the minimally invasive technique.

When we started our VATS thymectomy program, we preferred the left-sided approach with double-lumen intubation and single-lung ventilation. This choice offered us good access to visualize the thymic area and venous vessels.

With increasing experience, to perform a real extended operation and a safer dissection of the superior thymic horns, we have added an adjuvant cervicotomy similar to that used for transcervical thymectomy.

More recently we have also started also to take into consideration radiologic vascular imaging of the thymus to selectively choose left- or right-sided VATS access. We believe that using a tailored thoracoscopic approach with adjuvant cervicotomy, thymectomy can be safer and anatomically extended. Indeed, we consider our clinical results with this surgical strategy excellent.

Use of VATS and its variants for performing thymectomy in MG patients is now well established and will continue to evolve for further improvement in the results.

REFERENCES

1. Pascuzzi RM. The history of myasthenia gravis. Neurol Clin 1994;12:231–42.
2. Walker MB. Case showing the effect of prostigmin on myasthenia gravis. Proc R Soc Med 1935;28:759–61.
3. Blalock A, Mason MF, Morgan HJ, et al. Myasthenia gravis and tumors of the thymic region. Ann Surg 1939;110:544–61.
4. Drachman DB. Myasthenia gravis. N Engl J Med 1994;330:1797–810.
5. Gronseth GS, Barohn RJ. Practice parameter: thymectomy for autoimmune myasthenia gravis (an evidence-based review). Neurology 2000;55:7–15.

6. Mineo TC, Pompeo E, Ambrogi V, et al. Adjuvant pneumomediastinum in thoracoscopic thymectomy for myasthenia gravis. Ann Thorac Surg 1996;62:1210–2.
7. Mineo TC, Pompeo E, Lerut T, et al. Thoracoscopic thymectomy in autoimmune myasthenia: results of the left-sided approach. Ann Thorac Surg 2000;69: 1537–41.
8. Pompeo E, Tacconi F, Massa R, et al. Long-term results of thoracoscopic extended thymectomy in nonthymomatous myasthenia gravis. Eur J Cardiothorac Surg 2009;36:164–9.
9. Evoli A, Bianchi MR, Riso R, et al. Response to therapy in myasthenia gravis with anti-MuSK antibodies. Ann N Y Acad Sci 2008;1132:76–83.
10. Yim AP, Kay RL, Ho JKS. Video-assisted thoracoscopic thymectomy for myasthenia gravis. Chest 1995;108:1440–3.
11. Mack MJ, Landreneau RJ, Yim AP, et al. Results of video-assisted thymectomy in patients with myasthenia gravis. J Thorac Cardiovasc Surg 1996;112: 1352–60.
12. Rückert JC, Walter M, Müller JM. Pulmonary function after thoracoscopic thymectomy versus median sternotomy for myasthenia gravis. Ann Thorac Surg 2000;70:1656–61.
13. Tomulescu V, Ion V, Tulbure D, et al. Thymectomy by thoracoscopic approach in myasthenia gravis. Surg Endosc 2002;16:679–84.
14. Sakamaki Y, Kido T, Yasukawa M. Alternative choices of total and partial thymectomy in video-assisted resection of noninvasive thymomas. Surg Endosc 2008;22:1272–7.
15. Abel M, Eisenkraft JB. Anesthetic implications of myasthenia gravis. Mt Sinai J Med 2002;31:36.
16. Masaoka A, Yamakawa Y, Niwa H, et al. Extended thymectomy for myasthenia gravis patients: a 20-year review. Ann Thorac Surg 1996;62:853–9.
17. Masaoka A, Monden Y, Seike Y, et al. Reoperation after transcervical thymectomy for myasthenia gravis. Neurology 1982;32:83–5.
18. Miller RG, Filler-Katz A, Kiprov D, et al. Repeat thymectomy in chronic refractory myasthenia gravis. Neurology 1991;41:923–4.
19. Pompeo E, Nofroni I, Iavicoli N, et al. Thoracoscopic completion thymectomy in refractory nonthymomatous myasthenia. Ann Thorac Surg 2000;70:918–23.
20. Jaretzki A, Barohn RJ, Ernstoff RM, et al. Myasthenia gravis: recommendations for clinical research standards. Task force of the medical scientific advisory board of the Myasthenia Gravis Foundation of America. Ann Thorac Surg 2000;70:327–34.
21. Savcenko M, Wendt GK, Prince SL, et al. Video-assisted thymectomy for myasthenia gravis: an update of a single institution experience. Eur J Cardiothorac Surg 2002;22:978–83.
22. Manlulu A, Lee TW, Wan I, et al. Video-assisted thoracic surgery thymectomy for nonthymomatous myasthenia gravis. Chest 2005;128:3454–60.
23. Tumulescu V, Ion V, Kosa A, et al. Thoracoscopic thymectomy mid-term results. Ann Thorac Surg 2006;82:1003–8.
24. Bodner J, Wykypiel H, Greiner A, et al. Early experience with robot-assisted surgery for mediastinal masses. Ann Thorac Surg 2004;78:259–65.
25. Bachmann K, Burkhardt D, Schreiter I, et al. Long-term outcome and quality of life after open and thoracoscopic thymectomy for myasthenia gravis: analysis of 131 patients. Surg Endosc 2008;22:2470–7.
26. Papatestas AE, Alpert LI, Osserman KE, et al. Studies in myasthenia gravis: effects of thymectomy. Results on 185 patients with nonthymomatous and thymomatous myasthenia gravis. Am J Med 1971;38:580–5.
27. Bulkley GB, Bass KN, Stephenson GR, et al. Extended cervicomediastinal thymectomy in the integrated management of myasthenia gravis. Ann Surg 1997;226:324–35.
28. Stern LE, Nussbaum MS, Quinlan JG, et al. Long-term evaluation of extended thymectomy with anterior mediastinal dissection for myasthenia gravis. Surgery 2001;130:774–9.
29. Mantegazza R, Baggi F, Bernasconi P, et al. Video-assisted thoracoscopic extended thymectomy and extended transsternal thymectomy (T-3b) in non-thymomatous myasthenia gravis patients: remission after 6 years of follow-up. J Neurol Sci 2003;212:31–6.
30. Jaretzki A, Wolff M. "Maximal" thymectomy for myasthenia gravis. Surgical anatomy and operative technique. J Thorac Cardiovasc Surg 1988;96:711–6.
31. Masaoka A, Nagakoa Y, Kotabe Y. Distribution of thymic tissue at the anterior mediastinum – current procedure in thymectomy. J Thorac Cardiovasc Surg 1975;70:747–54.
32. Ashour M. Prevalence of ectopic thymic tissue in myasthenia gravis and its clinical significance. J Thorac Cardiovasc Surg 1995;109:632–5.
33. Özdemir N, Kara M, Dikmen E, et al. Predictor of clinical outcome following extended thymectomy in myasthenia gravis. Eur J Cardiothorac Surg 2003;23: 233–7.
34. Yu L, Li J, Ma S, et al. Different characteristics of nonthymomatous generalized myasthenia gravis with and without oropharyngeal involvement. Ann Thorac Surg 2007;84:1694–8.
35. Wright GM, Barnett S, Clarke CP. Video-assisted thoracoscopic thymectomy for myasthenia gravis. Intern Med J 2002;32:367–71.
36. Toker A, Tanju S, Sungur, et al. Videothoracoscopic thymectomy for nonthymomatous myasthenia gravis: results of 90 patients. Surg Endosc 2008; 22:912–6.

Surgical Approaches for Invasive Tumors of the Anterior Mediastinum

Antonio D'Andrilli, MD[a], Federico Venuta, MD[b], Erino A. Rendina, MD[a,*]

KEYWORDS

- Mediastinal tumors • Surgical approaches
- Vascular reconstruction

Mediastinal tumors develop with a higher incidence in the anterior compartment. About 50% to 55% of mediastinal neoplasms in adults and 40% to 45% in children originate in this site. Although more than two thirds of mediastinal masses are benign, predilection for malignancy is higher in the anterior compartment (60% of all mediastinal malignancies).[1–3]

Malignant tumors originating in the anterior mediastinum more frequently include thymoma comprising thymic carcinoma, germ cell tumors, lymphoma, and metastatic tumors. Most patients (about 85%) with invasive mediastinal diseases are symptomatic, since symptoms may be due to compression or direct invasion of the neighboring structures or may be related to paraneoplastic syndromes. Some of these tumors, because of their aggressive behavior, may extend to adjacent organs, such as the other mediastinal compartments (middle and posterior) or the cervical region, posing additional technical problems for the choice of the ideal surgical approach.

Surgery can be indicated in the presence of invasive masses of the anterior mediastinum either with diagnostic intent or for radical resection, more frequently as a part of a multimodality treatment.

SURGICAL APPROACHES WITH DIAGNOSTIC INTENT

Anterior mediastinal masses require precise histologic diagnosis to plan an adequate oncologic therapy. CT-guided fine-needle aspiration only occasionally provides diagnostic cytology. Core needle biopsy usually shows a higher diagnostic accuracy, but in many cases, especially in presence of lymphoma, a larger specimen is required to reach an accurate definition of the histology. For this reason, surgical biopsy still represents the gold standard for histologic diagnosis of invasive mediastinal tumors.

Several investigators[1,2] believe that preoperative biopsy should be avoided when the anterior mediastinal tumor has a well-demarcated border and could easily be resected completely. This strategy is principally justified by the increased risk of tumor seeding due to biopsy. However, for invasive tumors biopsy is always necessary because their complete resection requires simultaneous resection of involved vital organs and such procedures carry higher risks of morbidity and mortality.

Anterior Mediastinotomy

The parasternal anterior mediastinotomy was first described in 1966 by Chamberlain and McNeil.[4] This approach is most indicated for large masses located in the anterior mediastinum, especially when they show direct contact with the posterior aspect of the sternum and the adjacent chest wall. Moreover, this technique has been proposed and largely employed for the histologic definition of lymphadenopathies and masses located in the

[a] Department of Thoracic Surgery, Sant'Andrea Hospital, University of Rome La Sapienza, Via di Grottarossa 1035, Rome 00189, Italy
[b] Division of Thoracic Surgery, University of Rome La Sapienza, Policlinico Umberto I, Viale del Policlinico, Rome 155–00161, Italy
* Corresponding author.
E-mail address: erinoangelo.rendina@uniroma1.it

Thorac Surg Clin 20 (2010) 265–284
doi:10.1016/j.thorsurg.2010.02.002

paraortic region and in the aortopulmonary window.

This procedure is most frequently performed with the patient under general anesthesia. However, as the authors and other investigators have reported,[5,6] this technique can be performed safely and effectively also under local anesthesia. According to some investigators' experience,[7] the use of local anesthesia may provide significant advantages in patients with tumor compression of the distal trachea and main bronchi, in which critical airway collapse sometimes occurs after induction of general anesthesia.

With the patient placed in a supine position, a 2 to 4 cm parasternal skin incision on the side of the prevalent extension of the tumor is made. The level of the surgical access (usually between the second and the fourth intercostal space) has to be chosen based on radiological findings. Separation of fibers of pectoralis muscle and incision of the intercostal muscle is then made close to the sternum to allow direct access to the mediastinum preserving the internal mammary vessels. Removal of the costal cartilage is generally not necessary. An intraoperative histologic examination is usually required to assess whether the specimen is adequate for diagnosis. Pleural opening should be avoided whenever possible for the potential risk of tumor seeding.

Operative complications are reported ranging between 1% and 4%[3] and more frequently include hemorrhage due to injury to internal mammary vessels, pneumothorax, and wound infection. Dosios and colleagues[7] have reported a significantly increased perioperative morbidity in patients with tumors determining superior vena cava (SVC) obstruction with respect to patients without SVC obstruction.

In a Japanese series by Watanabe and colleagues,[6] the diagnostic accuracy in histologic definition of anterior mediastinal masses has been reported higher for parasternal mediastinotomy if compared with fine needle and core biopsy. Although the diagnostic yield of percutaneous needle biopsy has been reported in some experiences[7–9] between 71.3% and 100%, most investigators[10,11] conclude that this technique can be useful in many cases of carcinoma and thymoma, but is generally not sufficiently accurate for the characterization of lymphoma, thus advocating the need for a surgical approach.

In 2002, the authors reported a series of 46 patients with anterior mediastinal masses undergoing anterior mediastinotomy under local anesthesia with the use of mediastinoscope in case of tumors not abutting the anterior chest wall.[5] Diagnostic accuracy was 100% with a 4.3% non–life-threatening complication rate and no mortality. Histologic diagnosis showed lymphoma or thymoma in 43 of 46 patients. With this technique, care must be taken to infiltrate the periosteum of the sternal margin with the local anesthetic. Adherence to the bone when performing incision avoids injury to internal mammary vessels, which do not require exposure.

Cervical Mediastinoscopy (Conventional and Extended)

Conventional cervical mediastinoscopy is useful for the diagnosis of lesions located in the superior middle mediastinum at the level of paratracheal and pretracheal spaces and subcarinal lymph nodes. Therefore, the role of this technique in the histologic definition of anterior mediastinal masses is limited. The use of the latter approach in such cases is generally restricted to those tumors that extend outside the limits of the anterior mediastinum involving the peritracheal region. General anesthesia is required.

The possibility of anterior mediastinal biopsy through cervical incision was first mentioned by Specht[12] in 1965 and was further proved by Kirschner[13] who performed the first "extended mediastinoscopy." This technique, later modified by Ginsberg and colleagues,[14] and Lopez and colleagues,[15] allows access to the prevascular mediastinal space by sliding the mediastinoscope along the left anterolateral face of the aortic arch at the origin of the innominate artery after preparation of the retrosternal space. Although the abovementioned investigators have shown the safety and efficacy of this approach for the diagnosis of anterior mediastinal masses, and particularly for the histologic definition of lymphadenopathies in the aortopulmonary window and in the paraortic area, this technique has not gained wide diffusion due to its technical complexity and the related risk of vascular injuries. Therefore, there are very few published studies reporting the routine use of the extended mediastinoscopy for biopsy of anterior mediastinal tumors.

Metin and colleagues[16] have reported a 89% diagnostic yield with this technique, with no life-threatening complications and no operative mortality, in a limited series of patients with lymphoma or thymoma previously undergoing inconclusive needle aspiration or tru-cut biopsy of the anterior mediastinal tumor. However, in presence of invasive neoplasms of the anterior mediastinum, especially when the neighboring structures are invaded, this approach is rarely performed since the anterior mediastinotomy is generally considered more safe and effective.

Video-assisted Thoracic Surgery

Video-assisted thoracic surgery (VATS) does not have wide application for the histologic definition of invasive tumors located in the anterior mediastinum. It may be indicated in case of large masses protruding in the pleural cavity, especially when separate lesions involving the pleura are associated. In the literature, VATS has a diagnostic accuracy, when considering mediastinal tumors, ranging between 92% and 100%.[3,17,18]

The advantages of the thoracoscopic approach include a better evaluation of the relationship of the tumor with the adjacent structures and a higher efficacy in detecting neoplastic invasion or local metastatic spread. Disadvantages include the need for general anesthesia with one-lung ventilation, the need for a postoperative thoracostomy tube with possibly related chronic pain, and the longer hospital stay. There are few large series assessing the role of videothoracoscopy in the diagnosis of anterior mediastinal tumors. Roviaro and colleagues[19] have reported a series of 118 patients with mediastinal masses, 40% of whom underwent videothoracoscopy for diagnosis or staging. Thoracoscopic procedures yielded adequate diagnosis or staging in all the patients (47) undergoing operation for diagnostic purposes.

RADICAL SURGERY

Surgical Approaches, Type of Interventions and Results

Since invasive anterior mediastinal tumors usually do not present symptoms in the early stages, at the time of diagnosis they often appear locally advanced with invasion of the surrounding organs, including major blood vessels, lung parenchyma and pericardium, which may preclude a curative surgical resection.

Usually in the past, surgical resections of large masses along with the neighboring structures were not offered to patients because of related morbidity and mortality and limited information available on the prognostic advantage for long term. However, in the last decades, advances in surgical technique and perioperative management, as well as increased oncologic experience in this field, have allowed radical resection in selected patients with invasive tumors requiring resections extended to the surrounding structures and complex vascular reconstructions. Such aggressive surgical treatment has been proposed in association or not with adjuvant chemo- or radiotherapic regimens, achieving encouraging oncologic results with limited morbidity and mortality in experienced centers.

Moreover, some of these patients present with immediately life-threatening problems such as congestive heart failure or impending cardiovascular collapse due to the compression by the large mass. Since medical palliation is usually ineffective in this setting, an aggressive surgical treatment may remain the only option.

Surgical Approaches

Median sternotomy is the optimal approach for anterior mediastinal tumors, providing a good exposure even in presence of invasion of the adjacent structures such as the lung or the great vessels.[20,21] The standard incision is from the suprasternal notch to a point just below the xiphoid process (**Fig. 1**). The incision is generally carried to the pectoral fascia and linea alba with the scalpel. The interclavicular ligament can be divided sharply or with cautery. Blunt dissection is used to open superiorly and inferiorly the retrosternal space. The sternum is divided by the saw from top down or bottom up. Marrow bleeding can be controlled by judicious use of cautery and bone wax without increasing infectious complications.[22] Full control of the entire anterior mediastinal compartment is provided by this approach. Furthermore, upper lobectomy, bilobectomy, or pneumonectomy (eventually required along with the mediastinal mass removal), as well as pulmonary artery resection and repair, can be performed by this approach. Simultaneously, exploration of both the pleural cavities is allowed. This incision may be easily extended to the neck in case of cervicothoracic lesions.

Advantages of the sternotomic approach include the speed of opening and closing, the sparing of major thoracic muscles, and the relatively reduced postoperative pain. Main disadvantages are the limited exposure of the posterolateral compartment of the pleural cavities and of the pulmonary hili, and the risk for sternal infection, which is hard to manage.

The incidence of mediastinitis after sternotomy is reported around 1% to 2%. In addition to favorable anatomic characteristics of the patient, intraoperative hemostasis, proper sternal closure, and early extubation are the most significant factors preventing mediastinitis.[23] Delayed complications of median sternotomy include costochondral separation, occult rib fractures, chronic osteomyelitis of the sternum, rib cartilage necrosis, sternal nonunion and sternal wire erosion.[24]

As an alternative, a clamshell approach (bilateral anterior thoracotomy with transverse sternotomy)

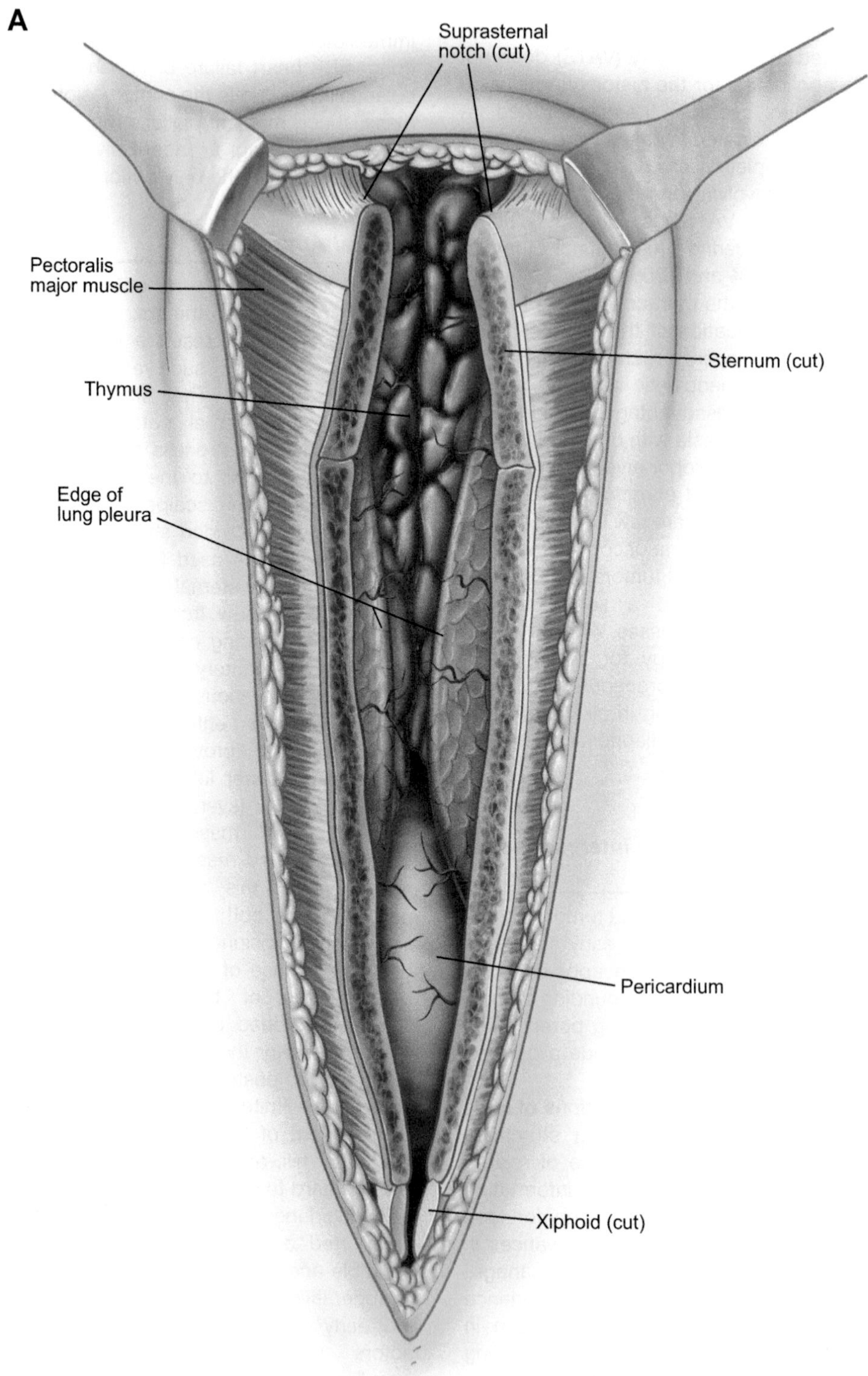

Fig. 1. (*A–B*) Median sternotomy.

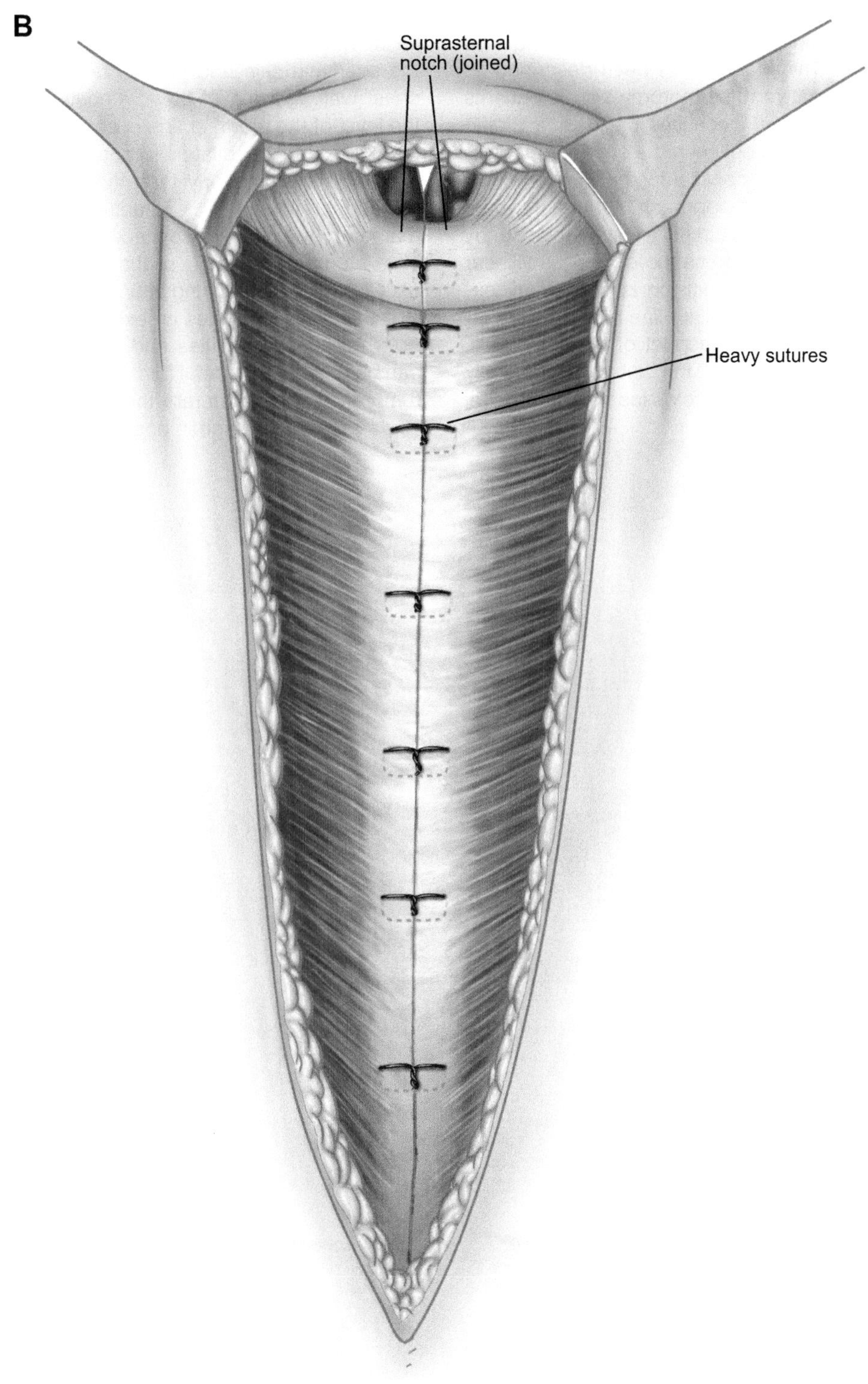

Fig. 1. (*continued*)

has been proposed for the excision of giant masses extending in both the pleural cavities (**Fig. 2**).[20,25] This incision has been described as a useful alternative to sternotomy also in patients with tracheostomy, because it allows avoiding the communication between the superior mediastinum and the lower cervical region.[26]

It was the standard approach in the early years of open heart surgery, until it was replaced by the less invasive median sternotomy. A curvilinear bilateral submammary incision is performed, extending from one midaxillary line to the contralateral across the anterior aspect of the chest wall. For cosmetic reasons, the incision generally follows the submammary folds located at the level of the sixth rib.

The pectoralis major muscle is separated from its inferior and medial attachments and lifted with the overlying skin and soft tissues exposing the chest wall. Incision of the intercostal muscles at the level of the fourth space is conducted starting from the sternum bilaterally and extended more laterally and posteriorly than the skin incision to allow increased rib spreading. The internal mammary vessels are isolated, tied, and divided. The sternum is then sectioned transversally, usually with an oscillating saw.

This incision provides an excellent exposure of both the pleural cavities and pulmonary hili and can be particularly useful for the treatment of giant tumors involving bilaterally the lungs. Main disadvantages include higher postoperative pain and

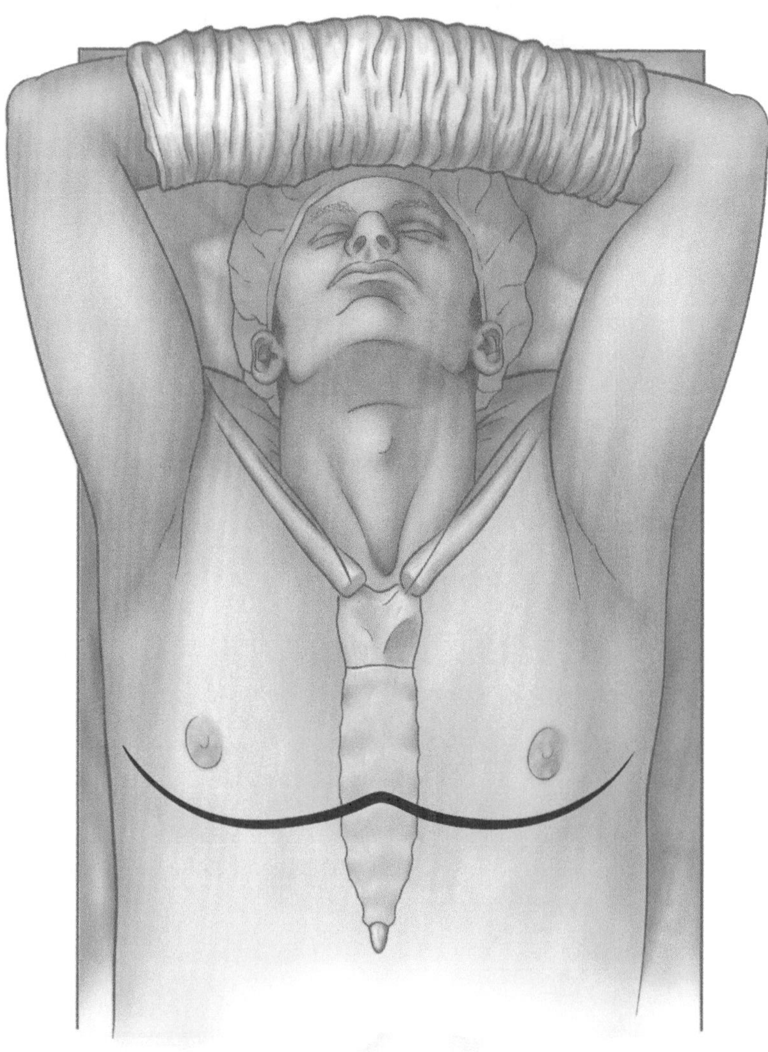

Fig. 2. Clamshell incision.

the increased risk of sternal complications (override or pseudoarthrosis).[27,28] Therefore, although the utility of this approach has been emphasized in an oncologic setting by some investigators,[25] its use in this field is still limited to very selected cases.

Some authors recommend the placement of several Kirschner wires in the reapproximated sternum to reduce override and shifts of the sternal wedges, although complications due to migration of wires have been reported.[29] Others suggest the offset of sternal tables by beveling the bone incision (tipping the saw at a 45° angle) to allow a more stable closure.[29]

Recently, a further extension of the clamshell approach has been described[30]—the so-called inverse-T incision (**Fig. 3**). This approach consists of a full clamshell incision together with a partial upper median sternotomy. This incision provides excellent access to the upper mediastinum and both the pulmonary hili. It thus allows an effective dissection of the entire upper third of the thorax. Moreover, this incision can be easily extended to the cervical region. Despite the magnitude of the incision, good results in terms of chest wall stability and preservation of the sternocostal arch functionality have been reported.[30] These technical results have allowed fast recovery and rapid postoperative respiratory rehabilitation.

Type of Vascular Resection and Reconstruction

Anterior mediastinal tumors infiltrating the surrounding vascular structures amenable for radical en bloc exeresis more frequently require the resection and reconstruction of the SVC and one or both of the innominate veins.

When the SVC is infiltrated for less than 30% of its circumference, a partial resection is possible and the vascular repair can be accomplished either by direct suture or by interposition of a patch (**Fig. 4**), usually of autologous material (pericardial or venous). If a larger circumferential involvement is present, a complete resection of the vessel with prosthetic replacement is required.

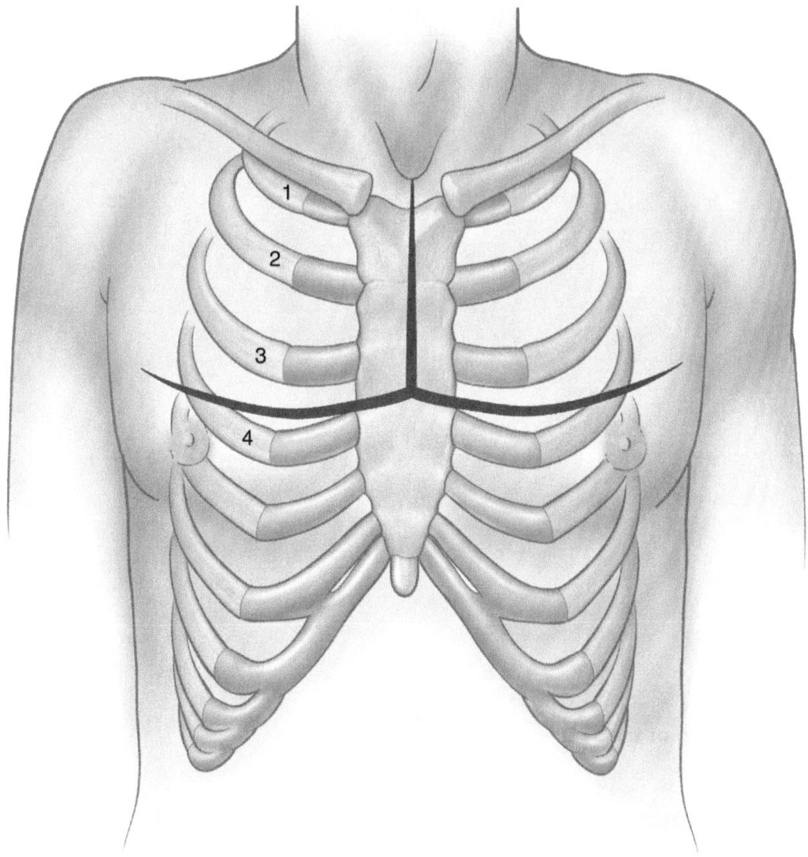

Fig. 3. Inverse-T incision.

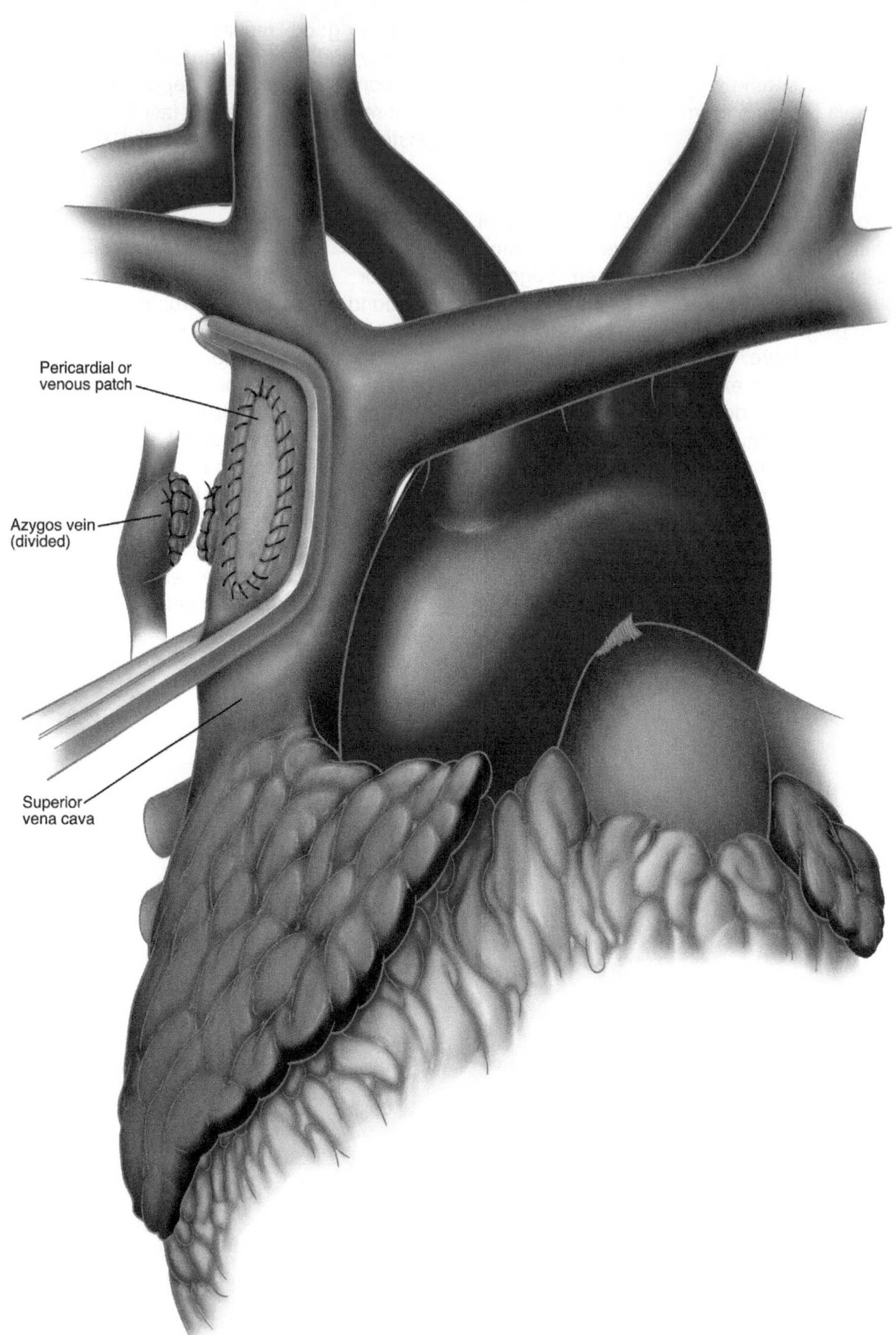

Fig. 4. Patch reconstruction of the SVC.

Extended operations including resection and reconstruction of the SVC represent a major technical challenge, especially for the potential detrimental effect of clamping a patent vessel.[31] Partial caval clamping or clamping of chronically obstructed SVC is usually well tolerated. On the contrary, during the complete clamping of a patent SVC, there is a marked hemodynamic imbalance, with an increase of mean venous pressure in the cephalic district and a decrease of mean arterial pressure with a consequent reduction of the brain arterial-venous gradient. This may produce cerebral edema and damage, intracranial bleeding, and potentially lethal reduction of the cardiac output.

This hemodynamic derangement can be minimized by several intraoperative technical and pharmacologic solutions. From the surgical point of view, the placement of intraluminal or extraluminal shunts (between the brachiocephalic vein or the internal jugular vein and the right atrium) may reduce the effects of clamping. However, thrombosis of the shunt may occur; furthermore, these devices occupy space in the operative field determining increased difficulties for the vascular sutures.

Intraoperative pharmacologic neuroprotection includes administration of steroids before clamping and optimization of circulatory parameters during clamping by fluid administration and vasoconstrictive agents to increase the mean arterial pressure. Anticoagulation with intravenous sodium heparin (0.5 mg/kg) is administered before clamping and it is continued in the postoperative period taking into account the characteristics of the graft material employed for reconstruction.

Vascular reconstruction can be performed by a SVC trunk replacement if a disease-free confluence of both the innominate veins is present. After clamping and vascular resection, the anastomosis between the superior caval stump and the prosthetic conduit is performed first (5-0 or 6-0 polypropylene suture).

To avoid kinking of the prosthesis, the length of the conduit is adapted so that the distal anastomosis could be under tension. In the case of neoplastic infiltration of the SVC origin at the confluence with the innominate veins, the revascularization is usually performed between the left innominate vein and the inferior SVC stump (or the right atrium) with closure of the right innominate vein (**Fig. 5**), or alternatively between the right innominate vein and the inferior SVC stump (or the right atrium) with closure of the left innominate vein, according to the local invasion.

These types of reconstruction are usually realized by synthetic materials (usually ringed polytetrafluoroethylene [PTFE] grafts) or bovine pericardium. Minimal dissection, especially at the left innominate vein, is mandatory to avoid its rotation above the anastomosis. The risk of kinking is lower for revascularization from the right innominate vein since the residual venous stump is shorter and the direction of the graft is almost vertical.

Revascularization of both the innominate veins implanted independently at the right atrium (**Fig. 6**) are generally not performed because the blood flow through the graft is too low and exposes at high risk of thrombosis. Total resections of the SVC and both the innominate veins and reconstruction with a Y-shaped synthetic prosthesis (Dacron or PTFE) have been successfully realized and reported in literature.[21]

Reconstructive Materials

Various materials have been proposed for these vascular reconstructions, including biologic (autologous or heterologous) or synthetic options.

Biologic materials, such as autologous or bovine pericardium, azygos vein, and saphenous vein have achieved large acceptance in the reconstruction of low-pressure thoracic vessels because of improved biocompatibility, lower risk of infection and thrombosis, and lower costs if compared with synthetic materials.

Among the biologic materials, autologous pericardium has been extensively used either for patch or conduit reconstruction. Although positive results have been obtained with both these options, the large amount of tissue required for the replacement of a long vascular tract makes this material unsuitable for most of cases of complete caval reconstruction. Conversely, autologous pericardium is generally considered the ideal option for patch reconstruction of the SVC, as well as of the pulmonary artery, since it shows a number of advantages: it has adequate thickness and resistance, is cost-free, and is available on both sides of the chest. Moreover, its harvesting does not require a separate procedure and offers a larger amount of tissue if compared with venous patches. However, fresh pericardium has some technical limits because it markedly shrinks and curls making the adaptation of the patch to the vascular wall defect more difficult to achieve. Therefore, uneven bites and bleeding sites may result when suturing it to the vessel.

For this reason, the authors have described an original method of fixation of the autologous pericardial patch by glutaraldehyde[32] that improves the technical features of this material. The glutaraldehyde rinsed autologous pericardial leaflet acquires stiffer edges and no tendency toward shrinkage and curling, making the tailoring of the patch and its suturing to the vascular wall easier.

Among the heterologous biologic materials, the bovine pericardium is currently the most used option. It displays some advantageous characteristics, such as the presence of even and stiff edges and the limited tendency to retract, facilitating its

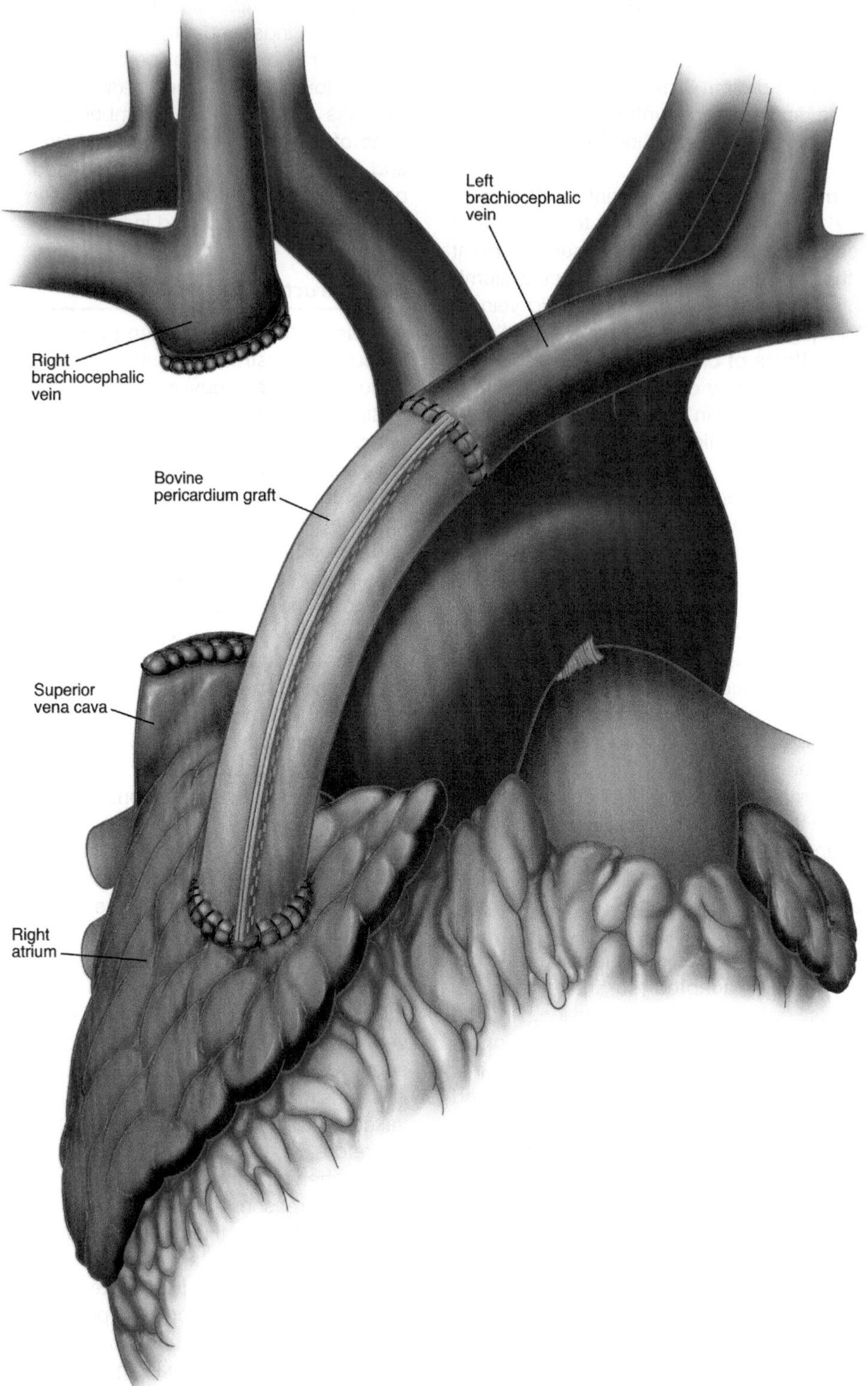

Fig. 5. Revascularization between the left innominate vein and the right atrium with closure of the right innominate vein.

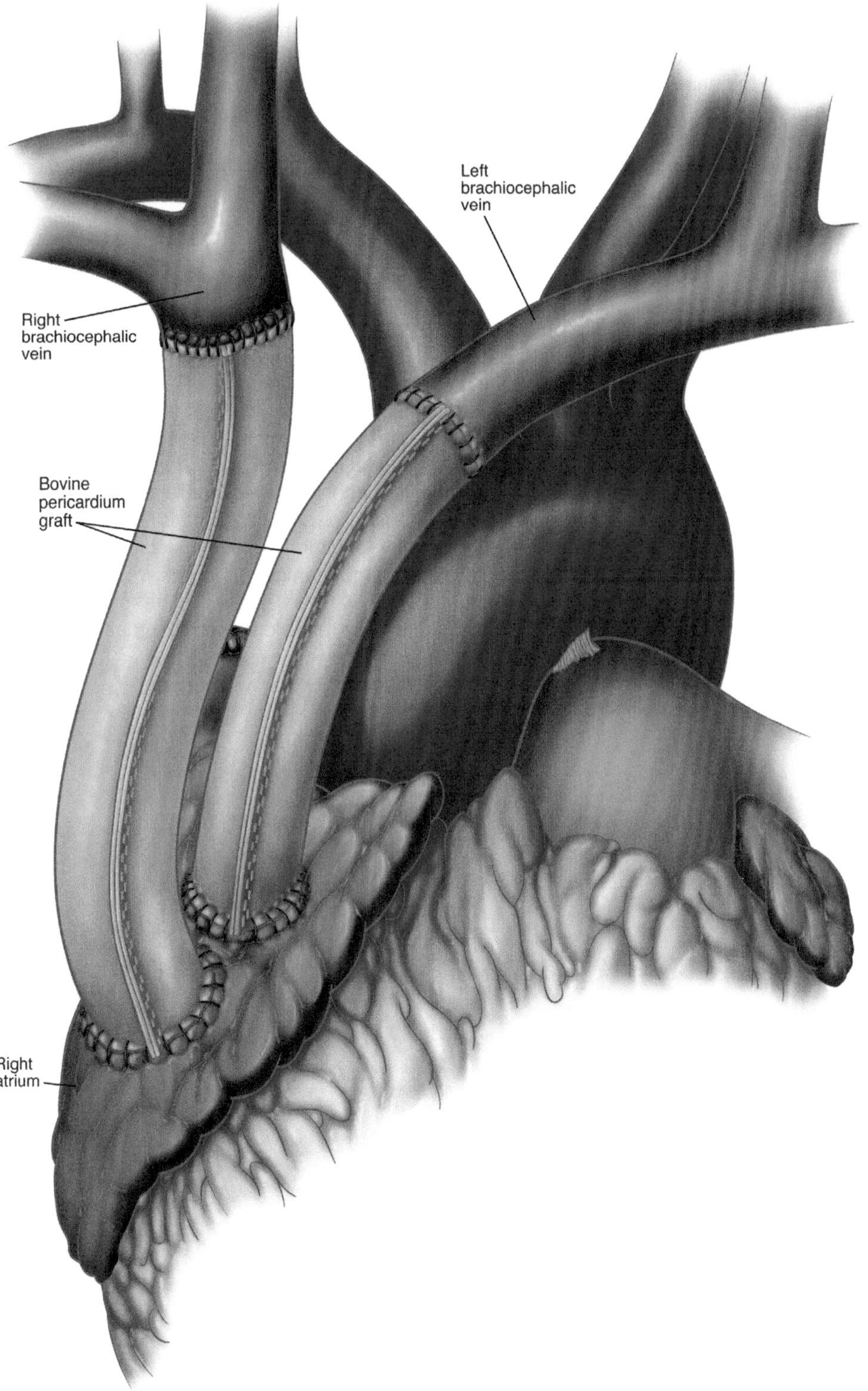

Fig. 6. Revascularization of both the innominate veins implanted independently at the right atrium.

adaptation and suturing to the vascular wall. However, in the patch reconstructive procedures it has lower diffusion with respect to the autologous pericardium because of inferior biocompatibility and higher costs. Conversely, when total SVC replacement is required, bovine pericardium is preferred because the autologous tissue is generally not sufficient to create a long conduit. The pericardial conduit has lower risk of infection and thrombosis and does not necessitate long-term anticoagulation if compared with synthetic materials.

The authors have devised and employed an original technique for the construction of a pericardial conduit to be used for SVC replacement.[33] The bovine pericardial leaflet is trimmed to a rectangular shape of the resected caval segment length, wrapped around a syringe (5 mL or 10 mL) to obtain the appropriate diameter, and sutured longitudinally by a linear reloadable stapler (**Fig. 7**A, B). In our previous experience, the longitudinal closure was performed with a running suture of 5-0 or 6-0 monofilament nonabsorbable material. The mechanical stapler recently introduced in this technique enables a quicker, easier, and more precise procedure and confers a more regular shape to the vascular graft, so that the anastomosis with the vascular stump is facilitated (see **Fig. 7**C; **Fig. 8**).

Autologous venous grafts (saphenous, jugular, superficial femoral) have a limited diameter that is sufficient only for the reconstruction of the brachiocephalic vein and is not suitable for SVC replacement. Saphenous vein graft of adequate diameter has been created by suturing the venous wall in a spiral fashion around a stent or a chest tube of appropriate size.[34]

Among the synthetic materials employed for graft reconstruction of the SVC (Dacron, PTFE, Gore-tex), the PTFE is the option of choice. It is the synthetic material showing the highest patency rate at long term and, shortly after its implantation, it becomes re-epitheliarized with autogenous epithelial cells in humans. PTFE grafts have low risk of infection, less platelet deposition, and less thrombogenicity of the flow surface if compared with Dacron grafts.[35] The synthetic grafts are usually reinforced with external rings.

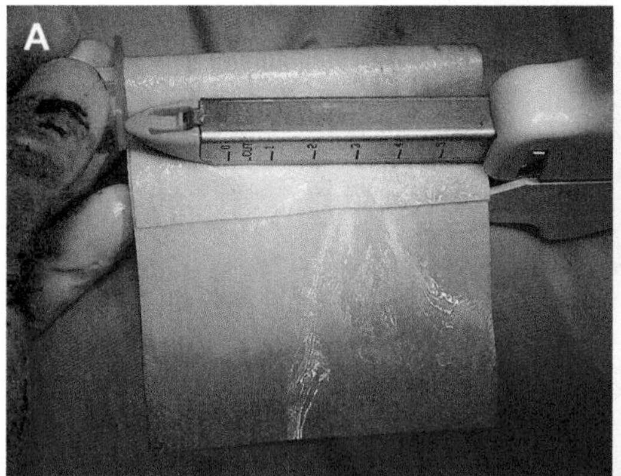

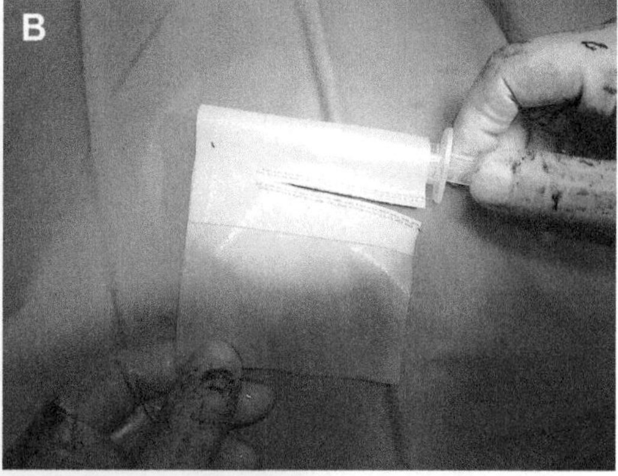

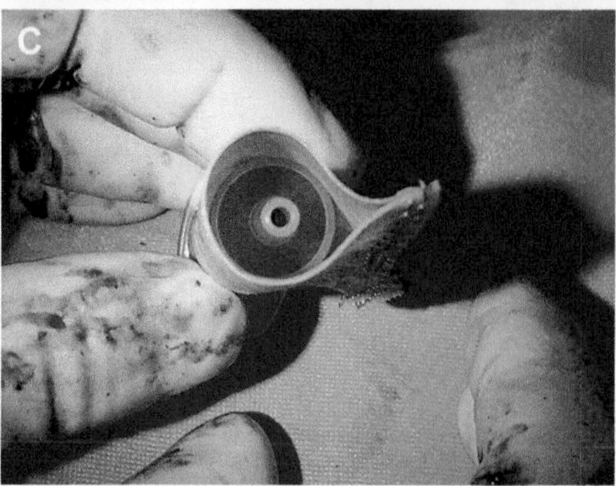

Fig. 7. Construction of the pericardial conduit: (*A*) The mechanical stapler is applied to the leaflet wrapped around a syringe. (*B*) The longitudinal mechanical suture is visible. (*C*) Construction of the pericardial conduit is completed.

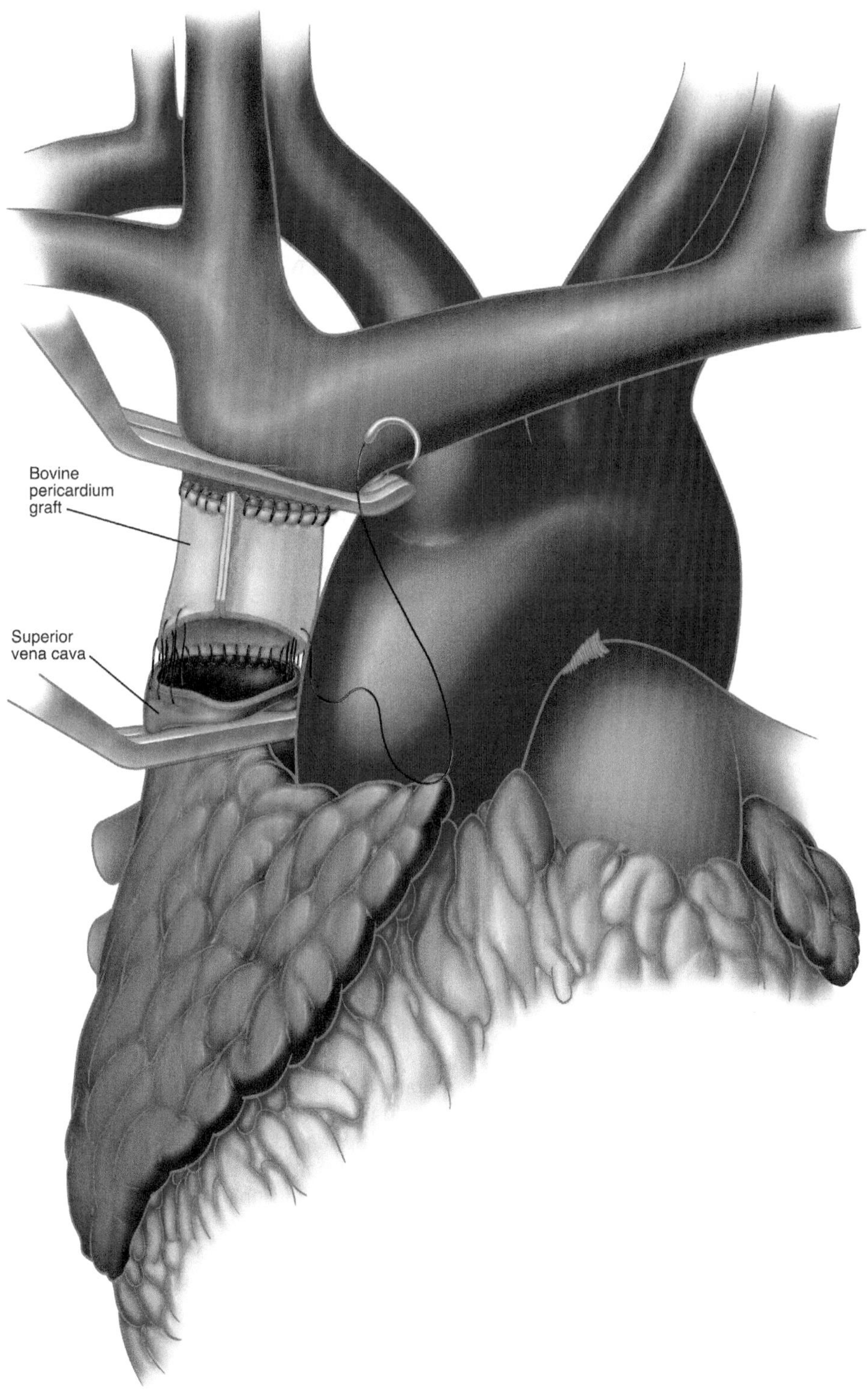

Fig. 8. The SVC replacement by bovine pericardial conduit is completed.

Results of Surgical Treatment

There are only few large experiences in the literature reporting the results of extended radical resections of invasive anterior mediastinal tumors invading the great vessels and the other neighboring structures. Moreover, some of these experiences provide cumulative data referring to results obtained with the treatment of different histologic neoplasms and heterogeneous oncologic multimodality protocols, so that the information acquired by these series does not always provide clear oncologic indications.

In 1998, the Marie Lannelongue Hospital group in Paris reported a 17-year experience including 89 patients with primary mediastinal tumors (74% of which located in the anterior mediastinum) resected with at least part of an adjacent structure.[20] There were 35 invasive thymomas, 12 thymic carcinomas, 17 germ cell tumors, 16 lymphomas, 3 neurogenic tumors, 3 thyroid carcinomas, 2 radiation induced sarcomas, and 1 mediastinal mesothelioma.

A median sternotomy was used in almost all the patients with an anterior mediastinal tumor and in some patients with tumor of the middle mediastinum (79% of all patients). A clamshell approach was chosen in three cases with large chemoresistant germ cell tumors.

The pericardium was the most frequently excised structure (73% of patients). Pulmonary resections (including 28 wedges, 16 lobectomies, and 5 pneumonectomies) were performed in 55% of cases. Forty percent of patients underwent resection of great vessels including SVC in 21 cases and innominate vein in 13. Replacement of SVC was performed in all cases by a PTFE graft. Vascular replacement was not done in patients undergoing innominate vein resection. Radical excision was achieved in 79% of patients. Major complications occurred in 17% of patients, requiring reoperation in four cases (4.5%). Surgical mortality was 6%. All SVC grafts but one were patent at 3 months. There was one late graft occlusion at 15 months, after the insertion of a central venous catheter.

Postoperative adjuvant radiation therapy was used in 85% of patients with thymoma and in 58% of those with thymic carcinoma. Postoperative chemotherapy was administered in 67% of patients with thymic carcinoma. Fourteen out of 17 patients with germ cell carcinoma underwent cisplatin-based combination preoperative chemotherapy. Ten of these patients underwent postoperative chemotherapy. Among the 16 patients with lymphoma, 8 with pretreatment diagnosis underwent preoperative chemotherapy and resection of the residual mass, and the other 8 patients without a preoperative diagnosis received chemotherapy postoperatively only.

Overall, 5-year survival was 63%. It was 69% for patients with thymoma (stage III or IV), 42% for those with thymic carcinoma, 48% for those with germ cell tumor, and 83% for those with lymphoma. Recurrence rate was higher in patients with thymic carcinoma (75%).

More recently, data from a Chinese experience has been published including 15 radically resected patients with malignant anterior mediastinal tumor invading the SVC or its branches.[21] There were nine patients with malignant thymoma and one patient each with thymic carcinoma, teratoma, embryonal carcinoma, Hodgkin's lymphoma, non-Hodgkin's lymphoma, and mixed teratoma with thymoma.

All the operations were performed through a median sternotomy. In two cases, the left innominate vein was removed and its distal end ligated without reconstruction. In seven patients, partial resection of the SVC or innominate vein was performed and repaired by direct suture with lateral SVC clamping. In three other patients, a pericardial patch reconstruction was performed using a total caval clamping. In the three remaining patients, complete resection of the SVC with both the innominate veins was performed with reconstruction by a Dacron graft. In one patient, a Y-shaped prosthesis was used. In the other two cases, a single lumen conduit was inserted between the right innominate vein stump and the right atrium with closure of the left innominate vein stump.

Major complication rate was 13%, without perioperative mortality.

Preoperative chemotherapy was administered in four patients (26%). At the time of publication, all patients but one were alive with a 35-months median follow-up and a disease-free survival ranging between 10 and 43 months.

In the last years, some interesting experiences have appeared in the literature reporting limited series of patients who have undergone resection of thoracic malignancies, mostly located in the anterior and middle mediastinum, requiring the use of cardiopulmonary bypass (CPB). The need for CPB was principally due to the direct invasion of cardiac structures or great vessels.

Vaporciyan and colleagues[36] have published a study of 19 patients with intrathoracic invasive tumors, most of which were metastatic lesions, showing direct involvement of cardiac chambers or great vessels, or significant cardiac compression requiring CPB to allow manipulation of the tumor during resection. Primary mediastinal tumors were present only in 20% of patients.

The operative approach was a median sternotomy in 68% of cases and a clamshell incision in 15%.

Reconstructive procedures were performed by direct suture whenever possible. In eight patients (42%), the vascular reconstruction included the use of autologous pericardium, bovine pericardium, Dacron graft, and Gore-tex patch or graft. Complications occurred in 58% of patients and perioperative mortality was 11%. The overall complete resectability (R0) rate from the cardiac structures was 79%. The overall median survival was 62.4 plus or minus 25.4 months and it was significantly higher in patients who underwent radical resection.

Another similar series from the Memorial Sloan Kettering Cancer Center has been reported in 2004 including 10 patients with malignancies invading the heart or great vessels, seven of which requiring CPB.[37] In three of these patients, the tumor was located in the anterior mediastinum and determined SVC obstruction. The anterior mediastinal tumors included one thymoma, one synovial cell sarcoma, and one malignant teratoma. These tumors were approached by median sternotomy in two cases and by a hemiclamshell incision in one (stage IV thymoma). SVC reconstruction was made by a ringed Gore-tex graft. Among these three patients, CPB was required only in the one with malignant teratoma. There were not postoperative deaths. Although the patient with thymoma received a radical (R0) resection, he died due to brain relapse of the disease after 29 months. On the contrary, the other two patients with anterior mediastinal malignancy were still alive at the time of publication after 69 months (synovial sarcoma) and 33 months (teratoma), although they presented microscopically infiltrated margins (R1). The latter two patients did not receive any postoperative oncologic treatment, while the patient with malignant teratoma received preoperative chemotherapy.

When considering only invasive thymic tumors (Masaoka stage III and IV) the completeness of surgical resection is generally reported as one of the most significant factors influencing prognosis.[38] Incomplete resections or surgical debulking usually do not modify long-term survival.[39–41]

Unfortunately, the presence of too-extended involvement of the surrounding anatomic structures makes radical surgery unfeasible in 30% for 40% of cases of invasive thymic tumors. In the largest published surgical experience from the Massachusetts General Hospital,[38] including 179 patients with thymoma and thymic carcinoma, the recurrence rate in patients with Masaoka stage III-IV tumors was definitively higher when compared with that reported in all other patients (stage III:31%, stage IV:45% vs other stages:2%).

Recent reports have suggested a survival advantage of induction therapy for stage III thymomas, if compared with adjuvant treatment.[39,40,42]

In 2003, the authors reported a series of 45 patients with stage III epithelial thymic tumors, 11 of whom with thymic carcinoma.[42] Thirty of these patients (66.6%) with a resectable stage III lesion (invasion of the SVC, pericardium, or limited invasion of the mediastinal pleura and lung) underwent primary surgery. The other 15 patients with tumors considered not completely resectable due to the extensive invasion of the surrounding organs underwent induction chemotherapy followed by surgical resection. All the operations were performed through a median sternotomy. After the operation, patients received adjuvant chemotherapy and radiotherapy at a dose of 40 Gy in case of complete resection or at a dose of 50 to 60 Gy in case of incomplete resection. A vascular reconstruction was performed in 11 patients by a bovine pericardial conduit interposition. In nine cases, it was made after resection of the SVC and, in two cases, after resection of the left innominate vein. Complete resection was feasible in 82% of patients with thymic carcinoma and in 91% of patients with other histologic diagnosis. Major complications occurred in 6.7% of patients. There was no operative mortality. The 10-year overall actuarial survival was 78%, whereas the cumulative disease-free survival was 53%. Ten-year survival for patients undergoing complete resection was 80%, while it was 60% for patients with incomplete resection (P = .3). Ten-year survival of patients receiving induction chemotherapy was 90%, compared with 71% for patients undergoing primary surgery (P = .2).

SURGICAL APPROACHES FOR INVASIVE CERVICOMEDIASTINAL TUMORS

In cases of tumors located in the anterior mediastinum and extending in the cervical region, the choice of an adequate surgical approach has to consider several additional technical aspects, since the mass may involve anatomic structures whose exposure may be limited with the conventional mediastinal approaches. In particular, for resection of some cervicothoracic masses, the division of sternoclavicular junction or partial or near complete resection of the clavicle or the first and second rib may become necessary.

Some of these approaches have been originally proposed for the resection of anterior Pancoast tumors, but they can be effectively applied also for the treatment of some cervicomediastinal neoplasms.

The median sternotomy may be an optimal approach also for many anterior cervicomediastinal tumors, since this incision can be easily extended to the neck either in a linear or in a curvilinear fashion. Advantages and limitation of this approach are substantially the same reported for the standard sternotomy employed for tumors confined to the mediastinal compartment.

The hemiclamshell approach consists of a partial median sternotomy combined with a neck incision and an anterior thoracotomy, usually performed in the second to the fifth intercostal space depending on the location and the extension of the mass (**Fig. 9**). Care must be taken to divide the pectoralis major muscle proximally to its insertion on to the ribs to allow reapproximation without tearing of this muscle. By this approach, the clavicle must not be divided as required by other approaches to the cervicomediastinal junction, and the sternoclavicular joint is left intact. This technical aspect improves shoulder stability and reduces postoperative discomfort. The vertical part of this incision can be prolonged to the neck along the anterior border of the sternocleidomastoid muscle, if required.

Korst and colleagues[43] have analyzed the results obtained using the hemiclamshell approach for the resection of cervicothoracic

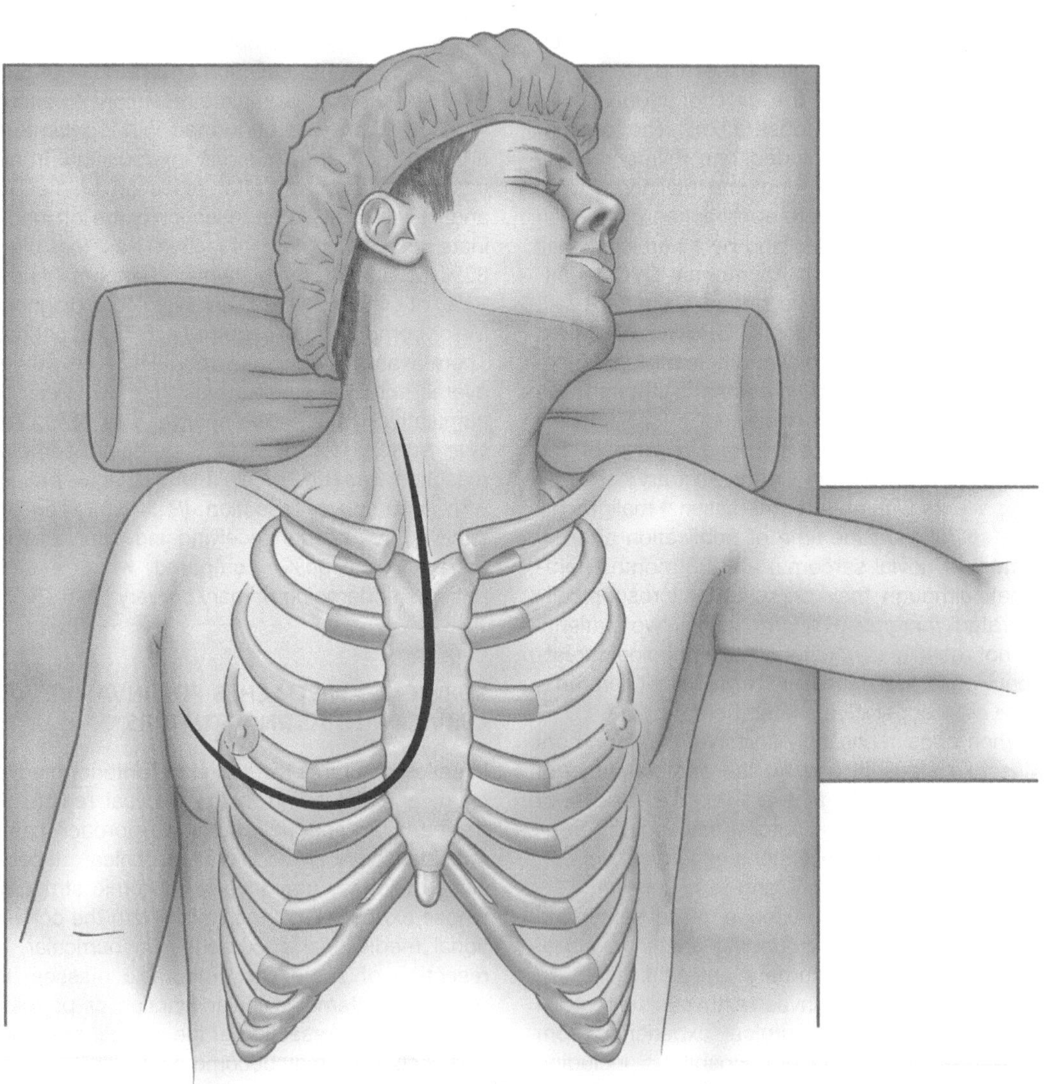

Fig. 9. Hemiclamshell incision.

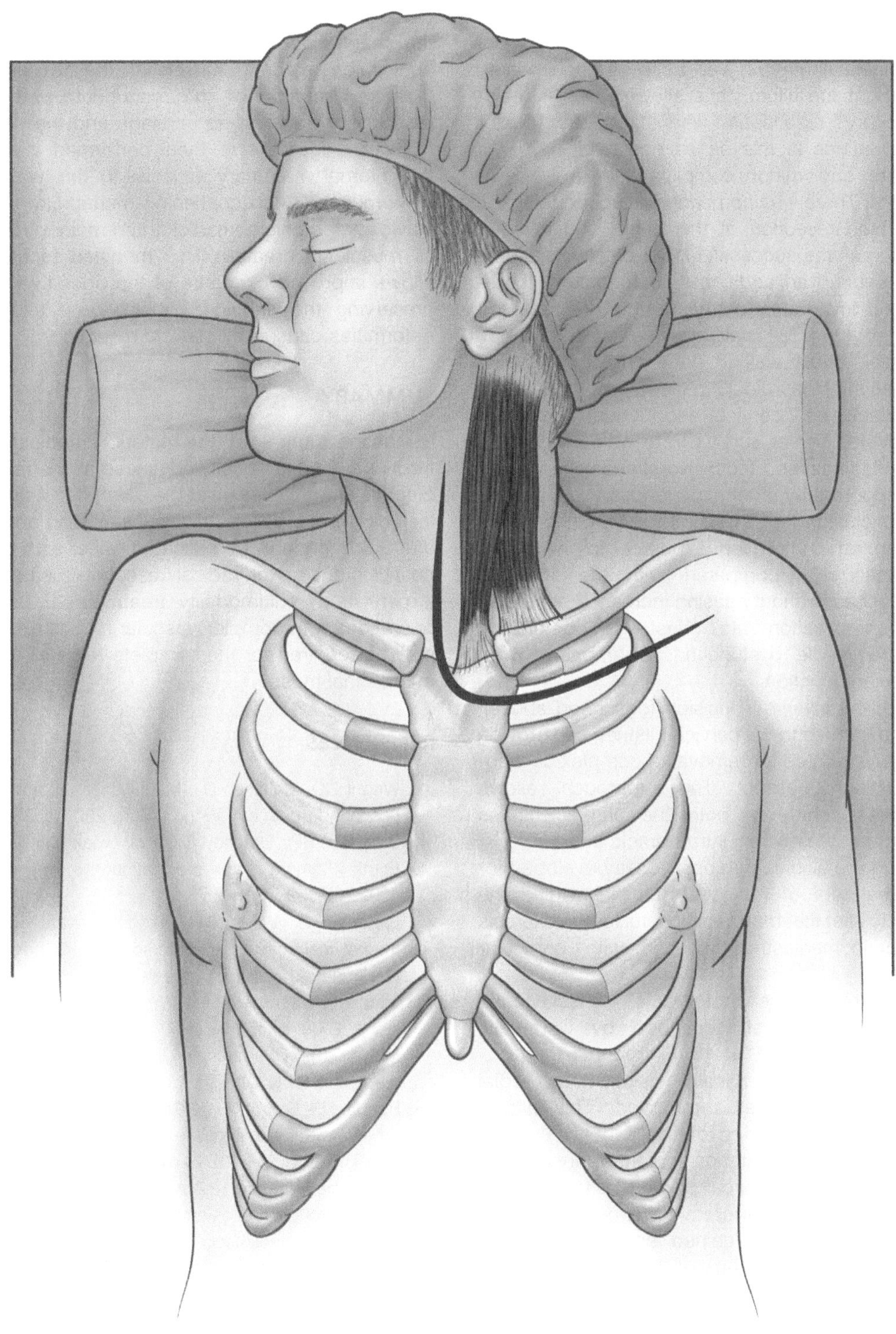

Fig. 10. Anterior transcervical thoracic approach.

primary or metastatic tumors on a series of 42 patients. They referred an excellent exposure of the mediastinum as well as of the pulmonary vessels at the hilum, thus allowing easier major pulmonary resections when required. Major complications in this series occurred in 7% of patients and minor complications in 19% of patients. There was no perioperative mortality.

En bloc resection of the tumor and invaded structures was successful in all but two patients who required an additional posterolateral thoracotomy. Invaded structures that were resected included lung (22 patients), vertebral body (7 patients), chest wall (8 patients), central veins (10 patients), thyroid (3 patients), carotid artery (1 patient), and cervical esophagus (1 patient). The overall 5-year survival rate was 67.4%.

The findings reported by Korst and colleagues[43] are supported by other experiences,[44] suggesting the conclusion that the hemiclamshell incision is able to offer improved exposure to the upper mediastinum if compared with the standard approaches, without causing increased postoperative complication rate, chest wall complaints, shoulder girdle dysfunction, or impairment of pulmonary function.

Also, the inverse-T incision (described above), when extended to the cervical district, can provide optimal exposure for removal of complex cervicomediastinal masses. This approach allows complete control of both the phrenic nerves throughout their whole intrathoracic course.

There are also some approaches developed for the treatment of Pancoast tumor invading the thoracic inlet that may result useful for the exeresis of cervicomediastinal masses with particular location.

The anterior cervicothoracic transclavicular approach was first described by Dartevelle and colleagues[45] (**Fig. 10**). Through a large L-shaped anterior cervical incision, the medial half of the clavicle is removed. This allows dissection or resection of the subclavian vein, sectioning of the anterior scalenus muscle and resection of the cervical portion of the phrenic nerve, if involved. Moreover, exposure of the subclavian artery is gained and dissection of the brachial plexus up to the spinal foramen can be done. The use of this approach is related with higher morbidity and its diffusion for surgery of cervicomediastinal masses is therefore limited.

A variation of the approach described by Dartevelle has been reported: the transmanubrial osteomuscular sparing approach.[46] This technique consists of an L-shaped skin incision along the sternocleidomastoid muscle and 2 cm below the clavicle. The incision has been modified allowing the sparing of insertions of sternocleidomastoid and major pectoralis muscle on the clavicle. An L-shaped section of the manubrium with the resection of the first-rib cartilage and the costoclavicular ligament is then performed dividing the internal mammary vessels. In this way, an osteomuscular flap containing manubrium edge, clavicle, sternocleidomastoid, and major pectoralis muscle is created. This modified technique allows improved exposure of the operative field, preserving the shoulder mobility and avoiding deformities caused by clavicle resection.

SUMMARY

Malignant tumors of the anterior mediastinum frequently appear locally advanced at the time of diagnosis, with invasion of the surrounding organs including major blood vessels, lungs, and pericardium. Surgery can be indicated either with diagnostic intent or for radical resection, usually as a part of a multimodality treatment. Extended operations with complex vascular reconstructions may be required for the complete removal of the mediastinal mass.

REFERENCES

1. Wright CD, Mathisen DJ. Mediastinal tumors: diagnosis and treatment. World J Surg 2001;25:204–9.
2. Whooley BP, Urschel ID, Antkowiak JG, et al. Primary tumors of the mediastinum. J Surg Oncol 1999;70:95–9.
3. Lardinois D, Weder W. Diagnostic strategies in mediastinal mass. In: Patterson GA, Cooper JD, Deslauriers J, et al, editors. Pearson's thoracic and esophageal surgery. New York: Churchill Livingstone; 2008. p. 1506–20.
4. McNeil TM, Chamberlain JM. Diagnostic anterior mediastinotomy. Ann Thorac Surg 1966;2:532–9.
5. Rendina EA, Venuta F, De Giacomo T, et al. Biopsy of anterior mediastinal masses under local anesthesia. Ann Thorac Surg 2002;74:1720–3.
6. Watanabe M, Takagi K, Aoki T, et al. A comparison of biopsy through a parasternal anterior mediastinotomy under local anesthesia and percutaneous needle biopsy for malignant anterior mediastinal tumors. Surg Today 1998;28:122–6.
7. Dosios T, Theakos N, Chatziantoniou C. Cervical mediastinoscopy and anterior mediastinotomy in superior vena cava obstruction. Chest 2005;128: 1551–6.
8. Zwischenberger JB, Savage C, Alpard SK, et al. Mediastinal transthoracic needle and core lymph node biopsy: should it replace mediastinoscopy? Chest 2002;121:1165–70.

9. Greif J, Staroselsky AN, Gernjac M, et al. Percutaneous core needle biopsy in the diagnosis of mediastinal tumors. Lung Cancer 1999;25:169–73.
10. Jahangiri M, Goldstraw P. The role of mediastinoscopy in superior vena caval obstruction. Ann Thorac Surg 1995;59:453–5.
11. Porte H, Metois D, Finzi L, et al. Superior vena cava syndrome of malignant origin: which surgical procedure for which diagnosis? Eur J Cardiothorac Surg 2000;17:384–8.
12. Specht G. Expanded mediastinoscopy. Thoraxchir Vask Chir 1965;13:401–7.
13. Kirschner PA. Extended mediastinoscopy. In: Jepsson O, Ruhbek-Sorensen H, editors. Mediastinoscopy. Odense: Odense University Press; 1971.
14. Ginsberg RJ, Rice TW, Goldberg M, et al. Extended cervical mediastinoscopy. A single procedure for bronchogenic carcinoma of the left upper lobe. J Thorac Cardiovasc Surg 1987;94: 673–8.
15. Lopez L, Varela A, Fleixinet J. Extended cervical mediastinoscopy. Prospective study of fifty cases. Ann Thorac Surg 1994;57:555–8.
16. Metin M, Sayar A, Turna A, et al. Extended cervical mediastinoscopy in the diagnosis of anterior mediastinal masses. Ann Thorac Surg 2002; 73:250–2.
17. Yim AP, Lee TW, Izzat MB, et al. Place of video-thoracoscopy in thoracic surgical practice. World J Surg 2001;25:157–61.
18. Gossot D, Girard P, de Kerviler E, et al. Thoracoscopy or CT-guided biopsy for residual intrathoracic masses after treatment of lymphoma. Chest 2001; 120:289–94.
19. Roviaro G, Varoli F, Nucca O, et al. Videothoracoscopic approach to primary mediastinal pathology. Chest 2000;117:1179–83.
20. Bacha EA, Chapelier AR, Macchiarini P, et al. Surgery for invasive primary mediastinal tumors. Ann Thorac Surg 1998;66:234–9.
21. Chen KN, Xu SF, Gu ZD, et al. Surgical treatment of complex malignant anterior mediastinal tumors invading the superior vena cava. World J Surg 2006;30:162–70.
22. Baskett RJ, McDougall CE, Ross DB. Is mediastinitis a preventable complication? A 10-year review. Ann Thorac Surg 1999;67:462.
23. Demmy TL, Park SB, Liebler GA, et al. Recent experience with major sternal wound complications. Ann Thorac Surg 1990;49:458.
24. Weber L, Peters RW. Delayed chest wall complications of sternotomy. South Med J 1986;79: 723.
25. Bains MS, Ginsberg RJ, Jones WG 2nd, et al. The clamshell incision: an improved approach to bilateral pulmonary and mediastinal tumors. Ann Thorac Surg 1994;58:30–3.
26. Marshall WG Jr, Meng RL, Ehrenhaft JL. Coronary artery bypass grafting in patients with a tracheostoma: use of a bilateral thoracotomy incision. Ann Thorac Surg 1988;46:465–6.
27. Wright C. Transverse sternothoracotomy. Chest Surg Clin N Am 1996;6:149–56.
28. Brown RP, Esmore DS, Lawson C. Improved sternal fixation in the transsternal bilateral thoracotomy incision. J Thorac Cardiovasc Surg 1996;112:137–41.
29. Durrleman N, Massard G. Clamshell and hemiclamshell incisions. MMCTS 2006. DOI: 10.1510/mmcts.2006.001867.
30. Marta GM, Aigner C, Klepetko W. Inverse T incision provides improved accessibility to the upper mediastinum. J Thorac Cardiovasc Surg 2005;129:221–3.
31. Gonzalez-Fajardo JA, Garcia-Yuste M, Florez S, et al. Hemodynamic cerebral repercussions arising from surgical interruption of the superior vena cava. Experimental model. J Thorac Cardiovasc Surg 1994;107:1044–9.
32. D'Andrilli A, Ibrahim M, Venuta F, et al. Glutaraldehyde preserved autologous pericardium for patch reconstruction of the pulmonary artery and superior vena cava. Ann Thorac Surg 2005;80:357–8.
33. D'Andrilli A, Ciccone AM, Ibrahim M, et al. A new technique for prosthetic reconstruction of the superior vena cava. J Thorac Cardiovasc Surg 2006; 132:192–4.
34. Doty DB. Bypass of superior vena cava: Six years' experience with spiral vein graft for obstruction of superior vena cava due to benign and malignant disease. J Thorac Cardiovasc Surg 1982;83:326.
35. Brewster DC. Prosthetic grafts. In: Rutheford RB, editor. Vascular Surgery. Philadelphia: WB Saunders; 1995. p. 492–521.
36. Vaporciyan AA, Rice D, Correa AM, et al. Resection of advanced thoracic malignancies requiring cardiopulmonary bypass. Eur J Cardiothorac Surg 2002; 22:47–52.
37. Park BJ, Bacchetta M, Bains MS, et al. Surgical management of thoracic malignancies invading the heart or great vessels. Ann Thorac Surg 2004;78: 1024–30.
38. Wright C, Wain J, et al. Predictors of recurrence in thymic tumors: importance of invasion, World Health Organization histology and size. J Thorac Cardiovasc Surg 2005;130:1413–21.
39. Jaxkson MA, Mall DL. Postoperative radiotherapy in invasive thymoma. Radiother Oncol 1991;21: 77–82.
40. Okumura M, Ohta M, Tateyama H, et al. The World Health Organization classification system reflects the oncologic behavior of thymoma. Cancer 2002; 94:624–32.
41. Wilkins KB, Sheikh E, Green R, et al. Clinical and pathological predictors of survival in patients with thymoma. Ann Thorac Surg 1999;230:562–74.

42. Venuta F, Rendina EA, Longo F, et al. Long-term outcome after multimodality treatment of stage III thymic tumors. Ann Thorac Surg 2003;76: 1866–72.
43. Korst RJ, Burt ME. Cervicothoracic tumors: results of resection by the "hemi-clamshell" approach. J Thorac Cardiovasc Surg 1998;115:286–95.
44. Lardinois D, Sippel M, Gupper M, et al. Morbidity and validity of the hemi-clamshell approach for thoracic surgery. Eur J Cardiothorac Surg 1999;16: 194–9.
45. Dartevelle PG, Chapelier AR, Macchiarini P, et al. Anterior transcervical-thoracic approach for radical resection of lung tumors invading the thoracic inlet. J Thorac Cardiovasc Surg 1993;105:1025–34.
46. Grunenwald D, Spaggiari L. Transmanubrial osteomuscular sparing approach for apical chest tumors. Ann Thorac Surg 1997;63:563–6.

Open Approaches to Posterior Mediastinal Tumor in Adults

Tetsuhiko Go, MD[a], Paolo Macchiarini, MD, PhD[b,*]

KEYWORDS

• Mediastinal tumors • Open approach • Surgery

Mediastinal tumors are usually classified into the three or four categories according to their original location in the thorax. Each tumor has some particular pathologic tendency, and methods of management are decided depending on tumor characteristics. Pathology of posterior mediastinal tumors (PMTs) differs between children and adults. Most of the PMTs in adults are benign lesions; they are mostly malignant in children. Obviously, surgery is curative for benign tumor, but plays an important role even in treating malignant PMTs in the context of a multimodality therapy. The indications for thoracoscopic surgery, including robotic surgery for the management of PMTs, have been extended with the improvement and refinements of the instruments.[1,2] However, thoracoscopic surgery remains a choice only for selected cases or a complementary therapeutic option for PMTs.[3–5]

This article discusses open approaches to PMTs in adults depending on tumor location and spinal involvement.

ANATOMY AND CLASSIFICATIONS

Several radiographic and surgical compartment models have been proposed according to the appearance of lateral view of chest radiograph. Most classification divides the mediastinum into four compartments—superior, anterior, middle, and posterior—or three, where superior and anterior mediastina are fused into one anterior compartment. Each has some overlapping portion and may cause some miss-leading.[6] Because of this, Shields[7] divided the mediastinum into three zones: prevascular, visceral, and retrovisceral. Although these distinctions are very useful for gross evaluation, they may give rise to the development of computerized imaging in terms of definite diagnosis, by which more accurate tumor characters and surgical information can be obtained.[8] In this article, the four compartment subdivisions are mainly used for anatomic explanation (**Fig. 1**).

Posterior mediastinum is defined as the area that lies between the back of the pericardium and vertebral bodies and includes costvertebral sulcus. This contains the tissues such as the descending thoracic aorta, esophagus, azygous vein, autonomic ganglia and nerves, thoracic lymph nodes, and fat.[9] PMT occasionally extends or involves the superior compartment tissue. Most of the tumors categorized into PMT are of neurogenic origin, including tumors from peripheral nerves (neurofibroma, neurilemoma [schwannoma], malignant schwannoma); tumors from the sympathetic ganglia (ganglioneuroma, ganglioneuroblastoma, neuroblastoma, paraganglioma, and others), gastroenteric cyst, and lymphoma.[9–11] Precise pathologic features and the explanations of each tumor are not the subject of this article.

SYMPTOMS AND DIAGNOSIS

PMTs are frequently and long asymptomatic, that is, only one third of adult patients complain of symptoms. However, about 50% of malignant

[a] General Thoracic and Breast-Endcrinological Surgery, Kagawa University Miki-Cho, Kita-gun, Kagawa 761-0973, Japan

[b] Department of General Thoracic and Regenerative Surgery and Intrathoracic Biotransplantation, University Hospital Careggi, Florence, Italy

* Corresponding author. Department of General Thoracic and Regenerative Surgery and Intrathoracic Biotransplantation, University Hospital Careggi, Florence, Italy.

E-mail address: pmacchiarini@thoraxeuropea.eu

Thorac Surg Clin 20 (2010) 285–295
doi:10.1016/j.thorsurg.2010.02.006
1547-4127/10/$ – see front matter

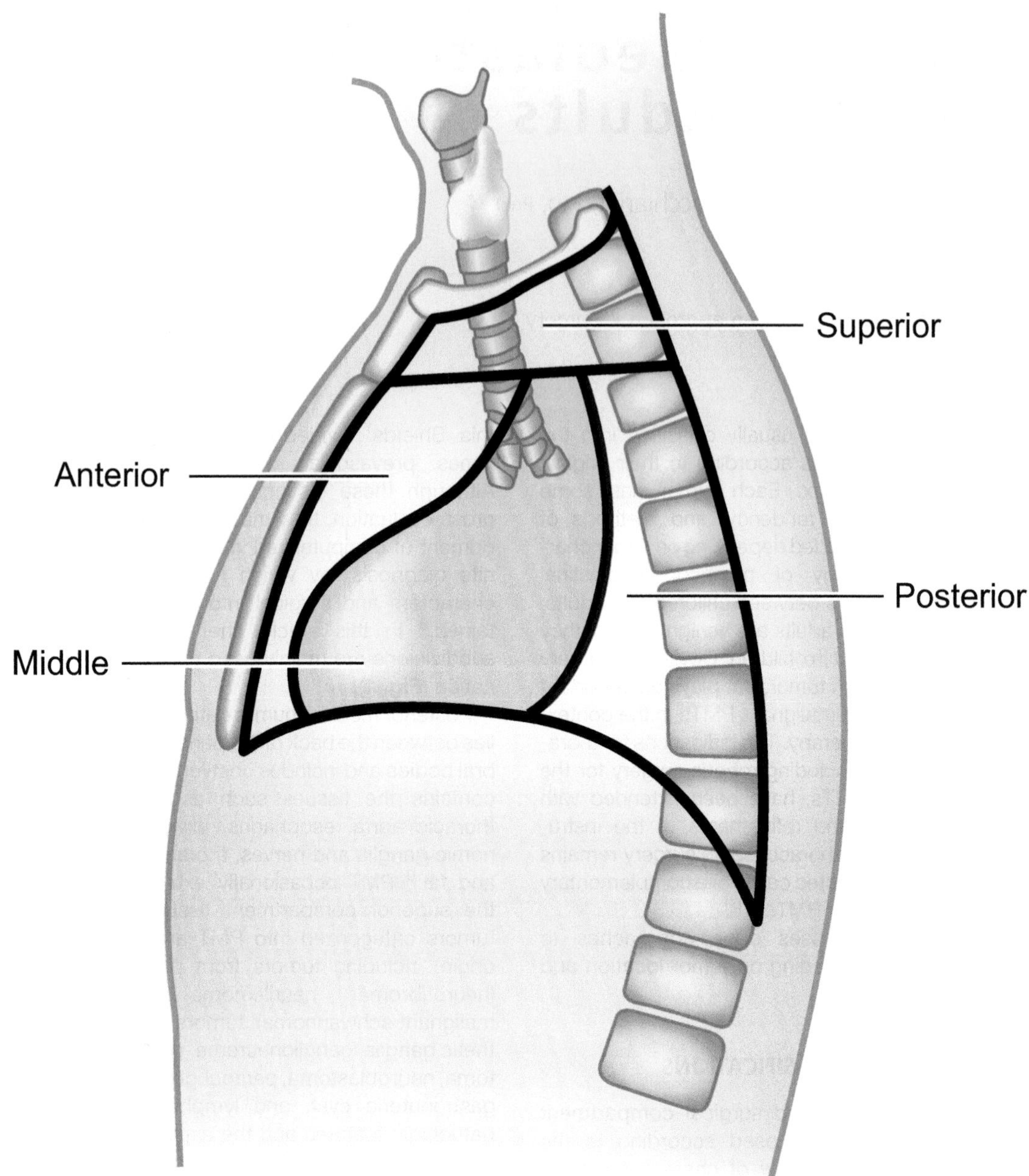

Fig. 1. The four mediastinal compartments. (*From* Warren WH. Anatomy of the mediastinum with special reference to surgical access. In: Pearson FG, editor. Pearson's thoracic and esophageal surgery, 3rd edition. Philadelphia: Churchill Livingstone Elsevier, 2008; with permission.)

PMTs display some sort of symptom.[3,6] Symptoms are divided in two categories: localized and systemic. Although localized symptoms such as cough and chest pain are often recognized as nonspecific respiratory symptoms, there are also symptoms secondary to the tumor invasion of surrounding organs such as dyspnea, pneumonia, dysphagia, hoarseness, paralysis, pain, and Horner syndrome.[3,5] Systemic symptoms are usually due to release of excessive hormones related to the tumor, such as pheochromecytoma.[9] Symptomatic patients are more likely to have malignancy compared with the patients with benign neoplasm. Davis and colleagues[12] reported that 16% of PMTs are malignant. Mass location, age, and symptoms are the important factors influencing the diagnosis of malignancy. Adult PMTs are mostly neurogenic and likely to be benign compared with PMT in children.[13]

The examination for diagnosis of PMT is started with posteroanterior and lateral chest radiograph. This is routinely performed for patients with respiratory symptoms; however PMTs are diagnosed incidentally with chest radiographs undertaken for unrelated or nonsymptomatic patients. This radiograph can give general information on a PMT in terms of size, location, and characteristics.[9] CT scan is a standard and essential imaging study, not only for the differential diagnosis, but also for understanding of tumor extension and relation to the surrounding tissues because they can distinguish tumor from fat tissue or cystic component and vascular structure. High-resolution CT scan or three-dimensional reconstruction is more useful for understanding tumor nature and behavior. MRI is recommended and useful in assessment of a tumor in the paravertebral area, especially for delineating spinal canal tumor extension and longitudinal extension. It is worthwhile to consider any possibility of tumor extension to the intraspinal region in the treatment of paravertebral lesion.[3–6]

Although other workups such as nuclear scans and biochemical markers are effective for diagnosis, histologic diagnosis is essential for planning treatments.

In a case of benign neoplasm being highly suggested after standard examinations, less invasive surgical excision of the tumor, including thoracoscopic surgery, is performed for simultaneous diagnosis and treatment. However if the tumor is likely to be malignant, biopsy including mediastinoscopy, thoracoscopy, and fine-needle aspiration (CT scan-guided, if necessary) are performed depending on the anatomic location and the radiographic appearance of PMT. Preoperative histologic definitive diagnosis is mandatory since malignant lesion of PMT requires multimodality treatment, including surgery, radiation, and chemotherapy. The fine-needle biopsy including CT san-guided aspiration is highly accurate on diagnosis, by more than 90%.[3,14]

TREATMENT

PMT pathologies are varied and they include cystic lesions (bronchogenic or enteric cyst of esophagus) and other unusual tumors.[15] However, treatments of these lesions are not discussed in this article because they have been already discussed extensively elsewhere.[16] Moreover, it seems appropriate to concentrate on the open approach for neurogenic tumors when discussing surgical treatment of PMT because more than 75% of PMTs in adults are neurogenic origin[3] and the principles of surgical approaches are in common within each PMT. Management of PMT differs depending on anatomic location, tumor size, and its pathologic nature. If a tumor is benign, simple excision will be done and, if it is malignant, multimodality treatment will be applied. Even on multimodality treatment, however, the role of surgery is very important. Complete surgical resection in the tumor-free margin contributes to better prognosis[3,6] and even reduction of tumor size or volume can provide the selected patients with the benefit of survival.[6,15]

When a tumor locates at the middle thorax, surgical approaches including open, thoracoscopic, or a combination is performed.[3,6,10,17] The preference of approach differs depending on tumor size or the surgeon's experience. However, the authors agree with Hoyos and colleagues[10] suggesting that PMTs larger than 3 cm or tumors that appear locally invasive should undergo open resection. When a PMT locates or occupies the apex of the thorax, including superior sulcus, or shows the appearance of so called dumbbell tumor, further attention will be needed. Although the same approaches are occasionally called by different names, the approaches discussed here are anterior, posterolateral, posterior, and the combination of anterior and posterior approach.

Surgery is performed under general anesthesia. This is maintained using a double-lumen endotracheal tube or a single-lumen tube with a bronchial blocker to allow ipsilateral lung deflation for optimal exposure. Standard managements of anesthesia for lung surgery such as hemodynamic monitoring with an arterial catheter are adopted.

Posterolateral Approach

Standard open surgical approach to PMT is through posterolateral thoracotomy (**Fig. 2**). The patient is placed at a lateral decubitus position and prepared and draped from the shoulder to below the costal arch, or iliac crest if necessary. A slightly curved sigmoid incision is made from the midpoint between the spine and the posterior border of the scapula to the anterior axillary line passing the one finger-width below the scapula tip. The scale of the incision can be flexibly extended to fit the location and size of the tumor. The incision is deepened by dividing the latissimus dorsi muscle in the middle and the trapezius muscle in part. The serratus anterior muscle is preserved and retracted anteriorly, detaching from its insertion in the rib cage by incising the serratus fascia. Retracting and lifting the scapula, the thorax is entered by cutting the intercostal muscles; depending on the tumor location, usually at the fourth or fifth intercostal space. To extend the intercostal incision, the paraspinous muscles are detached from the rib cage and preserved. Entering and exploring the thorax, resectability

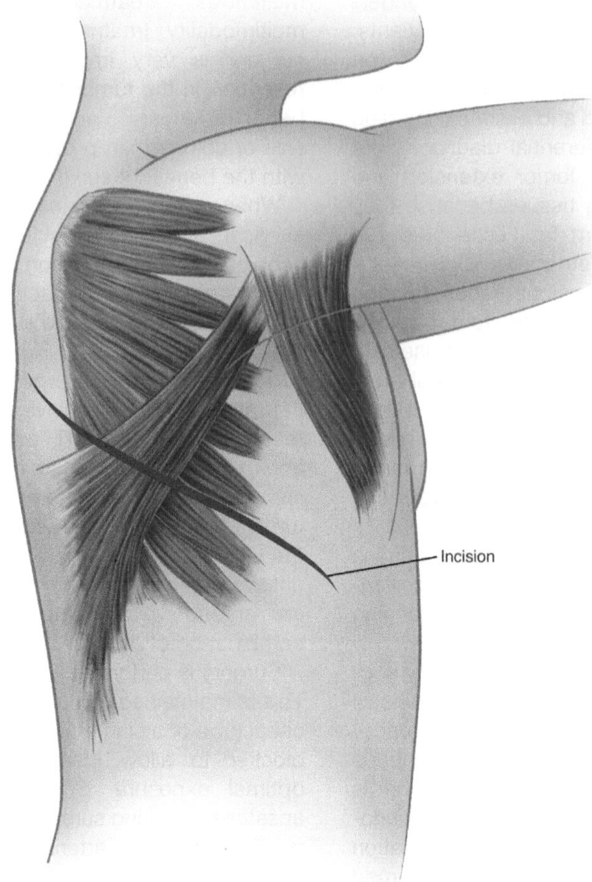

Fig. 2. Skin incision for posterolateral approach.

should be confirmed—especially if extended resection is needed.[3] For tumors of neurogenic origin, it is important to remember that excessive traction of a tumor may result in postoperative neurologic damage. Dissecting the parietal pleura or surrounding tissues a few centimeters away from the tumor margin, the surgery is performed step-by-step to identify the original nerve of the tumor and avoid injury of intercostal bundles by gently holding the tumor superiorly, laterally, and inferiorly. The indication for this approach is very wide and most PMTs are exposed and managed by this appropriate left- or right-sided approach. Even some of the tumor with intraspinal extension can be resected with this incision by rotating the patient slightly forward.[3,4] For PMTs at higher thorax locations, lateral or axillary approaches are another choice for surgery. However, a PMT at the very apex of the thorax, or a PMT involving superior sulcus, some paravertebral tumors, or dumbbell tumors sometimes cannot be managed only with this approach.

Posterior Approach

Depending on the tumor location or extension, especially the paravertebral lesion, posterior thoracotomy or incision will be chosen. In this approach, the patient is usually placed in the prone position (**Fig. 3**). Positioning the patient is very important, especially in the case that spinal cord compression or involvement is concerned. Consultations with a neurosurgeon might be helpful. Although this approach had been used for infectious lesion such as abscess drainage or biopsy,[18] it has been drawing focus extensively for the management of the paravertebral lesion such as dumbbell tumor through mid-vertical incision or paravertebral incision. In this case, most of the lesion is managed in the extrapleural space.[19,20]

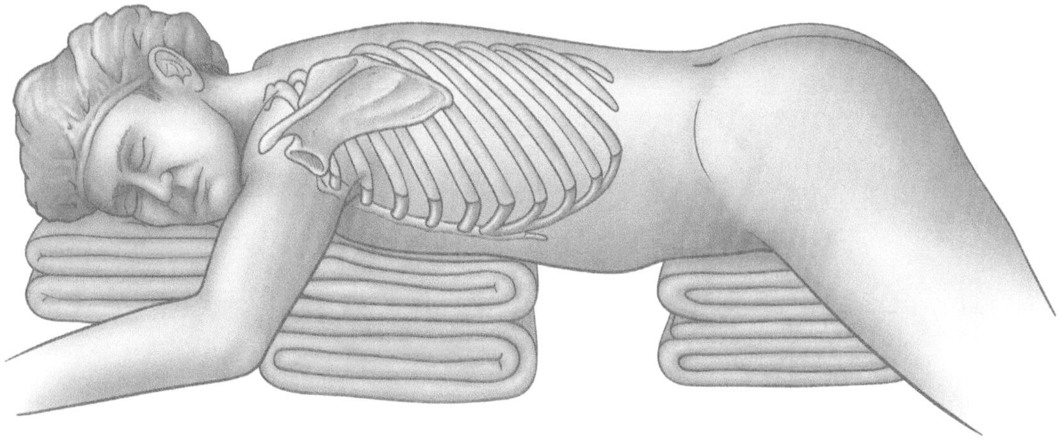

Fig. 3. Patient position for posterior approach.

However, the approach proposed by Grillo and colleagues[21] includes thoracotomy under an incision shaped like a hockey-stick.[4] In this sense, it may be appropriate for ihis method to be categorized into posterolateral approach.

Approaches to Dumbbell or hourglass tumor

Dumbbell tumors or hourglass tumors were first described by Heuer in 1929.[22] Love and Dodge[23] also used the name hourglass tumor. Naming of this tumor comes from its shape: two parts of paravertebral lesion and intraspinal lesion are connected with a narrow vertebral foraminal segment. Owing to its nature of intraspinal extension, about 60% of patients with a dumbbell tumor have neurologic symptoms related to spinal cord compression, in contrast to the 40% of patients with tumors with underestimated extension before surgery because of no symptoms.[10,21] For this reason, despite results of preoperative radiographic images, MRI should be performed when planning surgery of a paravertebral PMT or dumbbell tumor.

Furthermore, a dumbbell tumor locating at lower thorax requires extra attention in terms of its blood supply to the spinal cord. Thurer and Herskowitz[6] delineate the details of blood supply to the spinal cord and the needed attention for surgical intervention of the spine and the spinal cord (**Fig. 4**). They recommend that segmental arteries should be ligated over the vertebral body close to the aorta to preserve the collateral branches from intercostal arteries to the spinal cord to minimize the risk of ischemia. On treating the lesion locates below T6—especially between T7 and L2—surgeons must consider the location of Adamkiewicz artery because loss of this artery is likely to result in a spinal cord injury.[4,21,24] This artery is thought to be the largest feeder to anterior and posterior spinal artery at lumbar area. It arises on the left side in 70% of the patients,[24] between T7 and L4, mostly at the level of T8 to T10 intercostal arteries. It has been suggested that spinal angiography should be planned before the operation to identify Adamkiewicz artery if the PMT involves the area below T6, especially between T7 and L2.[6] Spinal angiography is not without risk and its indication for this small group of tumors is controversial. In his 480 patient's series, Kieffer and colleagues[25] reported that spinal angiography could detect 87.3% of Adamkiewicz arteries with low risk (1.6%) of major complications and mortality. There is an alternative to angiography suggested, which is use of somatosensory-evoked potentials.[26] By referring to this sensory monitoring, the surgeon can decide with confidence about dividing the large segmental vessels.

Two major approaches have been advocated for access to dumbbell tumor. One is the method described by Akwari and colleagues,[27] which is the combination of posterior and posterolateral approaches. The other is the posterior approach described by Grillo and colleagues[21] and others.[4,19,28]

In the Akwari method, first the intraspinal extension of the tumor is treated by posterior laminectomy followed by removal of the tumor via a posterolateral thoracotomy (**Fig. 5**). In Grillo's method, the patient is placed in the lateral decubitus position, rotating ventrally for simultaneous access to the thorax and spine. The incision begins with vertical midvertebral skin incision centering on the tumor location and extending horizontally to the tip of scapula with a hockey-stick shape. A flap of skin and subcutaneous tissue is prepared and raised over muscle layer and the thoracotomy is performed under this flap. They enter thorax first to control the thoracic portion and mobilize

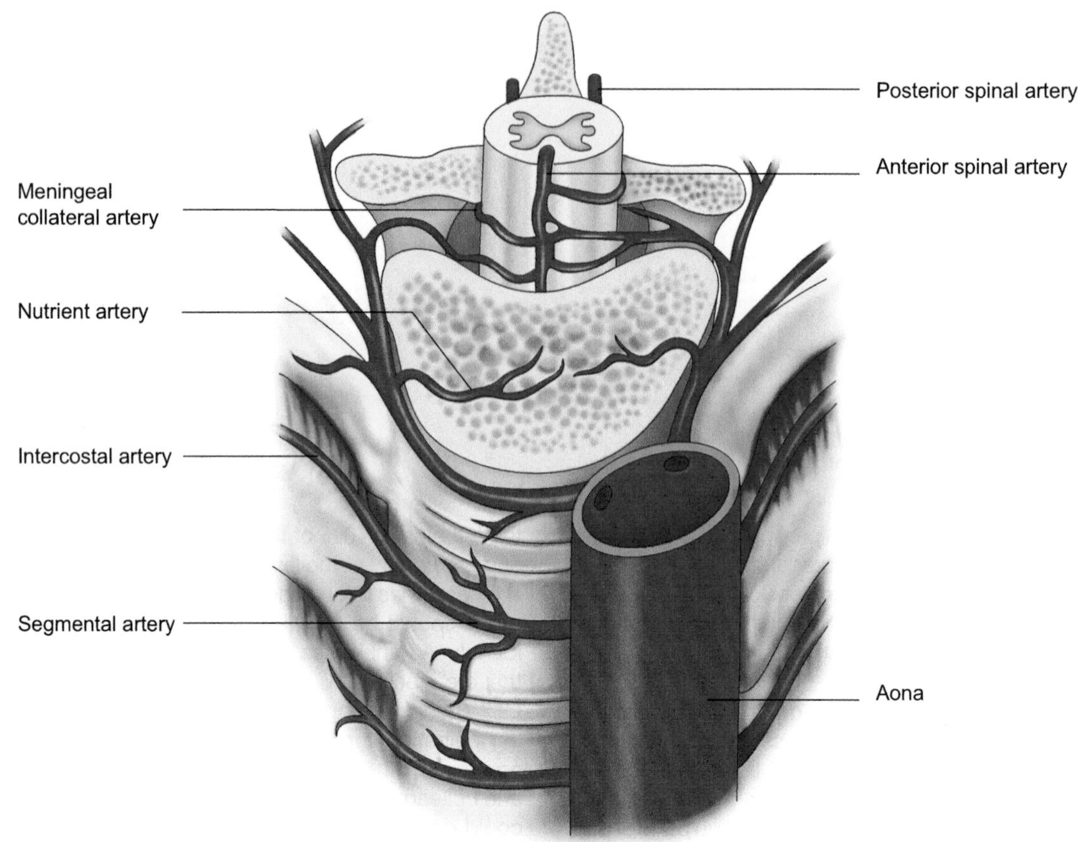

Fig. 4. Anatomy of the segmental arteries in relation to aorta and intercostal arteries. (*From* Anderson TM, Mansour KA, Miller JI. Jr. Thoracic approaches to anterior spinal operations: anterior thoracic approaches. Ann Thorac Surg 1993;55(6):1447–51; with permission.)

and left the tumor only attached by its intraforaminal extension to be resected later. Shadmehr and colleagues[4] reported on cases in which only foraminotomy with a high-speed drill was required to do en bloc resection of the tumor through thoracotomy incision.

McCormick[19] also describes the posterior approach to the spinal or paraspinal tumor, including dumbbell tumor. In this approach, the incision is made in the shape of hockey stick but not with the sharp angle of incision of Grillo's approach. After deepening the incision to the paraspinal muscle region, this muscle is dissected and retracted for the exposure of the spine, faucet joint, and ribs. The entire procedure for the resection of tumor and bony structures is performed in the extrapleural space.

The approaches to a dumbbell tumor are dependent on surgeon's preference. According to literature, however, one posterior approach incision is appropriate only for a "small" tumor. If a large tumor or multiple vertebral foramens are involved, an approach like the Akwari method is recommended.[3,5]

Whichever approach is chosen, the principles of surgery for the management of PMT—especially tumor with intraspinal extension—are resection in the tumor-free margin avoiding excess traction of the involving nerve and meticulous hemostasis. Hemostasis is particularly important because this not only contributes to better visualization during surgery, but also avoidance of postoperative spinal neurologic injury. For this purpose, however, absorbable gelatin sponges should not be packed and left in the neural foramen because they may swell, migrate, or collect the fluid, resulting later in spinal cord compression.[4]

There are other controversies such as whether thoracic portion or intraspinal portion should be managed first and whether the surgery should be done in one or two stages. Although there are still arguments on these issues, the authors believe

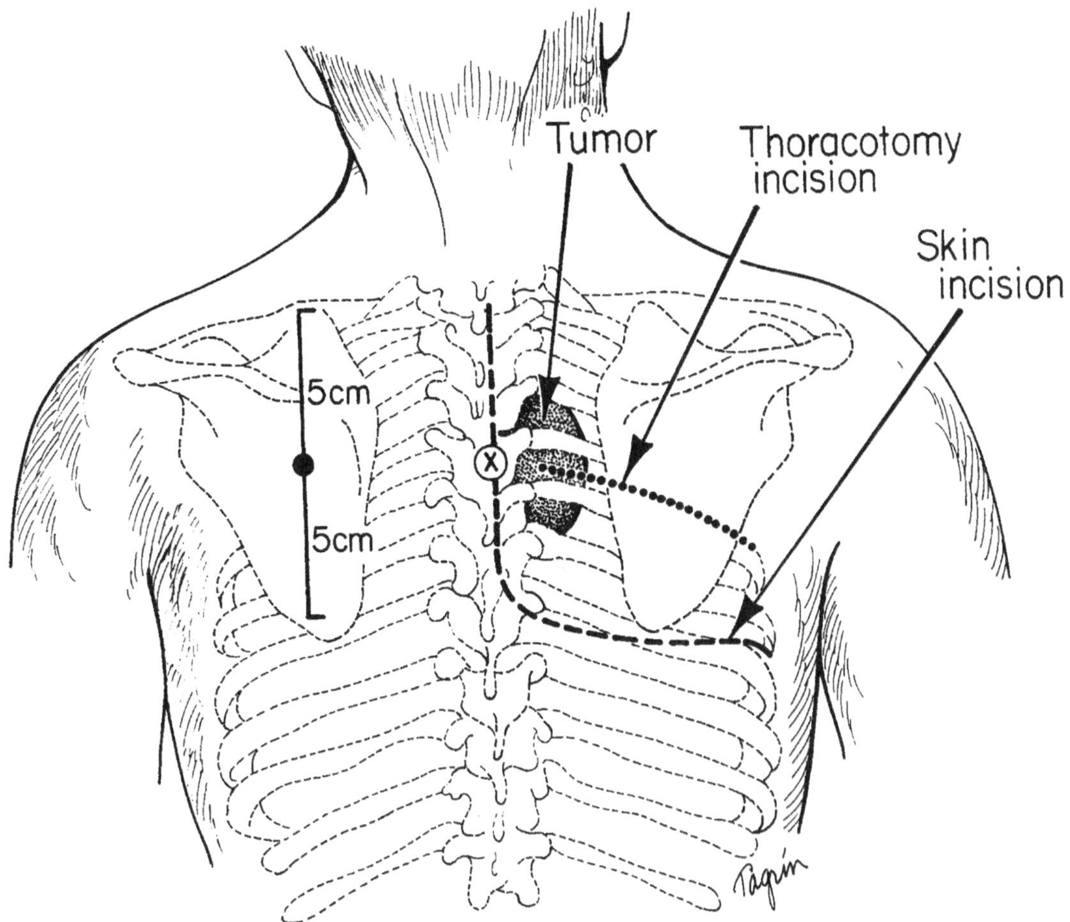

Fig. 5. Skin incision by Grillo and colleagues. (*From* Grillo HC, Ojemann RG, Scannell JG, et al. Combined approach to "dumbbell" intrathoracic and intraspinal neurogenic tumors. Ann Thorac Surg 1983;36:402–7; with permission.)

that one stage operation is preferable because this can reduce the risk of postoperative spinal cord injury due to bleeding and spinal edema from a two-stage operation.[4,5,21]

Anterior and Other Combined Approaches

Approaches to apical PMT and superior sulcus tumor

The approaches to the apical PMT and PMT involving superior sulcus show interesting variations. For a benign lesion or tumor that is not large, thoracoscopic[2] or limited resection through axillary thoracotomy or limited lateral thoracotomy are reported.[6] Akashi and colleagues[29] used thoracoscopic surgery combined with a supraclavicular approach to treat this type of PMT. The approach of using cervical incision alone[30] has been reported also. In these techniques, care must be taken to avoid injury to the recurrent laryngeal nerve.

Anterior transclavicular approach to a PMT invading the superior sulcus with suspicious involvement of vascular structures or brachial plexus is useful and the preferred choice of the authors. Several approaches to superior sulcus tumor, including PMT, have been extensively reported and discussed.[31–34] The authors' anterior approach is a modified version of Dartevelle's approach.[34,35]

An L-shaped incision of cervicotomy is made that includes an oblique incision along the anterior border of the sternocleidomastoid muscle extending horizontally below the clavicle or in the bed of the second intercostal space up to the deltopectoral groove. The myocutaneous flap of sternocleidomastoid muscle and upper part of the pectoralis muscle can be folded back to expose all the neck and thoracic inlet and upper part of the anterolateral chest wall. After confirming respectability of the tumor, the internal half of the clavicle is removed. The involved or related vascular structures, including the jugular vein and subclavian vein, are ligated and divided. The scalenus anterior muscle is divided on its insertion on the first rib. The subclavian artery is dissected and divided if the tumor invades it. This artery should be revascularized at the end of the procedure either with an end-to-end direct anastomosis or with a graft such as a polytetrafluoroethylene or a cryopreserved allograft.[36] The pleural space is usually opened by dividing the Sibson fascia. The middle scalenus muscle is divided above the insertion of the first rib or higher, according to tumor extension. The nerve root of C8 and T1 can be identified and dissected from outside inward, up to the confluence of the lower trunk of the brachial plexus. Then, the ipsilateral prevertebral or paravertebral area can be visualized and managed under direct exposure. Chest wall resection including the first and second ribs will follow the procedure if the PMT invades the chest wall.

An important point about this approach is the removal of the medial half of the clavicle. This allows the surgeon good control and deep dissection of underlying structures such as subclavian vein, anterior scalenus muscle, phrenic nerve, and subclavian artery. This can make it possible to resect PMT located at thoracic inlet with the whole tumor-bearing compartment.[35]

If this type PMT invades the spine, the tumor can be treated through the one-stage, combined anterior and posterior approach with the cooperation of neurosurgeons or orthopedic surgeons. After completion of removal of the tumor with all tumor-bearing structures through the transclavicular approach, the patient is placed in the prone position. The incision is made to access to the spinal or vertebral portion of tumor.[37] Macchiarini and colleagues[35] reported the case of a neurogenic PMT which was successfully treated by this approach (**Fig. 6**). Mazel and colleagues[38] also used this type of combination approach for resection of PMT involving superior sulcus and the spine. The extent of the spine resection, laminectomy alone, hemi-, or total vertebrectomy, varies with tumor infiltration.[38,39] An anterior spinal artery penetrating into the spinal canal through one of the invaded intervertebral foramina is a contraindication of this surgery.[35,37]

Because of its inherent scale of the surgery, indications of these techniques should be examined with attention. Thoracic surgeons must be familiar with the precise anatomy of thoracic inlet and be aware of the accompanying risk, including complications of surgery.[6,34,38] Although PMTs affecting

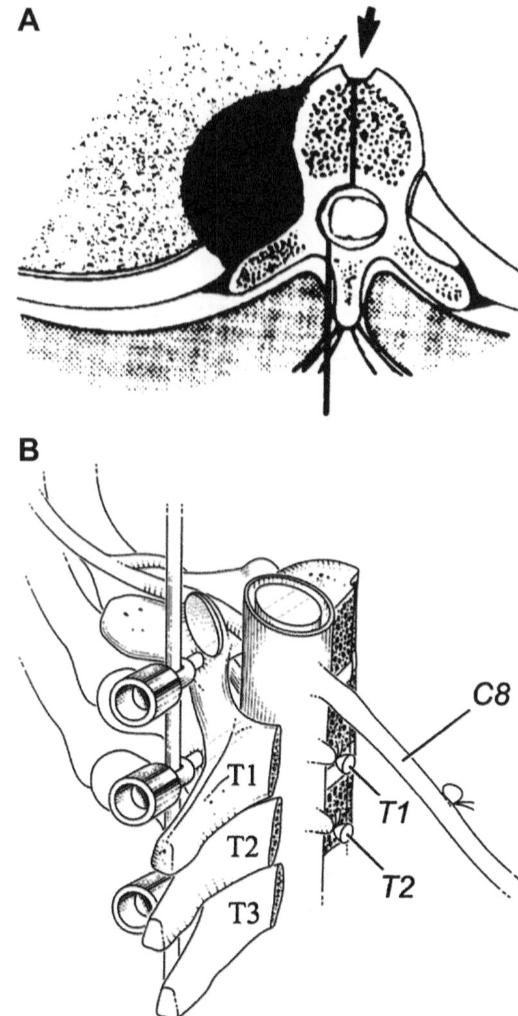

Fig. 6. (*A*) Transactional view of the pathway of resection of vertebral body for PMT involving superior sulcus. (*From* Dartevelle PG. Extended operations for the treatment of lung cancer. Ann Thorac Surg 1997;63:12–19; with permission). (*B*) Longitudinal view of the resection of vertebral body. (*From* Fadel E, Missenard G, Chapelier A, et al. En bloc resection of non-small cell lung cancer invading the thoracic inlet and intervertebral foramina. J Thorac Cardiovasc Surg 2002;123(4):676–85; with permission.)

the superior sulcus is rare, an anterior transclavicular approach offers the best approach for complete surgical resection of tumor.[6,35,38]

The surgical approaches described here are dependent on the patient's clinical status, the size, and the location of the tumor. Each technique has its pros and cons. They are summarized in the **Table 1**.

Table 1
Open approaches to PMT dependent on tumor locations

	Location of Tumor	Pro	Con
Anterior approach (transclavicular)	Apical or superior compartment	Good control of vascular structures and nerves	Learning curve Limited access to vertebra
Anterior (or posterolateral) and posterior	PMT with spinal extension including SST	General access to all PMT Good exposure	Change of patient position Learning curve Scale of incision
Posterolateral	PMT at mid-lower thorax	Single posture change Familiarity to thoracic surgeon	Limited access to apical and superior compartment Difficulty of vessel control in the superior compartment
Posterior	PMT with spinal extension or paravertebral tumor	Scale of incision	Limited access to thorax organ Tumor size

Abbreviation: SST, superior sulcus tumor.

POSTOPERATIVE MANAGEMENT AND COMPLICATIONS

The spectrum of complication is dependent on the type of surgery. The larger the scale of operation, the more complications may occur. Respiratory complications such as pneumonia and atelectasis are the most frequently encountered complication.[3,38] Appropriate and aggressive pain relief is mandatory for prevention of pulmonary complications, moreover preoperative cessation of smoking and nose and throat decontamination are important. Other complications such as Horner syndrome, esophageal fistula, hematoma, wound infection, and chylothorax are reported—although some of them are not frequently encountered.[3,5] Special attention is needed for PMTs involving superior sulcus and dumbbell tumors because of its inherent nature and the scale of surgery.[33,34,37,38] Collaboration with neurosurgeon or orthopedic surgeons is mandatory for the case with spinal resection, to prevent and detect neurologic injury because early mobilization of patients may cause instrumentation dismantling.[3–6,38]

SUMMARY

An open surgical approach to a PMT should be decided on based on the tumor location and pathology. In planning the surgical strategies, radiographic images are essential. Chest radiograph is a useful and simple examination to detect and diagnose the tumor according to the mediastinal distinctions.

Steps to be taken for surgery are;

1. CT images in high resolution should be taken to diagnose and assess the tumor extension to surrounding tissues. MRI is effective for evaluations of vessel and spinal extension and involvement.
2. Differential diagnosis should be done, including histologic examination with transcutaneous needle-aspiration biopsy, especially if malignant tumor is suspicious.
3. A surgical approach is decided on according to the tumor location, size, and type of resection. A combined surgical team with a neurosurgeon should be organized to treat the tumor involving the spine and the spinal cord.

Although classifications of PMTs are diversified, strategies, especially from the surgical point of view, are not complex but challenging. Surgery for treatment is apparent and this requires thoracic surgeons to be familiar with different available surgical approaches. This effort makes it possible to choose the best approach and contributes to better prognosis and patient quality of life.

REFERENCES

1. Bonder J, Wykypiel H, Greiner A, et al. Early experience with robot-assisted surgery for mediastinal masses. Ann Thorac Surg 2004;78:259–66.

2. Pons F, Lang-Lazdunski L, Bonnet PM, et al. Videothoracoscopic resection of neurogenic tumors of the superior sulcus using the harmonic scalpel. Ann Thorac Surg 2003;75:602–4.
3. Rahman A, Sedera M, Mourad IA, et al. Posterior mediastinal tumors: outcome of surgery. J Egypt Natl Canc Inst 2005;17(1):1–8.
4. Shadmehr MB, Gaissert HA, Wain JC, et al. The surgical approach to dumbbell tumors of the mediastinum. Ann Thorac Surg 2003;76:1650–4.
5. Yueksell M, Pamir N, Oeser F, et al. The principles of surgical management in dumbbell tumors. Eur J Cardiothorac Surg 1996;10:569–73.
6. Thurer RJ, Herskowitz K. Open approaches to posterior mediastinal tumors and the spine. Chest Surg Clin N Am 1996;6(1):117–38.
7. Shields TW. The mediastinum, its compartments and the mediastinal lymph nodes. In: Shields TW, Locicero J III, editors. General thoracic surgery. 6th edition. Philadelphia: Lippincott Williams and Wilkins; 2005. p. 2343–6.
8. Kennebeck SS. Tumors of the mediastinum. Clin Pediatr Emerg Med 2005;6:156–64.
9. Duwe BV, Sterman DH, Musani AI. Tumors of the mediastinum. Chest 2005;128:2893–909.
10. Hoyos A, Sundaresan RS. Videoscopic removal of mediastinal tumors. Operat Tech Thorac Cardiovasc Surg 2001;6(4):237–49.
11. Reynolds M, Shields TW. Neurogenic tumors of the mediastinum in children and in adults. In: Shields TW, Locicero J III, editors. General thoracic surgery. 6th edition. Philadelphia: Lippincott Williams and Wilkins; 2005. p. 2729–56.
12. Davis RD Jr, Newland Oldham H Jr, Sabiston DC Jr. Primary cysts and neoplasms of the mediastinum: recent changes in clinical presentation, methods of diagnosis, management and results. Ann Thorac Surg 1987;44:229–37.
13. Whooley BP, Urschel JD, Antkowiak JG, et al. Primary tumors of the mediastinum. J Surg Oncol 1999;70:95–9.
14. Bressler EL, Kirkham JA. Mediastinal masses; alternative appraoches to CT-guided biopsy. Radiology 1994;191:391–7.
15. Macchiarini P, Ostertag H. Uncommon primary mediastinal tumors. Lancet Oncol 2004;5(2): 107–18.
16. Prabhakar G, Murray GF. Benign tumors, cysts, and duplications of the esophagus. In: Shields TW, Locicero J III, editors. General thoracic surgery. 6th edition. Philadelphia: Lippincott Williams and Wilkins; 2005. p. 2251–61.
17. Miura J, Doita M, Miyata K, et al. Horner's syndrome caused by a thoracic dumbbell-shaped schwannoma: sympathetic chain reconstruction after a one-stage removal of the tumor. Spine 2003;28:33–6.
18. Shields TW. Posterior mediastinotomy. In: Shields TW, Locicero J III, editors. General thoracic surgery. 6th edition. Philadelphia: Lippincott Williams and Wilkins; 2005. p. 2453–4.
19. McCormick PC. Surgical management of dumbbell and paraspinal tumors of the thoracic and lumbar spine. Neurosurgery 1996;38:67–74.
20. Payer M, Radovanovic I, Jost G. Resection of thoracic dumbbell neurinomas: single postero-lateral approach or combined posterior and transthoracic approach? J Clin Neurosci 2006;13(6):690–3.
21. Grillo HC, Ojemann RG, Scannell JG, et al. Combined approach to "dumbbell" intrathoracic and intraspinal neurogenic tumors. Ann Thorac Surg 1983;36:402–7.
22. Heuer GJ. The so-called "hour-glass" tumors of the spine. Arch Surg 1929;18:935–81.
23. Love JG, Dodge HW Jr. Dumbbell (hourglass) neurofibromas affecting the spinal cord. Surg Gynecol Obstet 1952;94:161–72.
24. Koshino T, Murakami G, Morishita K, et al. Does the Adamkiewicz artery originate from the larger segmental arteries? J Thorac Cardiovasc Surg 1999;117:898–905.
25. Kieffer E, Fukui S, Chiras J, et al. Spinal cord arteriography: a safe adjunct before descending thoracic or thoracoabdominal aortic aneurysmectomy. J Vasc Surg 2002;35:262–8.
26. Naunheim KS, Barnett MG, Candell DG, et al. Anterior exposure of the thoracic spine. Ann Thorac Surg 1994;57:1436–9.
27. Akwari OE, Payne WS, Onofrio BM, et al. Dumbbell neurogenic tumors of the mediastinum. Mayo Clin Proc 1978;53:353–8.
28. Osada H, Aoki H, Yokote K, et al. Dumbbell neurogenic tumor of the mediastinum: a report of three cases undergoing single-staged complete removal without thoracotomy. Jpn J Surg 1991;21: 224–8.
29. Akashi A, Ohashi S, Yoden Y, et al. Thoracoscopic surgery combined with a supraclavicular approach for removing superior mediastinal tumor. Surg Endosc 1997;11:74–6.
30. Kido T, Nishi H, Nakao K. Transcervical paratracheal resection of a posterior mediastinal mass. J Thorac Cardiovasc Surg 1999;117(5):1036–7.
31. Paulson DL. Carcinomas in the superior pulmonary sulcus. J Thorac Cardiovasc Surg 1975;70: 1095–104.
32. Rusch VW. Management of Pancoast tumors. Lancet Oncol 2006;7:997–1005.
33. Macchiarini P. Resection of superior sulcus carcinomas (anterior approach). Thorac Surg Clin 2004; 14:229–40.
34. Dartevelle PG, Chapelier AR, Macchiarini P, et al. Anterior transcervical-thoracic approach for radical

resection of lung tumors invading the thoracic inlet. J Thorac Cardiovasc Surg 1993;105:1025–34.
35. Macchiarini P, Dartevelle P, Chapelier A, et al. Technique for resecting primary and metastatic nonbronchogenic tumors of the thoracic outlet. Ann Thorac Surg 1993;55:611–8.
36. Gómez-Caro A, Martinez E, Rodríguez A, et al. Cryopreserved arterial allograft reconstruction after excision of thoracic malignancies. Ann Thorac Surg 2008;86(6):1753–61.
37. Dartevelle PG. Extended operations for the treatment of lung cancer. Ann Thorac Surg 1997;63:12–9.
38. Mazel CH, Grunenwald D, Laudrin P, et al. Radical excision in the management of thoracic and cervicothoracic tumors involving the spine: results in a series of 36 cases. Spine 2003;28:782–92.
39. Bilsky MH, Vitaz TW, Boland PJ, et al. Surgical treatment of superior sulcus tumors with spinal and brachial plexus involvement. J Neurosurg 2002; 97(Suppl 3):301–9.

Technical Advances in Mediastinal Surgery: Videothoracoscopic Approach to Posterior Mediastinal Tumors

Calvin S.H. Ng, MD, FRCS (Edin) (CTh)[a],
Anthony P.C. Yim, MA, DM, FRCS[a,b,*]

KEYWORDS

- Videothoracoscopy • Mediastinal tumor
- Surgical procedure

The use of video-assisted thoracoscopic surgery (VATS) in the diagnosis and treatment of mediastinal conditions is now well established and continues to evolve. Its role extends from assessment of disease processes and diagnosis to definitive therapy. The extended application of VATS has been facilitated through advances in instrumentation and increasing experience. Over the years, VATS has become a promising therapeutic alternative to the open approach, and may be considered the standard of care in select conditions of the posterior mediastinum.

POSTERIOR MEDIASTINAL TUMORS

The mediastinum is compartmentalized into anterior, middle, and posterior divisions with important implications for diagnosing masses. Posterior mediastinum contains the descending thoracic aorta, esophagus, azygous vein, autonomic ganglia and nerves, thoracic lymph nodes, and fat. In general, the location of the mass in the mediastinum, age of the patient, and presence of symptoms are important factors in determining the likelihood of malignancy.[1,2] Out of the three compartments, posterior mediastinal tumors has the lowest percentage (16%) of tumors that are malignant.[1] However, the percentage of malignant posterior mediastinal tumors in children is much higher at 50%.[3] The differential diagnosis of posterior mediastinal mass include, neurogenic tumor, bronchogenic cyst, enteric cyst,[4] xanthogranuloma, diaphragmatic hernia, meningocele, and paravertebral abscess. Posterior neurogenic tumors can broadly be divided into those of nerve sheath origin (schwannoma, neurofibroma, granular cell, and malignant schwannoma), autonomic ganglia (ganglioneuroma, ganglioneuroblastoma, neuroblastoma), and paraganglionic systems (chemodectoma, pheochromocytoma, neuroectodermal tumors). Other unsuspecting lesions from extramedullary hematopoiesis, esophageal tumors, teratoma, lymphoma, angioleiomyoma, lipoma, lymphangioma, parathyroid adenoma, various sarcomas, and arteriovenous malformations have been reported.[5] In the pediatric population, neurogenic tumors are the most common, accounting for 34% to 58%.[2] Most paraspinal neurogenic tumors are incidental findings; however, chest symptoms such as cough, chest pain, dyspnea, dysphagia, as well as neurological symptoms associated with radiculopathy, myelopathy, and Horner syndrome can be present.[2,3] Very rarely, patients may have paroxysmal hypertension associated

[a] Division of Cardiothoracic Surgery, Department of Surgery, The Chinese University of Hong Kong, Prince of Wales Hospital, Shatin, N.T. Hong Kong SAR, China
[b] Minimally Invasive Centre, Union Hospital, Shatin, N.T. Hong Kong SAR, China
* Corresponding author. Minimally Invasive Centre, Union Hospital, Shatin, N.T. Hong Kong SAR, China.
E-mail address: yimap@cuhk.edu.hk

Thorac Surg Clin 20 (2010) 297–309
doi:10.1016/j.thorsurg.2010.02.003
1547-4127/10/$ – see front matter

thoracic.theclinics.com

with noradrenalin-producing pheochromocytoma,[6] or severe diarrhea caused by vasoactive intestinal peptide producing neuroblastoma.

Approach to Posterior Mediastinal Tumors

The video-thoracoscopic approach for resection of posterior mediastinal tumor was first reported by Landreneau and colleagues[7] from Pennsylvania in 1992. Subsequently, a number of series have been reported in both the adult and pediatric populations on the feasibility and safety of this approach.[8,9] The classic three-port approach has evolved with time into hybrid procedures combining utility thoracotomy with or without segmental rib resection,[10] posterior open laminectomy for tumors with intraspinal extension,[11,12] and supraclavicular approach in cases of cervicomediastinal tumors.[13] Furthermore, lower posterior mediastinal masses have been successfully approached by the transperitoneal laparoscopic transdiaphragmatic route by splitting the crural fibers.[14] More recently, the use of endoscopic robotic-assisted and total robotic approach for the management of mediastinal tumors has been performed.[15]

Owing to the absence of randomized controlled trials concerning videothoracoscopic approach to the treatment of posterior mediastinal mass, there is no consensus concerning the optimum surgical approach. Nevertheless, minimally invasive techniques have become increasingly popular because of their low procedural morbidity and mortality, improved cosmesis, lesser degree of access trauma[16] and postoperative pain,[17] and equivalent efficacy compared to conventional open techniques.

Diagnostic and Therapeutic Roles

The role of videothoracoscopy as a diagnostic tool is well established. The thoracoscope and camera allows magnified views of the mediastinal pathology, assessment of its distribution, and disease extent. In many cases, a percutaneous biopsy approach in obtaining tissue diagnosis can be technically difficult because of the specific location of the mass in the posterior mediastinum and its close association to major vascular structures. Furthermore, fine-needle aspiration often provides insufficient material for confirmatory cytological examination, particularly because of the relative acellularity of these tumors, and the result may even be misleading. Also, there is a significant risk of severe bleeding if the lesion is highly vascular. Videothoracoscopic surgery utilizing the same camera port site allows Tru-cut and incisional biopsy of the lesion under direct vision of the thoracoscope (**Fig. 1**).[5,18] An added advantage is that any hemorrhage that results from the biopsy can be better controlled compared with percutaneous approach. Furthermore, following intraoperative frozen section, the lesion can be resected in the same operation with minimal trauma.[5] Apart from excision of posterior mediastinal mass and tumors, the therapeutic role of VATS extends to the drainage of mediastinal abscess or infected cysts, as well as management of descending necrotizing mediastinitis.[4,19]

Patient and Preparation

Preoperative CT and MRI scans should be available for every patient to localize and define the nature of the tumor (**Fig. 2**). Erosion of the body or pedicle of the vertebrae or a widened intervertebral foramen suggests intraspinal involvement. Approximately 10% of posterior mediastinal neurogenic tumors include a spinal canal component and identification of these dumbbell (or hourglass) tumors preoperatively is important so that appropriate arrangements can be made to allow resection in a single-stage combined operation.[11] MRI can more accurately image any tumor extension into the spinal canal, the tissue plane, and relationship of the tumor to adjacent structures. Occasionally, MRI can help differentiate between neurogenic and rare (angiolipoma) dumbbell tumors.[20] Spinal arteriography may be considered

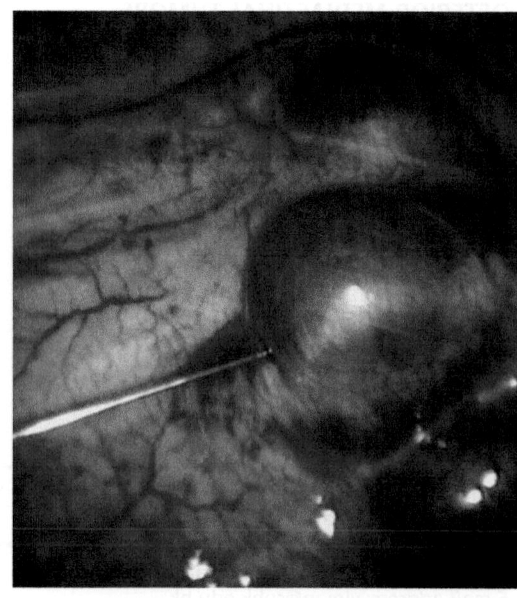

Fig. 1. Intraoperative photo of a VATS biopsy of intrathoracic paravertebral extramedullary hematopoiesis.

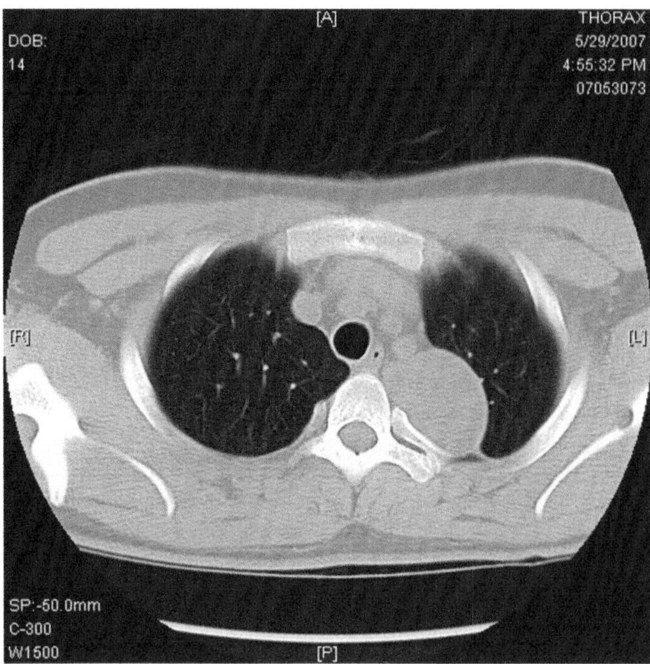

Fig. 2. CT scan of a large posterior mediastinal ganglioneuroma.

when the tumor is near the lower thoracic regions of T7-L1 to identify the artery of Adamkiewicz. The role of positron emission tomography in assessing posterior mediastinal tumors is unclear and can be misleading.[21]

Anesthesia

Selective one-lung ventilation is required to facilitate the operation. General anesthesia with a double-lumen endobronchial tube is used. Patients are induced with 2 mg/kg of propofol and 2 μg/kg of fentanyl, and intubated. Pretreatment of the tracheobronchial tree with local anesthetics can also facilitate intubation. Proper positioning of the endobronchial tube is confirmed with the use of the fiberoptic bronchoscope after intubation and reconfirmed after patient positioning. However, it is generally held that a body weight of at least 30 to 35 kg is necessary for the patient's airway to accommodate the smallest double-lumen device (28 French). This size limitation essentially precludes the use of these devices for patients younger than approximately 8 years of age. Other techniques to achieve one-lung ventilation such as placement of a bronchial blocker or intentional intubation of a main stem bronchus with an endotracheal tube (ETT) should be used. A technique that may improve the reliability of endobronchial blockers during one-lung anesthesia using a single-lumen ETT involves threading the stem of the blocker through the Murphy eye of the ETT and deliberately passing the tip of the ETT all the way to the carina. The tip of the ETT will then prevent any retrograde movement of the endobronchial blocker.[22]

Hypoxemia during one-lung ventilation is usually caused by shunting of blood. In case of hypoxemia, the position of the double-lumen endobronchial tube and hemodynamic stability should be confirmed. Low level of continuous positive airway pressure applied to the collapsed right lung may improve saturation. Applying positive end-expiratory pressure to the ventilated lung can also raise oxygen saturation during one-lung ventilation. Anesthesia is maintained with isoflurane 1% to 2%, 60% nitrous oxide in oxygen, and a single bolus of 0.1 mg/kg of morphine when motor evoked potentials monitoring is no longer required. Ventilation is controlled to achieve normocarbia.

The ECG, noninvasive blood pressure, pulse oximetry, end-tidal carbon dioxide, airway pressure, ventilatory volume, and inspired oxygen are routinely monitored and continuously displayed. Arterial line and central venous catheter for invasive pressure monitoring may be required for coexisting medical conditions. For neurogenic tumors, somatosensory evoked potentials and motor evoked potentials monitoring should be considered to avoid root avulsion injury to the spinal cord during tumor resection, even if most of the tumor appears to be confined to the chest cavity.

Positioning

Under general anesthesia with selective one-lung ventilation, the patient is positioned in the full lateral decubitus position for the approach to the posterior mediastinum. Some surgeons prefer the patient in a backward 45-degree lateral decubitus position while performing VATS; however, it would cause posterior displacement of the lung and reduce exposure to the posterior mediastinum. The operating table is flexed to 30° with the fulcrum just inferior to the level of the nipples, to open up the upper intercostals spaces for thoracoscope insertion and instrumentation.[17] Rotating the operating table forward may allow the lung to fall anteriorly and improve exposure to the posterior mediastinum.

Personnel and Equipment

The team of the principal surgeon, an assistant, scrub nurse, and the anesthesiologist, will usually remain in the same positions during the whole procedure. The operating room set-up consists of the anesthetic unit, video-thoracoscopy unit (television monitor, video image printer, video recorder, light source), television monitor, electrocautery, and instrument trolley (**Fig. 3**).

Mostly conventional instruments are utilized such as sponge-holding forceps and oval ring (for retraction), dental pledget mounted on a curved clamp (for dissection), and right-angled clamp (for dissection of vascular branches). The authors advocate the use of the conventional thoracic instruments such as the sponge-holding forceps whenever possible because they are less expensive and are more familiar to the surgeon (**Fig. 4**).[17] However, a few dedicated endoscopic instruments including; endoscissors for incising the mediastinal pleura, endograsper, and endoclip applier for vascular hemostasis (Endoclip, Autosuture, United States Surgical, Tyco Health Care, Norwalk, CT, USA) should be available to aid surgery.

Operative Principles

The chest is the most suitable body cavity for the minimal access approach because, once the lung is collapsed (with selective one-lung ventilation), there is plenty of room for instrument maneuvering. The use of carbon dioxide insufflation and, hence, valved ports, is unnecessary. There is evidence that thoracic carbon dioxide insufflation during VATS has an adverse effect on the patient's hemodynamics compared with selective one-lung ventilation. The creation of pneumoperitoneum is required in the transperitoneal laparoscopic transdiaphragmatic approach.[14]

There are a number of strategies in VATS that can assist in minimizing chest wall trauma, avoid intercostal nerve compression, and minimize postoperative pain. The use of trocar ports should be avoided by introducing instruments directly through the wound. Furthermore, when clinically allowed, a smaller (5 mm) and an angled lens thoracoscope (30° scope) can help reduce access trauma and avoid torquing of the scope. In addition, delivering specimen through the anterior port is facilitated by the wider anterior intercostals spaces.[17]

Port Strategies

Under general anesthesia, selective one-lung ventilation should be confirmed with the anesthesiologist prior to port incision. The position and number of ports used would depend on the type of procedure and pathology, as well as its relative position within the posterior mediastinum. Uniport technique is usually adequate for needle or Tru-cut biopsies with sharing of the port site by the thoracoscope and biopsy instrument. However, in selecting the position of the initial port, the surgeon should plan for the eventual need of the three-port approach for resection of the mass or for difficult hemostasis following the biopsy. These subsequent ports should be inserted under direct thoracoscopic vision. The port sites should be at a suitable distance from the target lesion to provide space for manipulation. Furthermore, the instrument and camera ports should be sufficiently far apart in a "triangulation" manner to prevent instrument "fencing", and be within the same 180° arc to avoid mirror imaging. Our general approach is to place the thoracoscope port incision at the fifth intercostal space along the anterior axillary line for the insertion of 10 mm port and 0° (or 30°) telescope. The second and third 5 mm instrument ports should be inserted by open technique under direct thoracoscopic vision at the third and seventh intercostals space midaxillary line (**Fig. 5**). In young girl patients, as far as possible, the instrument ports should be strategically placed over the submammary fold for cosmetic consideration. The positions of the thoracoscope and instrument ports may be exchanged during the procedure to allow better reach and different directions of approach to the tumor, particularly when conventional instruments are used.[3,11,23]

Exploration

The entire hemithorax is carefully examined using the videoscope with particular attention to the

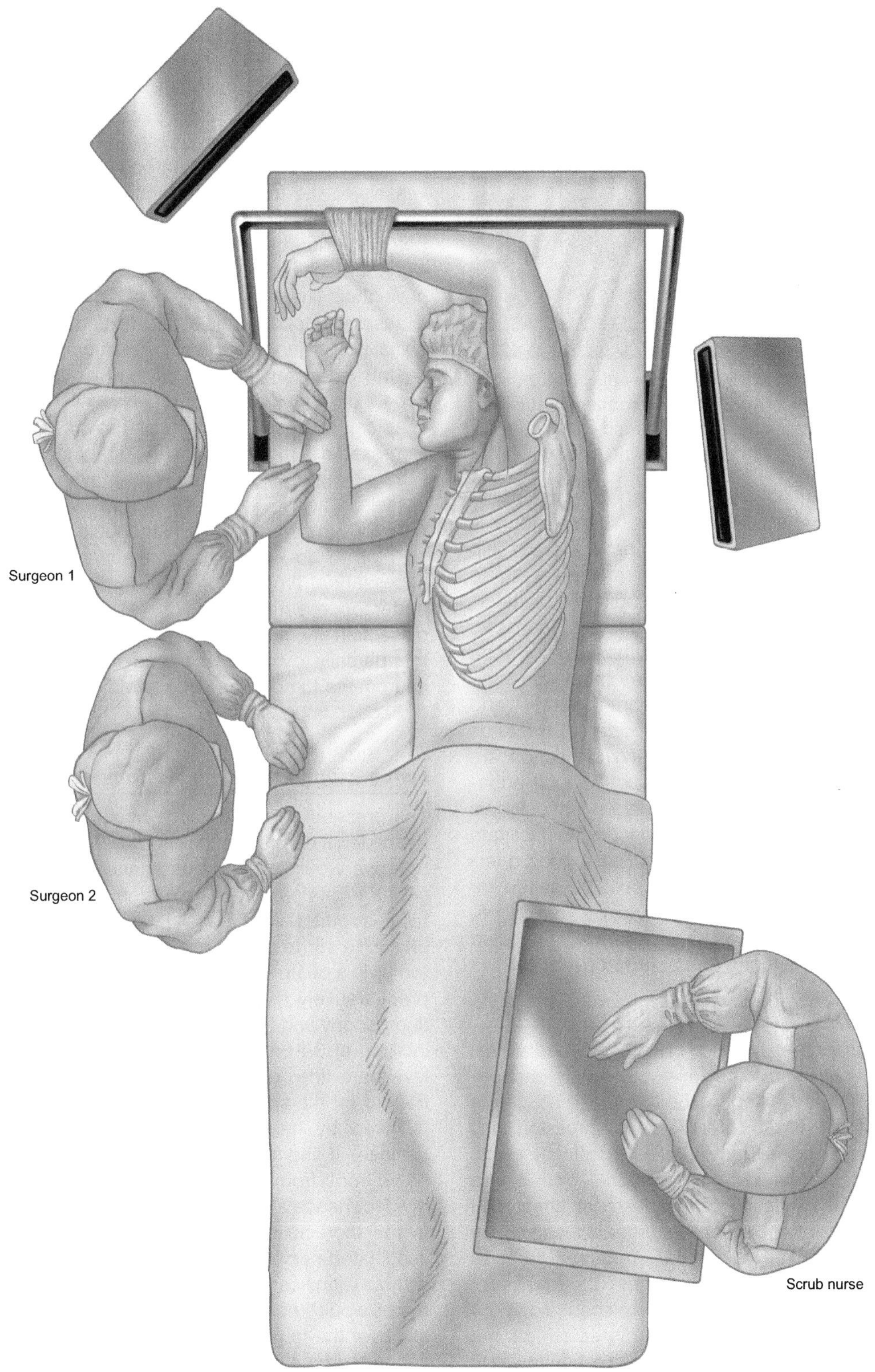

Fig. 3. Operating room setup VATS for posterior mediastinal lesions.

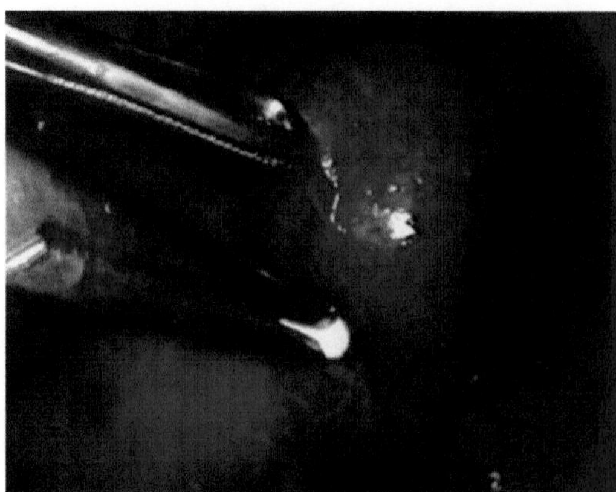

Fig. 4. Dissection of posterior mediastinal hemangioma using conventional instruments such as sponge-holding forceps and mounted pledget.

tumor and its relationship to the posterior mediastinum structures. Blunt instruments such as sponge-holding forceps may be used to help collapse the lung, and for manipulation to complete the exploration. Depending on the laterality, the following major structural landmarks should be identified, including the superior vena cava, azygos (and hemiazygos) vein, arch, and descending thoracic aorta, phrenic nerve and sympathetic trunk. Other important structures that may be encountered during dissection are the esophagus and thoracic duct. Pleural adhesions may be present and require adhesiolysis using diathermy or sharp dissection to facilitate complete lung collapse and achieve a good operating field. Pleural effusion should be saved for microbial culture and cytological examination, and any unsuspecting pleural deposits biopsied for frozen section and formal histology.

Dissection and Vascular Control

The surgical excision of posterior mediastinal neurogenic tumors are most commonly encountered. First, the extent of the tumor and its margin is identified (**Fig. 6**). Needle decompression may be considered for tumors with significant cystic component to facilitate dissection. The pleura covering the junction of the posterior chest wall with the lateral aspect of the tumor is then sharply incised, avoiding the deeper structures such as intercostal neurovascular bundle.[23] The tumor can then be lifted up and displaced aided by sponge-holding forceps, and dissected off the underlying chest wall in a medial direction towards the vertebrae with a combination of sharp and diathermy dissection (**Fig. 7**).[23] Some surgeons have found the harmonic scalpel (Ethicon Endosurgery, Cincinnati, OH, USA) to be an efficient alternative to the diathermy with production of less smoke and adjacent thermal dissipation injury, particularly to surrounding nerves. For areas with well-defined tissue plane, it may be useful to apply deliberate and gentle traction on the tumor to allow blunt dissection using a mounted pledget. Branches from the intercostal vessels and feeding vessels to the tumor are identified, clipped, and divided. It is important to obtain vascular control before further manipulation of the tumor. Tumors without extension into the spinal canal can simply have their (intercostal) nerve origin divided, but excessive traction should be avoided to prevent spinal cord injury. For dumbbell tumors, the intercostal nerve can first be divided at the lateral aspect of the tumor.

Apical posterior mediastinal tumors carry an increased risk of vascular injury and postoperative Horner syndrome due to the proximity to the great vessels, aorta, and sympathetic ganglion. Although, in general, the tumor should be excised en bloc in an extracapsular manner, it may be necessary at times to breach the capsule to gain better access and improve visualization during dissection in these difficult areas. Furthermore, the partially cystic and friable nature of some neurogenic tumors may make total extracapsular dissection impossible.

Laminectomy for Dumbbell Tumors

The presence of a dumbbell tumor should have been identified preoperatively by MRI. At our institute, we would elicit the assistance of neurosurgeons in performing the excision. The operating table is rotated from the full lateral position anteriorly up to 45° to facilitate access for hemilaminectomy via a posterior approach. The level is marked preoperatively and confirmed intraoperatively by fluoroscopy and the videoscope. Posterior midline incision of 3 to 4 inches (longer if multiple spinal levels are affected) is made and the muscles retracted off the spine exposing laminae bilaterally, followed by hemilaminectomy of two adjacent laminae. If the tumor is entirely extradural, the nerve root from which the tumor originates is divided, hence allowing mobilization of the tumor. In the thoracic spine between T4 and T11, the associated nerve root can be generally sacrificed without significant deficit. However, an intradural tumor would require the dura to be opened laterally over the tumor and its intraspinal component separated from the spinal cord using microsurgical techniques. The dissection is assisted by an ultrasonic dissector, CUSA (Cavitron Ultrasonic Surgical Aspirator, Tyco Healthcare, Mansfield, MA, USA). The edges of the involved dura are

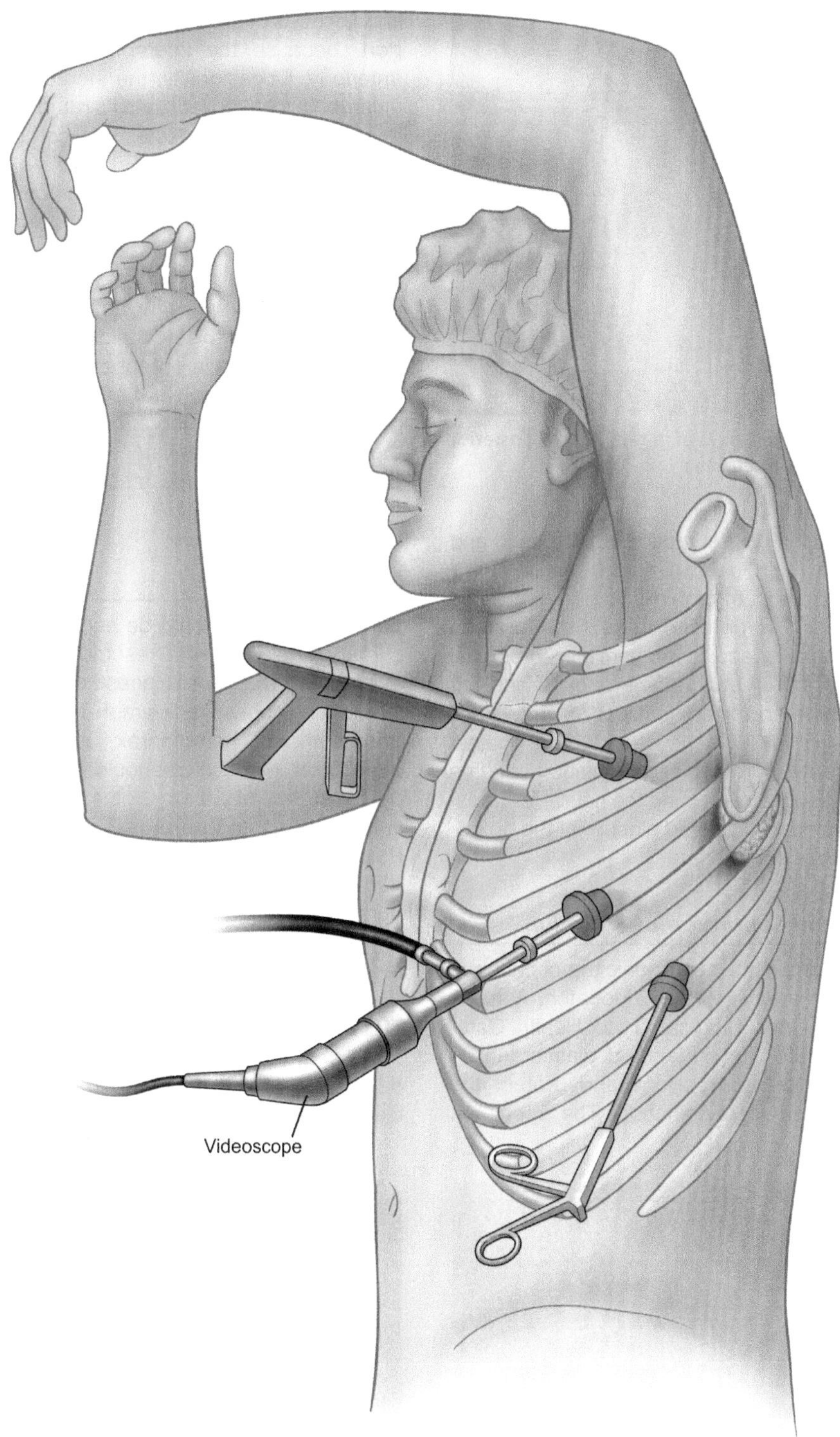

Fig. 5. Positions of the thoracic ports in VATS posterior mediastinal surgery.

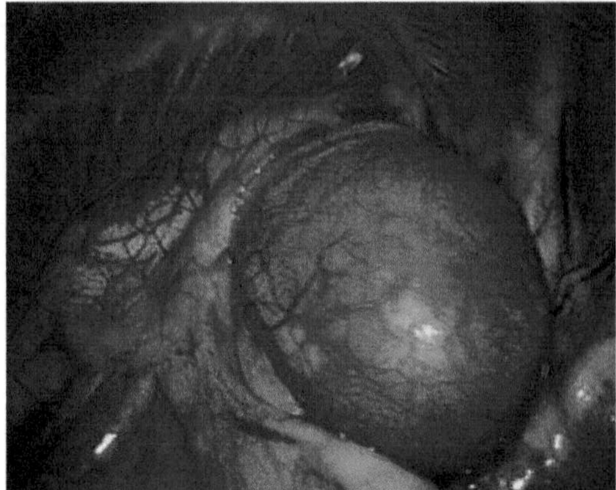

Fig. 6. Thoracoscopic view of a left 7.5 cm posterior mediastinal ganglioneuroma.

resected, and the dura is meticulously closed and covered with fibrin glue to avoid cerebrospinal fluid leak. A piece of thrombin-soaked absorbable gelatin sponge can be used to seal the foramen from the pleural space to prevent cerebrospinal fluid leakage, but should not be packed and left within the foramen for hemostasis as they swell postoperatively and can cause pressure against the spinal cord. Microbipolar coagulation ensures meticulous hemostasis around the neural foramen, which is paramount. Layered closure of the posterior wound is performed later.

Extraction and Conclusion of Procedure

As a free specimen, the neurogenic tumor can then be removed in a plastic bag (Endocatch, Autosuture, United States Surgical, Tyco Health Care, Norwalk, CT, USA, or a sterilized plastic "sandwich" bag) to prevent spillage and protect the incision site from contamination. The specimen should be brought out through the most anterior port, because the intercostals space is wider anteriorly. Occasionally, the incision needs to be enlarged slightly to facilitate its removal. The specimen should be inspected for completeness of resection (**Fig. 8**).

The posterior mediastinal tumor bed is inspected for hemostasis and completeness of resection (**Fig. 9**). Hemostasis of a diffusely oozing large tumor bed may be aided by spraying on fibrin-based glue with or without Surgicel covering. We have found this technique to be useful in reducing chest drain output and duration, as well as preventing late pleural effusion. A 28 French posterior basal tube thoracostomy is placed, and the lung is then reinflated under direct vision. Layered closure of the stab wounds completes the operation.

Postoperative Care

Early extubation should be encouraged following surgery. The patient can resume full diet when fully awake from the general anesthesia. A postoperative, sitting, chest radiograph is taken to detect pneumothorax, hemothorax, and any significant atelectasis. Mucolytics should be prescribed and postoperative chest physiotherapy and incentive spirometry should be provided and encouraged. Pain can usually be adequately controlled by standard oral analgesics. For dumbbell tumors, if the dura was opened intraoperatively, tube thoracostomy suction should be used briefly and the amount of suction minimized postoperatively to prevent perpetuating cerebrospinal fluid leakage. Tube thoracostomy can usually be removed on day 1 or 2 after confirming no air leak or bleeding, depending on the drainage. The patient may be discharged the following day after a chest

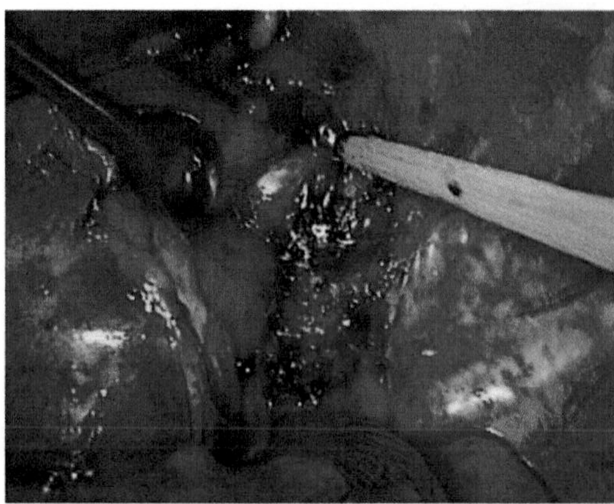

Fig. 7. Traction is applied by sponge-holding forceps and dissection off the chest wall with diathermy.

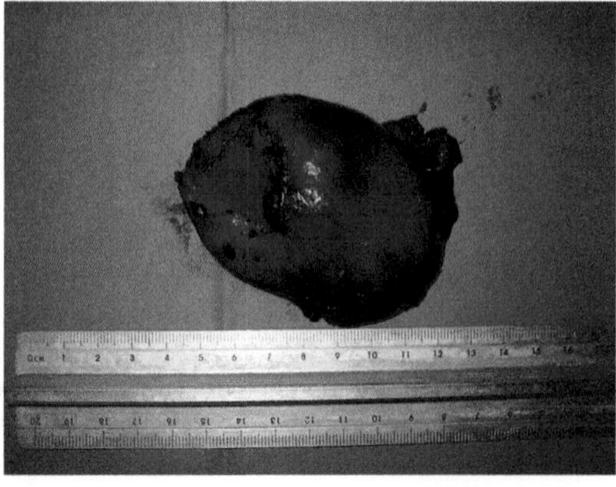

Fig. 8. The specimen is inspected for completeness of resection.

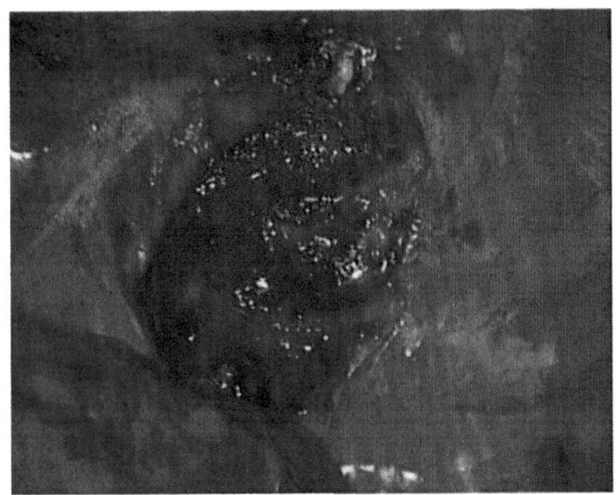

Fig. 9. Tumor bed following resection.

radiograph to confirm no delayed pleural effusion or pneumothorax.

COMMENT

The approach to the management of posterior mediastinal tumors has evolved considerably in the past decade and a half. Although controversies remain as to the best surgical approach, videothoracoscopic surgery has gradually gained acceptance as a safe and reliable minimal access alternative to thoracotomy for the management of posterior mediastinal tumor. Videothoracoscopic surgery has been shown to cause less access trauma, disturbance of native immune function, and pain and shoulder dysfunction.[16,24] Furthermore, numerous studies have shown a shorter hospital stay,[18,25,26] minimal postoperative morbidity, and more rapid recovery following VATS excision of posterior mediastinal tumors compared with open surgery (**Table 1**).[18,23,26–28] A more compelling result implicating greater morbidity with the open resection method was the longer time period before patients were able to return to work or full activity compared with VATS.[26] These benefits of VATS resection may translate into reduced heath care expenditure and socioeconomic burden, although cost savings may be offset by the need for specialized thoracoscopic equipment and operating rooms. Perhaps equally important is the improved patient acceptance for minimal access surgery leading to earlier diagnosis of posterior mediastinal mass and resection of the tumor compared with the conventional approach. It is also noteworthy that only occasionally is conversion from VATS to open approach required (0% to 17%) (see **Table 1**). Furthermore, VATS has additional advantages over the conventional thoracotomy approach because the visualization is much better and there is no crowding of instruments through a single access site. Video assistance provides a wide, magnified operative field, as well as allows the other team members to learn and appreciate the progress of the procedure. More importantly, we are performing the same operation thoracoscopically compared with the open approach, which is reflected in the very low tumor recurrence rates in the reported series up to follow-ups of more than 7 years (see **Table 1**). The cosmetic appearance of the surgical scars is seldom used to argue for a particular surgical approach. However, patients requiring posterior mediastinal tumor resection may be a notable exception considering that the majority of them are young, and the superior cosmetic appearance of VATS should not be dismissed.

For the surgical resection of dumbbell tumors, thoracotomy with laminectomy, VATS with laminectomy as a two-stage procedure,[23] and same-session VATS with laminectomy[11,23] have been described. Several reports advocate performing laminectomy and spinal dissection prior to VATS, citing the necessity for the patient to be in the prone position to permit the use of the neurosurgical operating microscope[12] and avoid spinal cord traction injury.[3] However, some recent series described VATS thoracic resection to be performed first to free up the tumor followed by posterior laminectomy with the operating table rotated from the full lateral position anteriorly up to 45° to facilitate posterior access and microscope use. In the authors' experiences with both approaches, we have found the latter sequence and positioning avoids the need to reposition the patient and to be more favorable should both neurosurgical and thoracic teams require simultaneous access during the procedure. Furthermore, with careful and gentle intrathoracic dissection, proximal nerve root avulsion and spinal cord injury should be avoided. Occasionally, neurogenic tumors thought to have intraspinal components preoperatively have turned out to be extraspinal during VATS intraoperative dissection; hence, the latter approach may avoid an unnecessary posterior laminectomy.

There are relatively few contraindications to VATS. In addition to the general contraindications such as severe coagulopathy, specific ones include pleural symphysis, and patients with severe underlying lung disease or poor lung function who are unable to tolerate the selective one-lung ventilation during general anesthesia. As previously discussed, VATS may not be the ideal approach for very young children. Their small airways are unable to accommodate the smallest double-lumen tube and other techniques to

Table 1
Results of videothoracoscopic approach to posterior mediastinal tumors

Author	Surgical Approach	Pathology	Median Age	Mean Size of Tumor (cm)	Mean Operative Time (min)	Intraoperative Mean Blood Loss (mls)	Chest Drainage (ml)	Mean Chest Drain Duration (Days)(Range)	Complications	Mean Hospital Stay (Days)(Range)	Mean Follow-up (Months)	Recurrence
Riquet, 1995[25]	18 VATS/ 8 Open	2 ganglioneuroma, 13 schwannoma, 3 neurofibroma/ 7 schwannoma, 1 neurofibroma	VATS 44.4[a] (13–70) Open 50.1[a] (23-78)	VATS 3.5 (1.5–6) Open 7.4 (3–14)	VATS: 92 (40–120)	NA	VATS: 170 (25–450)	VATS: 5.3 (2–9), Open 3 (2–5)	4 persistent pain, 1 left recurrent nerve palsy, 3 (17%) conversion to open for chest wall resection	VATS 5.3 (2–9), Open 7.7 (5–14)	VATS (2–24), Open (1–29)	NA
Vallières, 1995[12]	3 VATS-Lam/ 1 Open-Lam	3 schwannoma, 1 mesenchymal hamartoma	40 (35–56)	5.2 (3–8)	NA	NA	NA	NA	1 limited thoracotomy for bleeding control	NA	NA	NA
Bousamra, 1996[26]	6 VATS / 11 Open	Open: 8 schwannoma, 1 neurofibroma, 2 ganglioneuroma; VATS: 5 schwannoma, 1 ganglioneuroma	VATS 34.6[a] (20–64), Open 42.7[a] (19–68)	Open (2–7 cm); VATS (3–7)	VATS: 171 (120–270), Open: 112 (60–180)	NA	NA	NA	Open: 1 chylothorax, 1 hemothorax; VATS: 1 (17%) conversion to open, 1 needed 7 cm utility thoracotomy, 2 transient ptosis	VATS 2.6 (2–4) (return to work 4.3 weeks), Open 4.5 (3–8) (return to work 7.7 weeks)	NA	NA
Hazelrigg, 1999[18]	23 VATS	10 schwannoma, 8 neurofibroma, 1 granular cell, 1 malignant schwannoma, 1 ganglioneuroma, 1 ganglioneuroblastoma, 1 neuroblastoma	35 (1.2–70)	3[b] (0.7–13)	83[b] (30–120)	NA	NA	1[b] (1–4)	4 (17%) conversions to open to complete resection, 3 transient paresthesia, 2 ileus, 1 pleural effusion, 1 transient intercostal pain	2[b] (1–9) (2[b] VATS, 4[b] Open)	40	0

Liu, 2000[23]	139 VATS/ 4 VATS-Lam	72 neurofibroma, 33 neurilemmoma, 7 paraganglioma, 31 ganglioneuroma	40.8[a] (11–72)	3.5 (1.5–8)	40 (15–110)	<50	NA	NA	9 chest wall paresthesia, 1 empyema, 14 needed 6cm utility thoracotomy	4.1 (1–11)	29	0
Han, 2002[27]	6 VATS / 1 VATS-Lam	5 schwannoma, 1 paraganglioma, 1 ganglioneurofibroma	28 (7–52)	5.6 (4–7)	251 (120–540)	354 (50–1600)	NA	NA	1 Horner syndrome, 2 transient intercostal neuralgia	3.4 (2–6)	12.5 (1–30)	0
Takeda, 2004[2]	13 VATS/ 127 Open/ 6 Open-Lam	51 ganglioneuroma, 37 schwannomas, 30 neurofibromas, 18 neuroblastomas, 5 ganglioblastomas, 2 PNET, 3 Others	35.5 (0.5–73)	NA	NA	NA	NA	NA	Transient/mild Horner syndrome	NA	NA	1 recurrence for incomplete resection of benign tumor (recurrence for malignant tumors not included)
Barrenechea, 2006[11]	10 VATS/ 3 VATS-Lam	4 neurofibromas, 8 schwannomas, 1 granular cell tumor	44.9 (29–66)	(3–9)	229.5 (VATS: 102–317) (VATS-Lam: 320–340)	371 (VATS: 50–1500) (VATS-Lam: 450–500)	NA	NA	1 tongue swelling, 1 ulnar neuropathy, 1 intercostal hyperesthesia	2.8 (1–5)	31.7 (10–88)	1 (7.7%) at 2 years

Abbreviations: NA, not available; PNET, primitive neuroectodermal tumor; VATS, video-assisted thoracoscopic surgery; VATS-Lam: video-assisted thoracoscopic surgery and laminectomy.

[a] Mean.

[b] Median.

achieve one-lung ventilation are difficult. Furthermore, children with narrow rib space and small chest cavity often require significant enlargement of the port incision to facilitate tumor retrieval negating any minimal access advantage of VATS. Prior operation in the ipsilateral chest should not be regarded as a contraindication. Adhesions can usually be taken down using a combination of sharp and blunt dissection under videoscopic vision.

Evidence of invasion of chest wall, vertebrae and intraspinal extension, as well as close proximity to a spinal artery, have been considered contraindications for VATS resection in the past.[7,25] Furthermore, even if VATS resection was deemed suitable for particular dumbbell tumor, a staged VATS and laminectomy procedure was performed.[23,25] However, in many specialist centers, increasingly dumbbell tumors are being tackled by VATS and concomitant laminectomy.[11] The open approach may also be more appropriate for very large tumors (>8 cm).[18,23] Some have advocated the open approach even for tumors greater than 6 cm[25]; however, we would still perform VATS with utility minithoracotomy (with or without segmental rib resection) for tumor extraction.[23] Clearly, there comes a point when the extended incision required to remove a sizeable tumor is so large that any benefits of VATS is negated. In addition, those tumors located in the upper- (apex) and lowermost (costodiaphragmatic) reaches of the thoracic cavity, as well as those breeching the diaphragm may be more suited to the conventional approach.[11,25] The authors' contend that it is at these thoracic recesses where the magnifying videoscope with good illumination can provide the most advantages.

The authors' are careful in restricting VATS resection to benign tumors in the posterior mediastinum.[18,23] Neither CT nor MRI scans can completely accurately differentiate between benign and malignant tumors. As in other forms of tumors, the presence of invasion and local destruction of adjacent structures such as ribs and vertebrae (but not pressure atrophy or erosion), and pleural effusion or deposits would suggest a malignant lesion. In these cases, we would carefully examine the entire hemithorax using the videoscope before proceeding with open resection.

SUMMARY

Videothoracoscopic approach to posterior mediastinal tumors is a safe operation in experienced hands. The authors', as well as collective experience, so far shows that the VATS approach produces results comparable to the other conventional surgical techniques for posterior mediastinal tumor excision. Furthermore, by minimizing chest wall trauma, the thoracoscopic approach causes less postoperative pain, shortens hospital stay, and gives superior cosmesis. Compared to conventional surgery, VATS demands a new set of manual skills and hand-eye coordination. For someone who is experienced with open surgery, the learning curve is usually very steep.

Videothoracoscopic surgery is a safe and viable alternative technique for the management of patients with posterior mediastinal tumors. Its role has extended from assessment of disease processes and diagnostic to definitive therapy. The minimal invasive approach is well-suited for resection of posterior mediastinal tumors as most are benign, and neurogenic in origin. Surgical technique has evolved from the classic three-port access to better facilitate tumor removal, and dissection in the apical and inferior recesses of the posterior mediastinum. Dumbbell tumors should be identified preoperatively by CT and MRI imaging to allow resection in a single-stage combined operation. The sequence of either performing laminectomy first or following VATS dissection is largely a matter of surgeon preference; however, there are notable advantages and disadvantages to both approaches. Results from VATS posterior mediastinal tumor resection in terms of symptomatic improvement, recurrence, and survival are comparable to conventional surgical techniques. The VATS approach has shown to result in less postoperative pain, improved cosmesis, shorter hospital stay, and more rapid recovery and return to normal activities. Over the years, the VATS has become a promising therapeutic alternative to the open approach, and may be considered the standard of care in select conditions of the posterior mediastinum.

REFERENCES

1. Davis RD Jr, Newland Oldham H Jr, Sabiston DC Jr. Primary cysts and neoplasms of the mediastinum: recent changes in clinical presentation, methods of diagnosis, management and results. Ann Thorac Surg 1987;44:229–37.
2. Takeda S, Miyoshi S, Minami M, et al. Intrathoracic neurogenic tumors—50 years' experience in a Japanese institution. Eur J Cardiothorac Surg 2004;26:807–12.
3. Kan P, Schmidt MH. Minimally invasive thoracoscopic resection of paraspinal neurogenic tumors: technical case report. Neurosurgery 2008;63(1 Suppl 1):ONSE54.

4. Yim AP. Thoracoscopic resection of an esophageal cyst in a 4-year-old girl. Chest 1996;110:545–6.
5. Ng CSH, Wan S, Underwood MJ, et al. VATS and extramedullary haematopoiesis. Eur Respir J 2006; 28:255–6.
6. Sakamaki Y, Yasukawa M, Kido T. Pheochromocytoma of the posterior mediastinum undiagnosed until the onset of intraoperative hypertension. Gen Thorac Cardiovasc Surg 2008;56:509–11.
7. Landreneau RJ, Dowling RD, Ferson PF. Thoracoscopic resection of a posterior mediastinal neurogenic tumor. Chest 1992;102:1288–90.
8. Canvasser DA, Naunheim KS. Thoracoscopic management of posterior mediastinal tumors. Chest Surg Clin N Am 1996;6:53–67.
9. Patrick DA, Rothenberg SS. Thoracoscopic resection of mediastinal masses in infants and children: an evaluation of technique and results. J Pediatr Surg 2001;36:1165–7.
10. Shigemura N, Hsin MK, Yim AP. Segmental rib resection for difficult cases of video-assisted thoracic surgery. J Thorac Cardiovasc Surg 2006;132:701–2.
11. Barrenechea IJ, Fukumoto R, Lesser JB, et al. Endoscopic resection of thoracic paravertebral and dumbbell tumors. Neurosurgery 2006;59:1195–202.
12. Vallières E, Findlay M, Fraser RE. Combined microneurosurgical and thoracoscopic removal of neurogenic dumbbell tumors. Ann Thorac Surg 1995;59: 469–72.
13. Yamaguchi M, Yoshino I, Kameyama T, et al. Thoracoscopic surgery combined with a supraclavicular approach for removing a cervico-mediastinal neurogenic tumor: a case report. Ann Thorac Cardiovasc Surg 2006;12:194–6.
14. Chowbey PK, Vashistha A, Khullar R, et al. Laparoscopic excision of a lower posterior mediastinal paraspinal mass: technique and feasibility of the laparoscopic approach. Surg Laparosc Endosc Percutan Tech 2002;12:378–81.
15. Yoshino I, Hashizume M, Shimada M, et al. Video-assisted thoracoscopic extirpation of a posterior mediastinal mass using the da Vinci computer enhanced surgical system. Ann Thorac Surg 2002; 74:1235–7.
16. Ng CSH, Whelan RL, Lacy AM, et al. Is minimal access surgery for cancer associated with immunologic benefits? World J Surg 2005;29:975–81.
17. Yim AP. Minimizing chest wall trauma in video assisted thoracic surgery. J Thorac Cardiovasc Surg 1995;109:1255–6.
18. Hazelrigg SR, Boley TM, Krasna MJ, et al. Thoracoscopic resection of posterior neurogenic tumors. Am Surg 1999;65:1129–33.
19. Nakamura Y, Matsumura A, Katsura H, et al. Successful video-thoracoscopic drainage for descending necrotizing mediastinitis. Gen Thorac Cardiovasc Surg 2009;57:111–5.
20. Negri G, Regolo P, Gerevini S, et al. Mediastinal dumbbell angiolipoma. Ann Thorac Surg 2000;70: 957–8.
21. Hsu CH, Lee CM, Wang FC, et al. Neurofibroma with increased uptake of [F-18]-fluoro-2 deoxy-D-glucose interpreted as a metastatic lesion. Ann Nucl Med 2003;17:609–11.
22. Ho AM, Karmakar MK, Critchley LA, et al. Placing the tip of the endotracheal tube at the carina and passing the endobronchial blocker through the Murphy eye may reduce the risk of blocker retrograde dislodgement during one-lung anaesthesia in small children. Br J Anaesth 2008;101:690–3.
23. Liu HP, Yim AP, Wan J, et al. Thoracoscopic removal of intrathoracic neurogenic tumors: a combined Chinese experience. Ann Surg 2000;232:187–90.
24. Li WW, Lee TW, Yim AP. Shoulder function after thoracic surgery. Thorac Surg Clin 2004;14:331–43.
25. Riquet M, Mouroux J, Pons F, et al. Videothoracoscopic excision of thoracic neurogenic tumors. Ann Thorac Surg 1995;60:943–6.
26. Bousamra M 2nd, Haasler GB, Patterson GA, et al. A comparative study of thoracoscopic vs open removal of benign neurogenic mediastinal tumors. Chest 1996;109:1461–5.
27. Han PP, Dickman CA. Thoracoscopic resection of thoracic neurogenic tumors. J Neurosurg 2002;96: 304–8.
28. Yim AP. VATS major pulmonary resection revisited—controversies, techniques, and results. Ann Thorac Surg 2002;74:615–23.

Videothoracoscopic Approach to the Spine in Idiopathic Scoliosis

Eugenio Pompeo, MD[a,*], Federico Mancini, MD[b], Ernesto Ippolito, MD[b], Tommaso C. Mineo, MD[a]

KEYWORDS

• Idiopathic scoliosis • Surgical approaches • Thoracoscopy
• Video-assisted thoracoscopic surgery • Discectomy

Idiopathic scoliosis accounts for about 80% of all types of scoliosis in the adolescent population, and more than 50% of these conditions are thoracic in location. Surgical treatment of idiopathic scoliosis has classically included posterior, anterior, or combined open surgical techniques. The goals of surgical correction are to fuse the minimum number of motion segments needed to safely prevent curve progression, to correct the deformity, and to achieve a balanced spine over the pelvis.[1–3]

In recent years, a videothoracoscopic approach to the spine has been increasingly employed either in combination with the posterior open approach or as a stand-alone treatment including anterior release and fusion. This has stimulated the development of multispecialty surgical teams entailing dedicated thoracic and orthopedic surgeons working together to optimize results.

Proponents of videothoracoscopic approaches believe that they allow clinical outcomes comparable to those of open surgery with minimized surgical trauma and postoperative pain, superior cosmetic effects, and less impairment of respiratory function.[4–6] Furthermore, periodic technological refinements continue to be proposed and are likely to contribute toward rendering these surgical options simpler, safer, and more effective.

This article reports on the current state of the art of the videothoracoscopic approaches most commonly employed for the surgical treatment of thoracic idiopathic scoliosis.

ANTERIOR APPROACH TO THE SPINE

The anterior approach to the thoracic spine has been traditionally performed through a thoracotomy, first reported by Hodgson and Stock[7] in 1956 for the treatment of Pott disease. Subsequently, Cook in 1971[8] and Richardson and colleagues[9] in 1976 emphasized the role of the thoracic surgeon in joining the orthopedic surgeon to provide anterior access to the thoracic spine.

VIDEOTHORACOSCOPY

The history of thoracoscopy dates back to 1865, when the Irish physician Francis Richard Cruise employed a modified Désormeaux cystoscope to perform a binocular thoracoscopy in an 11-year-old girl with empyema.[10] Nonetheless, the Swedish internist Hans Jacobaeus deserves to be called the father of thoracoscopy because he successfully disseminated this minimally invasive technique that he initially employed to sever pleural adhesions and help lung collapse during a Forlanini artificial pneumothorax.[11] Subsequently, thoracoscopy remained underused for many decades until 1990 when the introduction of video technology and magnified imaging led to the birth of the modern videothoracoscopic surgery. The videothoracoscopic approach to the spine was first reported by Mack and colleagues[12] in 1993. Videothoracoscopic surgery has since

[a] Department of Thoracic Surgery, Fondazione Policlinico Tor Vergata, Tor Vergata University, Viale Oxford, 81, Rome 00133, Italy
[b] Department of Orthopedic Surgery, Fondazione Policlinico Tor Vergata, Tor Vergata University, Viale Oxford, 81, Rome 00133, Italy
* Corresponding author.
E-mail address: pompeo@med.uniroma2.it

Thorac Surg Clin 20 (2010) 311–321
doi:10.1016/j.thorsurg.2010.01.004
1547-4127/10/$ – see front matter

thoracic.theclinics.com

played a considerable role in the treatment of spinal deformities requiring anterior release.[13]

SPINE FUSION INSTRUMENTATION

There has been a considerable evolution in dedicated instrumentation for spinal fusion since the introduction of the Harrington rod system. In fact, with third generation Cotrel-Debousset implants, the concept of segmental pedicle screw constructs with multiple fixation points has been proposed to overcome typical shortcomings related to the use of former systems and including suboptimal fixation, loss of correction, hook dislodgement, and induction of lumbar kyphosis.[14] Increased segmental bony purchase and better 3-dimensional control on the posterior spinal elements have improved coronal spinal correction from nearly 20% up to a range of 40%–67% while preserving more normal sagittal alignment.[14–17] Yet, hybrid constructs using pedicle screws, hooks and wires are also increasingly chosen today.[18]

INDICATIONS

Indications for videothoracoscopy are the same as for the open thoracotomy procedure, and include single thoracic curves that are also regarded as type I curves according to the classification system proposed by Lenke and colleagues[19] (**Fig. 1**). Overall, surgical treatment of idiopathic scoliosis is usually indicated when the curve exceeds 45° or 50° by the Cobb method. This limit is based on some accepted findings. First, curves larger than 50° progress even after skeletal maturity. Second, thoracic curves with magnitude between 50° and 75° at skeletal maturity (Risser IV or V) have been reported to progress about 29° through a 40-year follow-up period.[20] Third, curves larger than 55° at skeletal maturity are expected to progress more than 0.5° per year.[21]

According to the classification of Lenke, the sagittal plane should have either a hypokyphotic or normal (N) sagittal thoracic modifier. Hyperkyphosis with T5 to T12 Cobb equal to or greater than 40° indicating a "+" sagittal thoracic modifier is a relative contraindication to an anterior thoracic approach, due to a high pseudoarthrosis rate and progressive kyphosis reported over time, particularly in skeletally immature patients.[22,23] The videothoracoscopic approach is also appropriate for skeletally immature patients with a type I curve at risk of crankshaft, since anterior discectomy and fusion should eliminate anterior growth.[24,25]

Curves of magnitude greater than 75° can cause loss of pulmonary function and even respiratory failure in extreme cases. In particular, it has been reported by Bjure and colleagues[26] that with curves between 60° and 100°, total lung capacity decreases to 68% of predicted values whereas nearly half of the patients with thoracic curve larger than 80° have some degree of dyspnea at the average age of 42 years.[27] In addition, vital capacity of less than 45% predicted and a Cobb angle greater than 110° proved to be risk factors for respiratory failure and early mortality. As a rule, the greater the curve progresses, the more difficult is surgical treatment because more surgical anchors may be necessary, operative time is longer, there is more blood loss, and higher morbidity rate may be expected. For these reasons it has been suggested that, provided adequate training with thoracoscopic release and fusion has been undergone, type I curves of less than 75° can be treated by the sole thoracoscopic approach, whereas curves of 75° or greater are better suited for anterior thoracoscopic release followed by posterior open fusion and instrumentation.[28]

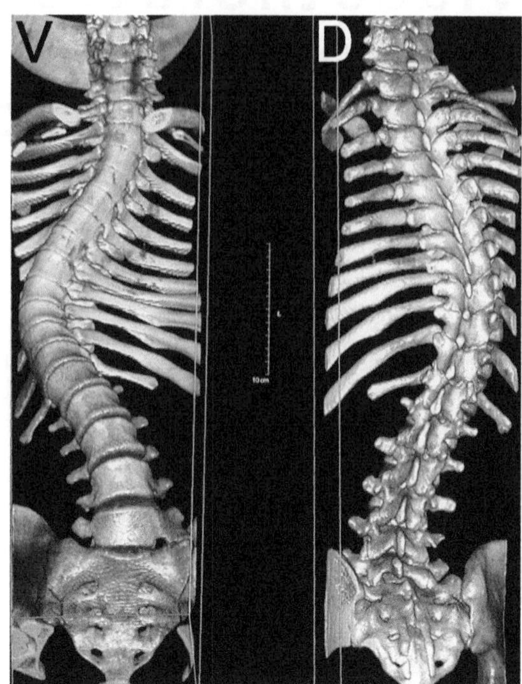

Fig. 1. Computed tomographic, 3-dimensional reconstruction imaging of the spine showing ventral (V) and dorsal (D) aspects of the spine deformity.

Relative contraindications for videothoracoscopy include extremely severe scoliosis when the spine is nearly touching the rib cage, previous thoracotomy on the side targeted for operation, and patients with severe restrictive functional defect who would not tolerate single-lung ventilation. These conditions, though rare, are in any event better suited for an open approach.

PREOPERATIVE STUDY

Routine preoperative workup is always performed, including blood gas analysis, electrocardiogram, and spirometry. Radiologic study includes full-length standing posteroanterior and lateral radiographs of the spine to document characteristics and extension of the spinal deformity. Moreover, the fulcrum-bending radiograph, obtained with the patient lying sideways hanging over a fulcrum, provides a simple and reproducible technique for the in vivo assessment of spinal flexibility and can accurately predict before surgery the amount of correction that can be achieved by surgical treatment. The authors also advocate utility of computed tomography with standard axial images and 3-dimensional reconstruction algorithms that respectively provide additional information on distribution of main perispinal anatomic structures and longitudinal axial rotation of the spine (**Fig. 2**). In selected instances magnetic resonance imaging is also performed because it can provide additional information on perispinal vascular structures and soft-tissues, particularly when they are involved with associated comorbid conditions.

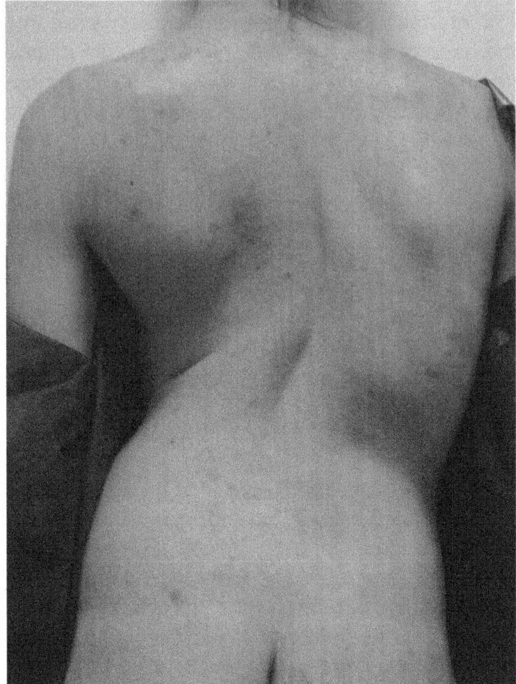

Fig. 2. A 23-year-old patient with a classic type I curve according to the classification of Lenke. *Data from* Lenke LG, Betz RR, Harms J, et al. Adolescent idiopathic scoliosis: a new classification to determine extent of spinal arthrodesis. J Bone Joint Surg 2001;83:1169–81.

SURGICAL TECHNIQUES

In their experience, the authors have preferred a combined videothoracoscopic and posterior open approach. Patients who are candidates for surgical intervention are informed fully on the characteristics of the different surgical approaches, and written informed consent is obtained.

Combined Videothoracoscopic Anterior Approach with Posterior Open Instrumentation

The patient is placed in the full lateral decubitus position (**Fig. 3**). The surgical team entails participation of 2 thoracic surgeons and 2 orthopedic surgeons. In contrast to other videothoracoscopic procedures in which the surgeon and assistant are positioned on opposite sides of the operating table, in spinal surgery procedures both surgeons are positioned on the anterior side of the patient while the monitor is positioned on the dorsal side.

A double-lumen endotracheal tube for single-lung ventilation is employed. The patient is prepared and draped in a standard manner as for a full thoracotomy and the spine is approached from the side of convexity. Videothoracoscopic access includes use of 4 flexible trocars placed through 2-cm skin incisions. A camera is inserted through a trocar placed along the mid-axillary line while operative trocars are placed in a linear fashion along the anterior axillary line (**Fig. 4**). The authors prefer to use a 30° angled, 10-mm

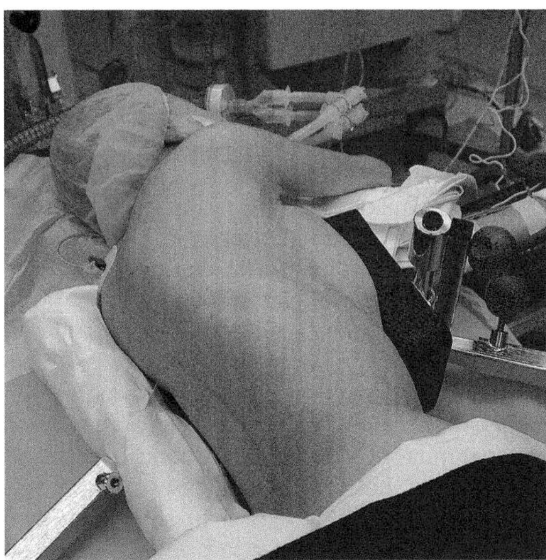

Fig. 3. Position of the patient for videothoracoscopic discectomy.

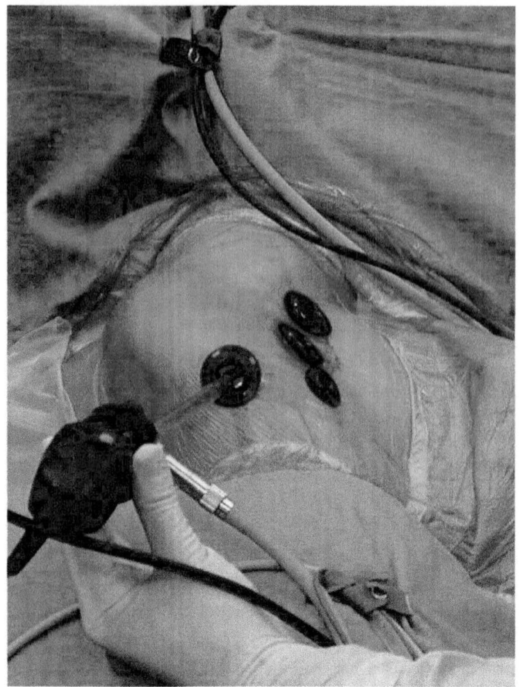

Fig. 4. Trocars' positioning for videothoracoscopic approach to the spine.

camera that facilitates an oblique vision deep into the intervertebral space during discectomy.

The operative setup includes presence on the nurse's table of full instrumentation for emergency thoracotomy in case of technical difficulty or uncontrolled bleeding.

The pleura is divided transversally at each targeted intervertebral space, and intercostal vessels are preserved by working between them (**Fig. 5**A, B). In their most recent patients the authors have successfully employed the 5-mm harmonic scalpel (Ultracision, Ethicon Endosurgery, Cincinnati, OH, USA) that produces less smoke and minimizes thermal dispersion during coagulation (**Fig. 5**C). The annulus fibrosus and the anterior longitudinal ligament are incised by either electrocautery or the harmonic scalpel. A thorough discectomy extended back to the posterior annulus is performed on each disc excised, starting from lumbar vertebrae (**Fig. 5**D) and proceeding in an upward direction. The apical levels should have the annulus released superficially and anteriorly, and released or thinned in the deep portion. Disc material must be thoroughly cleaned off the end plate back to, but not through the posterior longitudinal ligament. It is critical to limit intradiscal bleeding because this jeopardizes visualization during surgical maneuvering. Approximately 60% of the cartilage endplates, nucleus, and annulus are routinely excised. During discectomy, the rib head must be identified because it is an extremely important landmark to prevent migration through the posterior longitudinal ligament, which will always lie posterior to the rib head. Once all disc excisions are completed, mobility of vertebral bodies between excised discs is tested. Finally, autogenous bone grafting can be performed if available. This procedure can decrease intradiscal bleeding but has the disadvantage that it must be harvested before discectomy, eventually increasing operating time.

Subsequently, hemostasis is accurately revised and the parietal pleura is left open (**Fig. 6**). One chest tube is inserted in the paravertebral space and the lung is progressively reventilated. Finally, the trocar incisions are sutured.

In their early thoracoscopic discectomy procedures, the authors employed a halofemoral traction for an average of 12 days followed by open posterior instrumental spinal fusion (**Fig. 7**).

Posterior spinal fusion is undertaken through a standard posterior approach with the patient in the prone position. Following longitudinal skin incision over the thoracic column, segmental pedicle screw fixation is used bilaterally at each level. The authors prefer polyaxial pedicle screws because they have more freedom at the screw-rod interface that facilitate seating of the rod into the head of the screw. Pedicle screws are placed segmentally along the concavity of the curve and approximately at every other level along the convexity. The screws on the top and bottom of the construct are placed in a fairly neutral position, with the apical screws placed in the most posterior position due to vertebral rotation. The screws should start in the same position on the lateral vertebral body just anterior to the rib head. Yet it is theoretically advisable that a bicortical screw position be achieved particularly in the proximal screws, which are at highest risk of pullout and plowing. However, because this can expose to the risk of injuring the thoracic aorta, is advisable to have screws with 2.5-mm variable length options available in the operating theater.

A left-sided rod is contoured to the desired sagittal contour and is placed in the pedicle screws on the concave side. A rod derotation maneuver is performed, and the rod is fixed by tightening firstly the superior screws and then the inferior ones. Manipulation of the concave and convex screws simultaneously can allow additional correction by performing a derotation maneuver. Subsequently a second rod is placed and further derotation, distraction, and compression maneuvers are performed to finalize the correction (**Fig. 8**A). Finally, demineralized bone

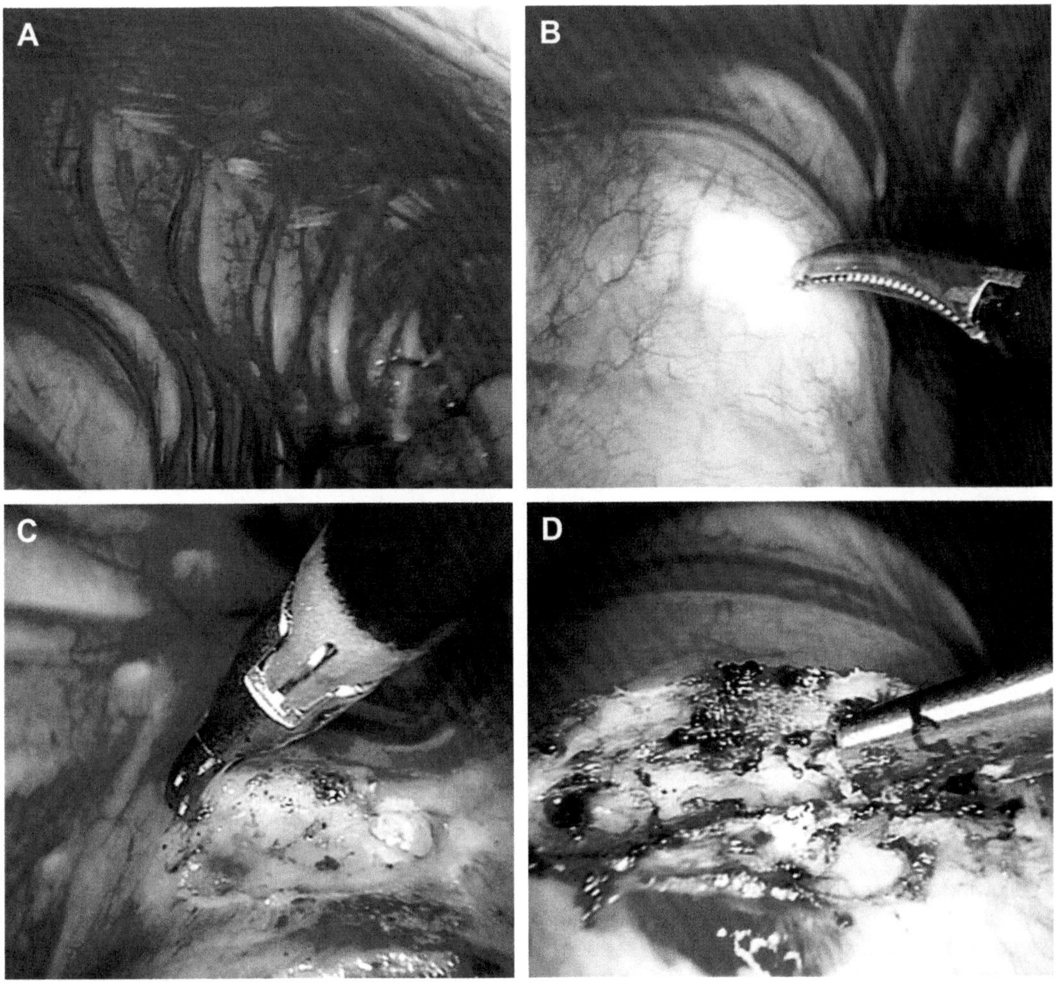

Fig. 5. (*A*) Thoracoscopic view of right pleural cavity and thoracic spine before discectomy. (*B*) The mediastinal pleura is incised transversally over the intervertebral space with respect to the intercostal vessels. (*C*) A harmonic scalpel is used to coagulate a small vessel and incise the pleura over the third intervertebral space. (*D*) Discectomy is accomplished over a lumbar vertebra with a thoracoscopic Kerrison forceps.

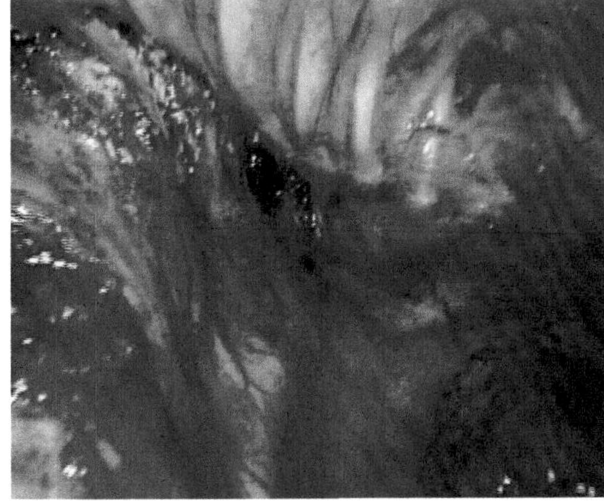

Fig. 6. Intraoperative thoracoscopic view of a completed 6-level discectomy.

matrix is released over the entire instrumented area to facilitate fusion (**Fig. 8**B).

Single-Stage Videothoracoscopic Anterior Discectomy, Fusion, and Instrumentation

The use of anterior instrumentation systems means that anterior discectomy and fusion can be performed as a stand-alone videothoracoscopic procedure, avoiding the need for posterior open surgery.[28–31]

The type of anesthesia and patient positioning is the same as for anterior thoracoscopic release, whereas positioning of the trocars is somewhat different in that operating ports are usually placed posteriorly along the posterior axillary line while the camera port is placed anteriorly along the mid-axillary line in an L-shaped disposition.

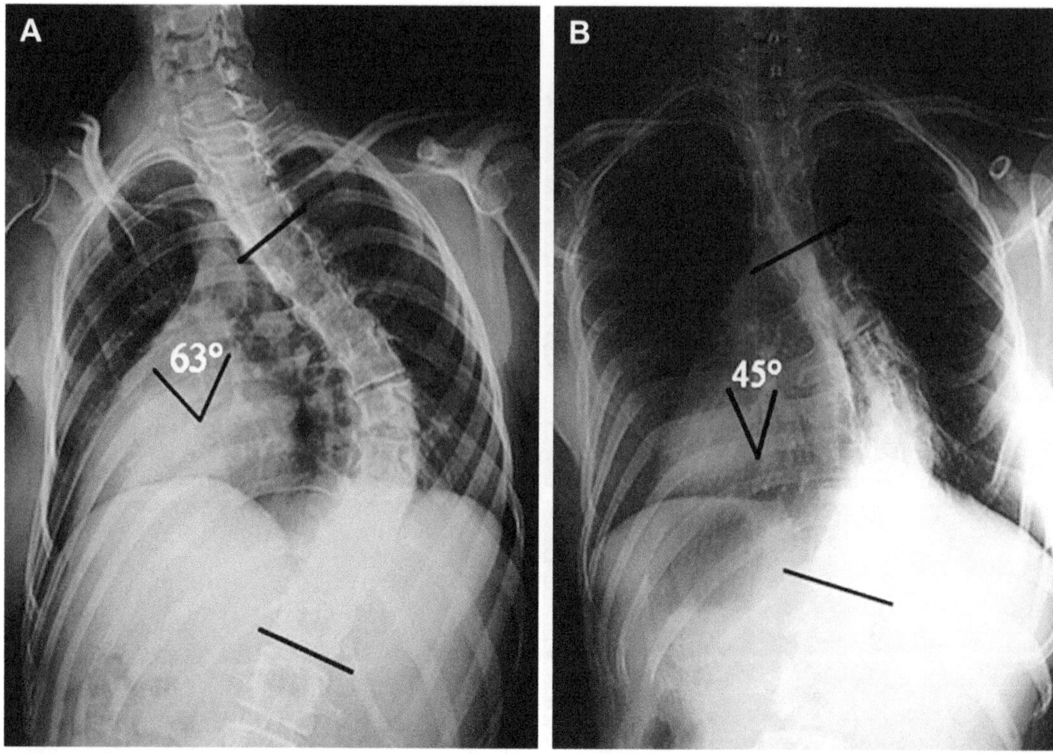

Fig. 7. Preoperative radiograph (*A*) compared with radiograph performed 12 days after thoracoscopic discectomy and subsequent halotraction showing improvement in spinal deformity (*B*).

Following discectomy according to the surgical steps described above, screws are placed in the proximal vertebrae first, sequentially moving inferiorly. A standard 15-mm trocar is employed for screw placement. The rib head is maintained without other rib disruption. The screw hole is started usually with an awl placing the screw in the midlateral vertebral body, parallel to the endplates, just anterior to the rib head. A calibrated tap, followed by a depth gauge can be used to determine exact screw length with bicortical purchase attempted. Two to 3 screws are placed through each trocar incision, moving the portal into the appropriate rib interspace to align each screw parallel to its corresponding vertebral body. The exact screw position is then verified by the image intensifier in anteroposterior and lateral views, and rod length measured with a calibrated template. A 4- to 4.75-mm diameter titanium stainless steel system is preferred. The rods are contoured to the appropriate sagittal plane, and some degree of scoliosis placed in the rod based on the ultimate scoliosis correction that is thought to be achievable. The rods are placed in the proximity screws first, capturing these screws and bone-grafting the intervertebral space with previously harvested bone graft. With the proximal 3 levels captured, bone-grafted, and compressed, the rod is then sequentially cantilevered into the lower screws. Each of subsequent levels is similarly grafted and compressed. Following the instrumentation, pleural closure can be performed by an Endo Stitch device or left open. The chest is irrigated by saline with antibiotics and the chest tube placed.

IMAGE-GUIDED SURGERY

Image-guided systems are commonly used in intracranial surgery, and have been adapted to assist with screw placement since the mid-1990s.[32,33] The use of image-guided systems relies on precise localization of the pedicles by using computed tomography scanning, and is aimed at improving placement of pedicle screws and reducing extent of surgical exposure, operative time, and blood loss.

Foley and Gupta[34] described the use of "virtual fluoroscopy" in various spinal procedures including pedicle screw insertion. Nolte and colleagues[33] detailed the principles of computer-assisted pedicle screw fixation that included an infrared camera to track specific

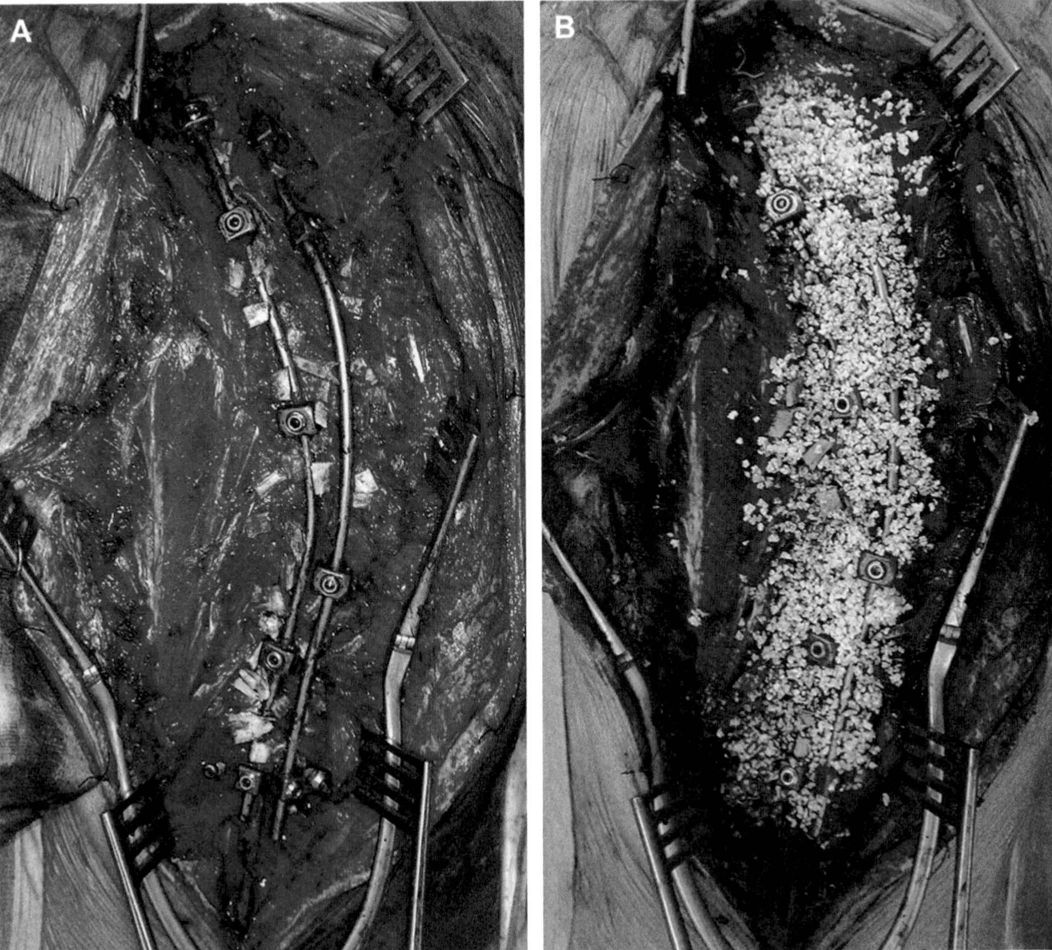

Fig. 8. Intraoperative view of the posterior open approach employed after thoracoscopic discectomy, showing instrumentation (*A*) and demineralized bone matrix released over the spine (*B*).

instruments equipped with light-emitting diodes. The dynamic reference was fixed to the spinous process of the vertebra to receive instrumentation, and accuracy of calibration was confirmed by normal bone landmarks and their correlations with images. Computer-assisted fluoroscopic targeting for pedicle screw fixation has also been reported,[35] although a comparison of the accuracy of pedicle screw placement accompanied by the fluoroscopy-guided system with the image-guided system revealed no significant difference. More recently, isocentric C-arm fluoroscopy has been developed. With this system, computed tomography images generated with the aid of an intraoperative fluoroscope may offer new means of 3-dimensional intraoperative navigation by using a 2-dimensional imaging source.[36]

RESULTS

Learning Curve

The learning curve for videothoracoscopic spinal surgery is steeper than for other procedures. Two separate studies[37,38] have shown that approximately 25 to 28 cases are needed to reduce the learning curve. This result has to be taken into account particularly when the technique is taught. Indeed it has been emphasized that in an academic institution, each clinical fellow may assist on approximately 2 to 5 videothoracoscopic spinal procedures throughout their fellowship. Nevertheless Lonner and colleagues[38] have suggested that before introducing this demanding technique into practice, in-depth comfort with open anterior spinal approaches is helpful. In the authors' experience, creation of a multidisciplinary team including a dedicated thoracic surgeon experienced in advanced thoracoscopic procedures and orthopedic surgeons experienced in open surgical treatment of idiopathic scoliosis permitted safe management even in their early cases, at least in minimizing perioperative risks.

Complications

In a meta-analysis of 10 videothoracoscopic series, the overall complication rate was 18% with most being pulmonary complications in patients with neuromuscular disorders.[13]

More recently, Bomback and colleagues[29] reported a rate of minor complications of 41% including pneumonia, pneumothorax, pleural effusion, pancreatitis, and urinary tract infection; and a rate of major complications of 29% including reintubation, cardioversion, junctional degeneration requiring extension of the fusion at 2 and 8 years of follow-up, respectively, and dislodged hook requiring surgical revision. In another series[30] the most frequent complications included atelectasis and pneumonia, although pulmonary embolus, myelomeningocele, and contralateral tension pneumothorax have also been described.

In patients undergoing thoracoscopic release and instrumentation, complications include implant failure due to intraoperative vertebral body fracture or postoperative break of the steel rod, inappropriate length of vertebral fusion, loss of correction of more than 10° or hyperkyphosis of 40° or greater. Other less frequent and yet potentially life-threatening complications include contralateral tension pneumothorax, major bleeding, or neurologic damage. In a series of 50 patients from Newton and colleagues,[31] implant failure occurred in 3 patients (6%) whereas revision surgery was needed in 2 (4%).

Correction of Deformity

In a series of patients undergoing thoracoscopic anterior release with discectomy, Al-Sayyad and colleagues[30] reported a final correction in the scoliosis population of 68%. Newton and colleagues[31] reported postoperative scoliosis correction of 80% whereas in a previous meta-analysis by Arlet,[13] correction rates varied from 55% to 63%.

Weinzapfel and colleagues[39] compared correction rate and radiographic fusion rate after thoracoscopic release with either allograft bone or demineralized bone matrix, and found that correction rates were 68% and 67%, respectively, whereas fusion rates were 82% and 92%. The conclusion reached was that demineralized bone matrix should be considered to be an effective bone graft substitute in thoracoscopic surgery for idiopathic scoliosis.

Bomback and colleagues[29] compared thoracoscopic versus thoracotomy spinal release in patients undergoing subsequent instrumented posterior spinal fusion. There was a nonsignificant trend in reduced blood loss in the thoracoscopic group while the percentage curve correction was almost identical (52% vs 51%).

Picetti and colleagues[6] reported on one-stage videothoracoscopic discectomy, fusion, and instrumentation in 50 patients with thoracic scoliosis. Initial curve correction averaged 50%, improving to over 68% in the last 10 patients. In a recent series comparing thoracoscopic spinal fusion and with posterior spinal fusion, Lonner and colleagues[40] reported that operative time was higher in the thoracoscopic group; correction of the major curve was 57% versus 64% with no significant difference, although the average blood loss and number of fused levels were lower in the thoracoscopic group. The investigators concluded that for single thoracic curves less than 70° thoracoscopic spinal fusion can produce equivalent radiographic results, clinical outcomes, and complication rates in comparison with posterior spinal fusion. However, in another study the same investigators[41] reported that based on the Scoliosis Research Society's outcome measures (SRS-22) scores, patients treated by videothoracoscopy scored higher in the self-image, mental health, and total score than those treated by the posterior approach, and concluded that this might be due to the smaller surgical scar and less invasive nature of thoracoscopic procedures.

Furthermore, Lenke[28] reported that by thoracoscopic anterior release with a mean preoperative Cobb measurement of 82°, postoperative correction reached 70° whereas in patients undergoing thoracoscopic release and instrumentation, with a mean preoperative curve of 53°, correction rate averaged 51°.

Finally, in an analysis by Luhman and colleagues[42] comparing anterior-posterior spinal fusion with posterior spinal fusion alone in patients with large 70° to 100° thoracic idiopathic scoliosis curves, the anterior-posterior approach allowed greater coronal correction of the thoracic curve when using a thoracic hook construct but not with the use of pedicle screw constructs.

SUMMARY

Videothoracoscopic spine surgery has been widely performed over the past 15 years, and interest in this approach continues to grow as both surgeons and patients strive to minimize risks of surgical-related morbidity. Theoretical advantages over open thoracotomy include decreased incisional pain and intercostal neuralgia, fewer pulmonary complications, improved view of the thoracic spine, avoidance of rib spreading, and improved cosmesis. Possible disadvantages are the steep learning curve and difficulties with endoscopic distraction, compression, and rod rotation when anterior instrumentation is accomplished. Several encouraging results have suggested that thoracoscopic anterior release is as safe and effective as open thoracotomy for the treatment of idiopathic thoracic scoliosis, and can offer similar curve correction with decreased blood loss and complication rate (**Fig. 9**). However, long-term prospective data on videothoracoscopic treatment of idiopathic scoliosis are still lacking, and to be widely adopted these techniques must prove safe and reproducible with an acceptable learning curve and a real advantage in cost-to-benefit ratio.

Thus far, enthusiasm of surgeons advocating videothoracoscopic spinal surgery has been mitigated by other surgeons who emphasize the efficacy of the sole posterior open approach due to the excellent corrective power of 3-column stabilization afforded by pedicle screws[42–44] and the potential improvement in coronal and sagittal plane correction through the use of osteotomies.[45,46] Nonetheless, the authors believe that thoracic and orthopedic surgeons involved in surgical treatment of idiopathic scoliosis should be aware of the currently available minimally invasive procedures and their outcomes.

In conclusion, the goals of videothoracoscopic surgery are certainly laudable, although uncertainty that these goals may be all achieved will persist until well-designed prospective studies prove that what can be done in a safe, effective, and reproducible manner by open surgery can be done at least as well by the videothoracoscopic approach. Despite these open issues, the authors are sure that continuing technical refinements will increasingly help surgeons to "hit the home run" of minimal invasiveness, safety, and efficacy in surgical treatment of idiopathic scoliosis.

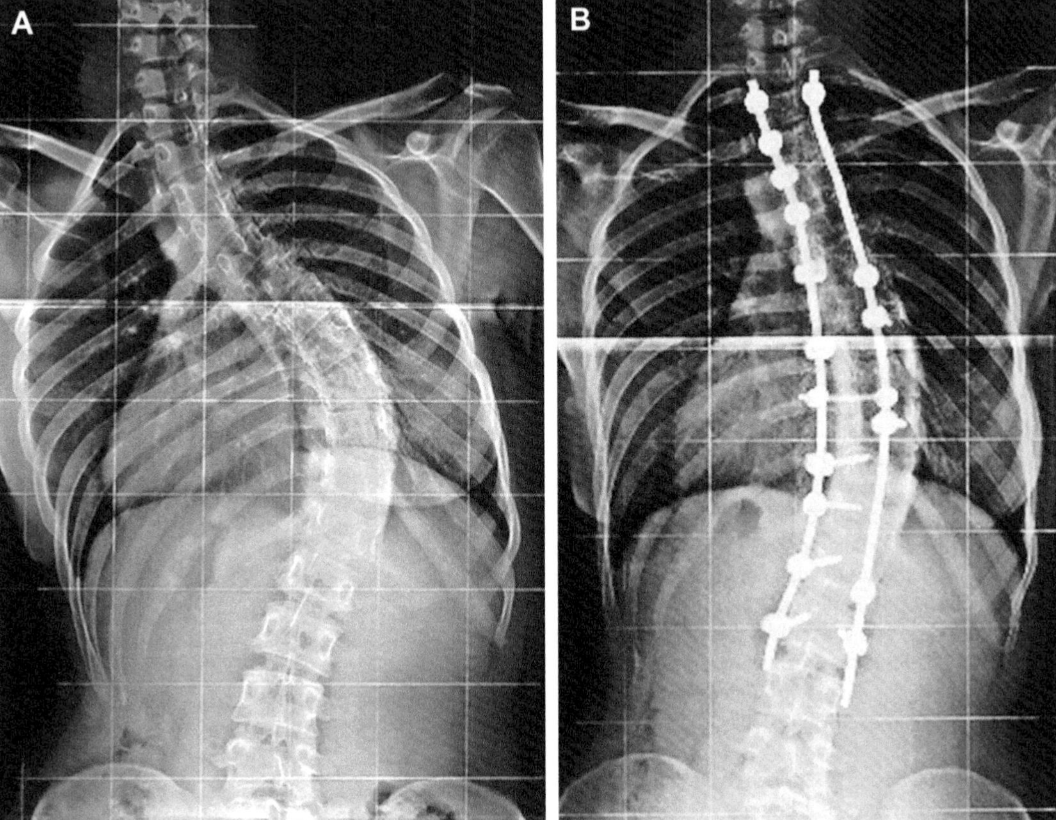

Fig. 9. Preoperative (*A*) and postoperative (*B*) radiographs of a patient undergoing one-stage thoracoscopic discectomy and posterior open approach for instrumentation.

REFERENCES

1. Kuklo TR, Lenke LG, Won DS, et al. Spontaneous proximal thoracic curve correction after isolated fusion of the main thoracic curve in adolescent idiopathic scoliosis. Spine 2001;26:1966–75.
2. Kuklo TR, O'Brien MF, Lenke LG, et al. Spinal Deformity Study Group: AIS Section. Comparison of the lowest instrumented, stable, and lower end vertebrae in "single overhang" thoracic adolescent idiopathic scoliosis: anterior versus posterior spinal fusion. Spine 2006;31:2232–6.
3. Lenke LG, Betz RR, Bridwell KH, et al. Spontaneous lumbar curve coronal correction after selective anterior or posterior thoracic fusion in adolescent idiopathic scoliosis. Spine 1999;24:1663–72.
4. Dickman CA, Mican C. Thoracoscopic approaches for the treatment of anterior thoracic spinal pathology. BNI Q 1996;12:14–9.
5. Mack MJ, Regan JJ, McAfee PC, et al. Video-assisted thoracic surgery for the anterior approach to the thoracic spine. Ann Thorac Surg 1995;59: 1100–6.
6. Picetti GD, Blackman RG, O'Neal K, et al. Anterior endoscopic correction and fusion of scoliosis. Orthopedics 1998;21:1285–7.
7. Hodgson AR, Stock FE. Anterior spinal fusion: a preliminary communication of radical treatment of Pott's disease and Pott's paraplegia. Br J Surg 1956;44:266–75.
8. Cook WA. Transthoracic vertebral surgery. Ann Thorac Surg 1971;12:54–68.
9. Richardson JD, Campbell DL, Grover FL, et al. Transthoracic approach for Pott's disease. Ann Thorac Surg 1976;21:552–6.
10. Gordon S. Clinical reports of rare cases, occurring in the Whitworth and Hardwicke Hospitals. Dublin Q J Med Sci 1866;41:83–90.
11. Jacobaeus HC. The cauterization of adhesions in artificial pneumothorax treatment of pulmonary tuberculosis under thoracoscopic control. Proc R Soc Med 1923;16:45–62.
12. Mack MJ, Regan JJ, Bobechko WP, et al. Application of thoracoscopy for diseases of the spine. Ann Thorac Surg 1993;45:736–8.
13. Arlet V. Anterior thoracoscopic spine release in deformity surgery: a meta-analysis and review. Eur Spine J 2000;9(Suppl):17–23.
14. Helenius I, Remes V, Yrjonen T, et al. Harrington and Cotrel-Dubousset instrumentation in adolescent idiopathic scoliosis: long-term functional and radiographic outcomes. J Bone Joint Surg Am 2003;85: 2303–9.
15. Bridwell KH, Hanson DS, Rhee JM, et al. Correction of thoracic adolescent idiopathic scoliosis with segmental hooks, rods, and Wisconsin wires posteriorly: it's bad and obsolete, correct? Spine 2002;27:2059–66.
16. De Jonge T, Dubousset JF, Illes T. Sagittal plane correction in idiopathic scoliosis. Spine 2002;27: 754–60.
17. Lenke LG, Bridwell KH, Baldus C, et al. Cotrel-Dubousset instrumentation for adolescent idiopathic scoliosis. J Bone Joint Surg Am 1992;74: 1056–67.
18. Maruyama T, Takeshita K. Surgical treatment of scoliosis: a review of techniques currently applied. Scoliosis 2008;3:1–6.
19. Lenke LG, Betz RR, Harms J, et al. Adolescent idiopathic scoliosis: a new classification to determine extent of spinal arthrodesis. J Bone Joint Surg 2001;83:1169–81.
20. Weinstein SL, Ponseti IV. Curve progression in idiopathic scoliosis. J Bone Joint Surg Am 1983;65: 447–55.
21. Edgar M. The natural history of unfused scoliosis. Orthopedics 1987;10(6):931–9.
22. Betz RR, Lenke LG, Harms J, et al. Anterior spinal fusion and instrumentation for adolescent idiopathic scoliosis. Semin Spine Surg 1998;10:88–94.
23. D'Andrea LP, Betz RR, Lenke LG, et al. The effect of continued spinal growth on sagittal contour in patients treated by anterior instrumentation for adolescent idiopathic scoliosis. Spine 2000;25: 813–8.
24. Dubousset J, Herring JA, Shufflebarger HL. The crankshaft phenomenon. J Pediatr Orthop 1989;9: 541–50.
25. Hefti FL, McMaster MJ. The effect of the adolescent growth spurt on early posterior spinal fusion in infantile and juvenile idiopathic scoliosis. J Bone Joint Surg 1983;65:247–54.
26. Bjure J, Grimby G, Kasalicky J, et al. Respiratory impairment and airway closure in patients with untreated idiopathic scoliosis. Thorax 1970;25: 451–6.
27. Collis DK, Ponseti IV. Long-term follow-up of patients with idiopathic scoliosis not treated surgically. J Bone Joint Surg Am 1969;51:425–45.
28. Lenke L. Anterior endoscopic discectomy and fusion for adolescent idiopathic scoliosis. Spine 2003;28:s36–43.
29. Bomback DA, Charles G, Widmann R, et al. Video-assisted thoracoscopic surgery compared with thoracotomy: early and late follow-up of radiographical and functional outcome. Spine J 2007; 7:399–405.
30. Al-Sayyad MJ, Crawfrod AH, Wolf RK. Early experience with video-assisted thoracoscopic surgery: our first 70 cases. Spine 2004;29:1945–51.
31. Newton PO, Parent S, Marks M, et al. prospective evaluation of 50 consecutive scoliosis patients

surgically treated with thoracoscopic anterior instrumentation. Spine 2005;30:s100–9.

32. Glossop ND, Hu RW, Randle JA. Computer-aided pedicle screw placement using frameless stereotaxis. Spine 1996;21:2026–34.
33. Nolte LP, Zamorano LJ, Jiang Z, et al. Image-guided insertion of transpedicular screws. A laboratory set-up. Spine 1995;20:497–500.
34. Foley KT, Gupta SK. Percutaneous pedicle screw fixation of the lumbar spine: preliminary clinical results. J Neurosurg 2002;97:7–12.
35. Choi WW, Green BA, Levi AD. Computer-assisted fluoroscopic targeting system for pedicle screw insertion. Neurosurgery 2000;47:872–8.
36. Thongtrangan I, Le H, Park J, et al. Minimally invasive spinal surgery: a historical perspective. Neurosurg Focus 2004;16:1–10.
37. NIH Consensus Statement on total knee replacement. NIH Consens State Sci Statements 2003; 20:1–34.
38. Lonner BS, Scharf C, Antonacci D, et al. The learning curve associated with thoracoscopic spinal instrumentation. Spine 2005;30:2835–40.
39. Weinzapfel B, Son-Hing JP, Armstrong DG, et al. Fusion rates after thoracoscopic release and bone graft substitutes in idiopathic scoliosis. Spine 2008; 33:1079–83.
40. Lonner BS, Auerbach JD, Estreicher M, et al. Video-assisted anterior thoracoscopic spinal fusion versus posterior spinal fusion. Spine 2009; 34:193–8.
41. Lonner BS, Auerbach JD, Estreicher M, et al. Video-assisted thoracoscopic spinal fusion compared with posterior spinal fusion with thoracic pedicle screws for thoracic adolescent idiopathic scoliosis. J Bone Joint Surg Am 2009;91:398–408.
42. Luhman SJ, Lenke LG, Kim YJ, et al. Thoracic adolescent idiopathic scoliosis curves between 70° and 100°. Spine 2005;30:2061–7.
43. Dobbs MB, Lenke LG, Kim YJ, et al. Anterior/posterior spinal instrumentation versus posterior instrumentation alone for the treatment of adolescent idiopathic scoliotic curves more than 90 degrees. Spine 2006;31:2386–91.
44. Suk SI, Chung ER, Kim JH, et al. Posterior vertebral column resection for severe rigid scoliosis. Spine 2005;30:1682–7.
45. Ahn UM, Ahn NU, Buchowski JM, et al. Functional outcome and radiographic correction after spinal osteotomy. Spine 2002;27:1303–11, 37.
46. Kishan S, Bastrom T, Betz RR, et al. Thoracoscopic scoliosis surgery affects pulmonary function less than thoracotomy at 2 years postsurgery. Spine 2007;32:453–8.

Thoracoscopic Sympathectomy

Mark J. Krasna, MD

KEYWORDS

• Sympathectomy • Hyperhydrosis • Renaud disease

Sympathectomy has been performed for various conditions since the turn of the twentieth century. With the advent of videotechnology, it has assumed a more important role in the armamentarium of managing diseases of the autonomic system. Currently it is used primarily for hyperhydrosis, although sympathectomy for reflex sympathetic dystrophy (RSD), Raynaud disease and other diseases still are performed, but less frequently.

HISTORICAL PERSPECTIVE

Sympathectomy first was performed by Alexander in 1889.[1] The posterior approach, described by Adson in 1908, involved a rib resection with concurrent removal of the sympathetic ganglion.[2] Kotzareff[3] first noted that sympathectomy resulted in ipsilateral anhydrosis in 1920. In 1935, Telford[4] identified the supraclavicular approach as a less invasive procedure to perform for a sympathectomy. Thoracoscopic sympathectomy (TSSYM) has been used for the treatment of sympathetic dysfunction since it first was described by Kux[5] in the 1940s using a standard eyepiece cystoscope. The modern era of video-assisted sympathectomy (VATS SYM) using newer optics and videotechnology was ushered in by the group in Boras, Sweden, by Claes and Drott.[6]

INDICATIONS

Thoracic sympathectomy is indicated for various sympathetic disorders. These include, but are not limited to hyperhydrosis (HH), reflex sympathetic dystrophy (RSD), upper extremity ischemia, Raynaud disease, and splanchnicectomy for pancreatic pain.[7,8] The most common indication, and the indication in which the results are most satisfactory, is hyperhydrosis. The worldwide incidence of hyperhydrosis has been reported around 1% to 2%. Other, more unusual and rare indications that have been described in the past include hypertension, asthma, various psychiatric disorders, cardiac arrhythmias, and facial blushing (7A). Most of this article will refer primarily to hyperhydrosis patients.

It generally is felt that patients undergoing TSSYM should previously have completed a trial of nonoperative therapy as much as can be tolerated. Nonsurgical management of diseases of the sympathetic chain depends on the primary symptom. Patients with hyperhydrosis (HH) generally are offered topical agents such as aluminum chloride. Occasionally, a trial of iontophoresis is appropriate if the patient can tolerate the adverse effects of tingling and electrical shocks. This can be useful for both hand and feet sweating and may have a lasting impact for up to 6 to 12 hours. Unfortunately, the effects generally wane over time, and patients often complain of inability to tolerate the sensation of shocks at the skin. Oral agents have been used with some success in patients with HH. Medications like beta-blockers and cholinergics do have some chance of success with improvement in HH; however, the duration of these effects may be short. This may be helpful if patients can anticipate situations that will aggravate their condition. Propanolol at 10 mg two to four times a day can be quite helpful to these patients. Alternatively, glycopyrrolate 0.5 to 1 mg may help patients who can tolerate the most frequent adverse effect of dry mouth. Although Botulinum toxin injections have been required by

Program of Health Policy, St Joseph Cancer Institute, University of Maryland, 7501 Osler Drive, Suite 104, Towson, MD 21204, USA
E-mail address: markkrasna@catholichealth.net

Thorac Surg Clin 20 (2010) 323–330
doi:10.1016/j.thorsurg.2010.02.008
1547-4127/10/$ – see front matter

many insurers, this technique is not yet approved by the US Food and Drug Administration (FDA) and has not proven to be of significant benefit consistently. Although some physicians attempt a trial of antidepressants or other psychotropic medications, the author and colleagues generally have not found these medications to be of significant benefit. Instead they may allow the patient to deal with the psychological trauma caused by the socially debilitating symptoms of HH. In fact, most psychotropic medications actually cause hyperhydrosis to some degree as a common adverse effect. Many patients stop medications because of the adverse effects of these drugs.

DEFINITIONS AND NOMENCLATURE

Many different terms have been used to describe the actual procedure that is performed in different reports of sympathectomy. Unfortunately, the terminology is generally inconsistent and often leads to confusion. The following glossary has been proposed and corresponds to the most common surgical approaches to TSSYM. The reader is referred to the International Sympathetic Surgery Society (ISSS) Web site, which lists the current rib-oriented and ganglion-oriented nomenclature. This has been adopted by consensus in the ISSS meetings in 2005 and 2007 and instituted as standard as of the March 26, 2009 meeting (www.isss.net).[9] In addition, a recent consensus paper of the Society of Thoracic Surgery (STS) General Thoracic Surgery Workforce (GTSU) on sympathectomy has been developed. The terms are as follows:

Thoracoscopic—done with any means of thoracoscopy including video and standard eyepiece-assisted procedures

VATS (video-assisted thoracic surgery)—refers only to those procedures using a video camera to help with visualization of the intrathoracic cavity

Sympathectomy—refers to procedures in which the sympathetic chain is resected, ablated, or divided

Sympathicotomy—refers to the division of the sympathetic chain without removal of any section thereof. Unless otherwise specified, this would exclude ablation techniques that are done without a directed resection of the chain.

ETS (endoscopic thoracic sympathectomy)—another common term for VATS sympathectomy used more often in the nonthoracic surgery literature for sympathectomy

Ablation—refers to procedures where the chain is destroyed using electrocautery or laser without directed division

G2 sympathectomy—resection of the G2 ganglion, generally achieved by resecting the sympathetic chain between the middle of the second rib (R2 rib) and the third rib (R3); requires careful identification of the ganglial swellings

R2/R3 sympathicotomy—division of the sympathetic chain over the middle of the second rib and division of the sympathetic chain over the middle of the third rib. This accomplishes isolation of the G2 ganglion that is found in between the two incisions. This standard nomenclature should be used for all subsequent levels (ie, R3/R4 sympathectomy).

Sympathicotomy—involves resection/ division of the nerve chain over the third and fourth ribs achieving T3 ganglion isolation and so on.

One-lung ventilation—involves isolating each lung in turn using a double-lumen endobronchial tube or a bronchial blocker.

A detailed description of definitions and nomenclature can be found on the ISSS Web site. According to this nomenclature, further description with modifiers such as u (upper), m (middle), l (lower) can be done. The general consensus is now to describe the surgical procedure according to rib (R) level. This is due in part to the inconsistent location of the sympathetic ganglia in relation to the corresponding ribs.

PREOPERATIVE CONSIDERATIONS

Dermatologists, neurologists, endocrinologists, and cardiologists involved in diagnosing or treating hyperhydrosis should be consulted to evaluate the patients before referral to surgical treatment as needed. Contraindications before surgery are rare but include: severe cardiovascular insufficiency or pulmonary insufficiency; severe pleural diseases (tuberculosis, pleuritis, empyema) or uncontrolled diabetes. Prior thoracic surgery, although perhaps more challenging, is not an absolute contraindication.

LEVEL OF SYMPATHECTOMY

There are many different options used for level of transaction, technique of division or ablation, and anesthetic technique. An attempt has been made to describe the most common options used in the literature and to offer the author's preferences when appropriate.

Transection Level

The choice of the appropriate level is primarily dependent on the location of the primary symptoms, although it also may depend on the etiology. In patients with HH, the level of division of the sympathetic chain generally is accepted as follows:

For patients undergoing thoracoscopic sympathectomy for facial sweating or blushing, division of the chain high over the R2 rib, taking great care to avoid injuring the stellate ganglion, is needed. It is possible to perform a sympathectomy and include up to the lower third of the stellate as well without a Horner's resulting. Likewise, patients being operated upon for thoracic outlet syndrome/RSD are generally undergoing a R2-R3 sympathectomy. The G2 ganglion level is isolated by dividing over or resecting between the R2 and R3 ribs. Some authors just make one cut over the middle or top of the R2 rib without attempting to isolate the nerve further below.

For patients with hand sweating (the most common indication) the R2,3 levels are isolated by division or resection; or more recently R3 alone is cut and the G2 or G3 is isolated.

For axillary sweating, the R3,4 levels are divided. Recent series have emphasized the importance of including the R4 level in patients with axillary sweating or G4 isolation.[10]

Patients referred for splanchnicectomy for chronic pancreatic pain will need division of the R4 to R10 levels. Alternatively, these patients can undergo division of the splanchnic nerve distal to the actual chain.

For Long QT syndrome, the sympathetic chain is sectioned from the level of the inferior third of the stellate ganglion (G1) to the sympathetic ganglia of T5, together with any branch that courses to the caudal region or in the lateral direction.[11]

ANATOMY AND PHYSIOLOGY OF THORACIC SYMPATHETIC NERVES

The thoracic sympathetic chains are visualized readily in each hemithorax during thoracoscopy in its posterior paravertebral location (**Fig. 1**). The sympathetic nerve chain is an elongated white-colored structure often visible underneath the parietal pleura, running parallel to the vertebral column and just lateral to the heads of the thoracic ribs. Although the location of the sympathetic chain is generally constant, the width and size of the sympathetic chain can be variable; the cephalad caudal course of the chain can be straight or meander somewhat also.

Proper identification of chain level is determined by counting the ribs from an intrathoracic approach at the time of surgery. Commonly, each ganglion is located within the intercostal space of its paired rib; hence, the second thoracic ganglion is found below the second rib in the second intercostal space. This is not consistent, however. Therefore some surgeons prefer a ganglion-oriented approach to a rib-oriented approach. The recent ISSS consensus statement is that rib levels must be reported, whereas ganglion level can be reported if so desired by the surgeon. In most people, the first thoracic ganglion fuses with the inferior cervical ganglion to form the stellate ganglion, and it is located high above the level of the second rib. At thoracoscopy, the stellate ganglion often is surrounded or hidden by a fat pad at the apex of the hemithorax. Careful cadaver dissections of the sympathetic chain have confirmed that there are occasionally normal anatomic variations to the sympathetic chain that are important to appreciate in sympathetic nerve surgery. For example, Singh and colleagues[12] found in their series that although the second thoracic ganglion lies within the second intercostal space over 90% of the time, in the small number of remaining cases, the second thoracic ganglion may lie over the neck of the second rib and cross into the first intercostal space (2.5%), be fused to a discrete and separate first thoracic ganglion (2.5%), or fuse directly to the stellate ganglion and span both the first and second intercostal spaces (5%). A comparable distribution of normal anatomic variation also was found by Chung and colleagues,[13] where in their series, the second thoracic ganglion was fused to the stellate ganglion in approximately 7% of cases. Noteworthy in the latter series, was that a discrete second thoracic ganglion was not identifiable in 7% of cases.

Functionally, the thoracic sympathetic chains are part of the body's autonomic nervous system and provide sensorimotor innervation to the visceral organs of the chest. Structurally, the source of the nerve fibers comprising the sympathetic chain is from preganglionic sympathetic fibers that arrive via white rami communicantes of the ventral primary rami of spinal nerves T1 to L2. The preganglionic cell bodies are located in the intermediolateral gray matter of the spinal cord of the corresponding levels. Within the

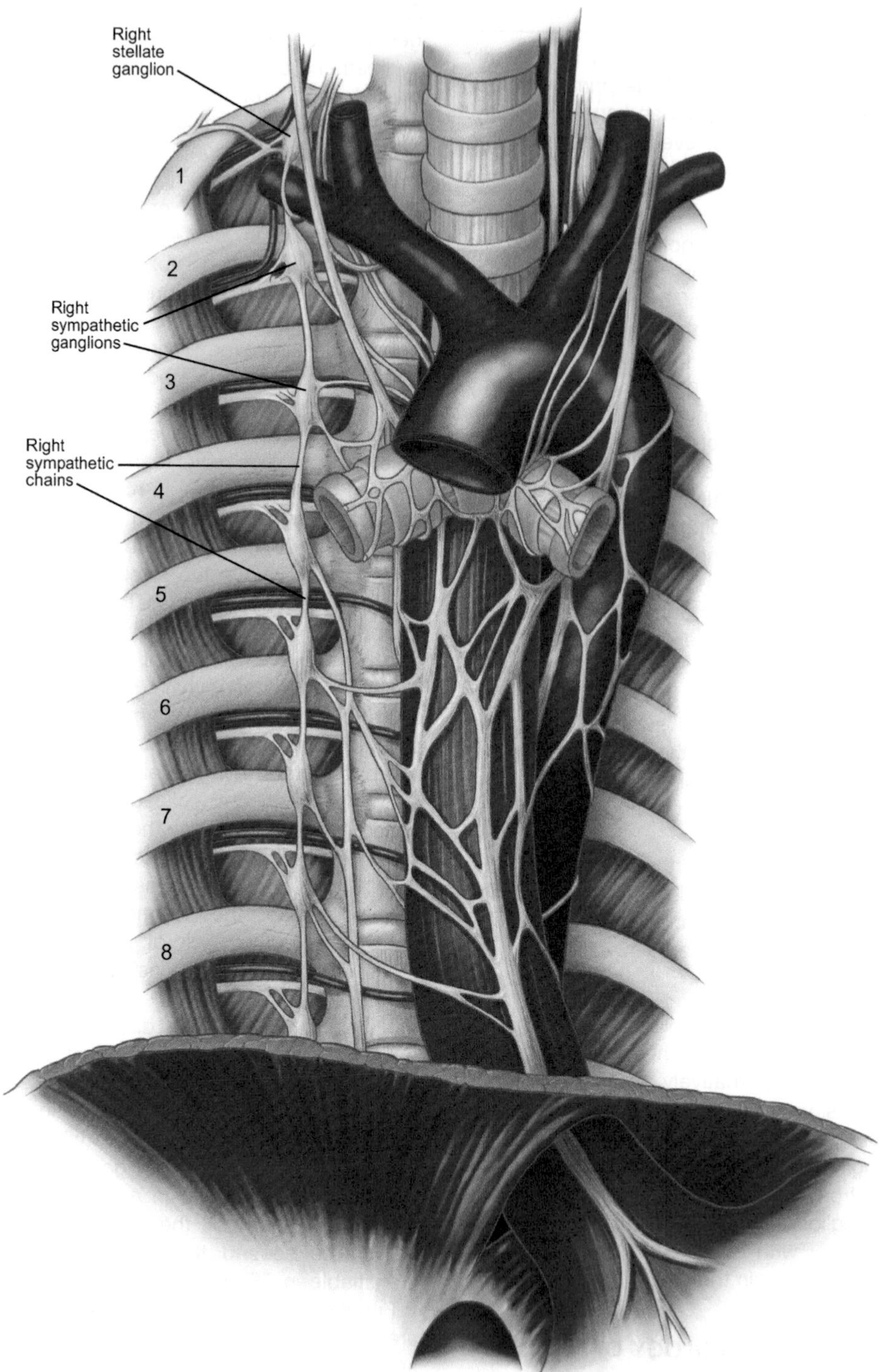

Fig. 1. Schematic sympathetic chain showing ganglia and nerve roots.

sympathetic chain, preganglionic fibers synapse (or may pass through to synapse higher, lower, or peripherally), and postganglionic sympathetic fibers depart via gray rami communicantes at all spinal cord segments. The sensory component is responsible for detection of pain from the viscera, while the motor component innervates organs such as the vascular smooth muscle, errector pili muscles, and sweat glands of the skin, the heart, and the lungs.

At the level of the stellate ganglion, the oculosympathetic pathway can be interrupted as a result of trauma, where neurons project postganglionic axons to the eye to innervate the dilator of the iris, the Muller muscle of the eyelid, and follow the external carotid artery to regulate the sweat glands of the face. When only the lower half of the ganglion is removed as a treatment for hyperhydrosis, symptoms generally are relieved without the development of a Horner syndrome. Of note, a parallel sympathetic chain may be identified.

TECHNIQUE FOR DIVISION

There are many methods by which one can achieve a sympathectomy. These include cautery ablation using a spatula or round tip. Careful division of the nerve over the ribs can be achieved by using a shears cautery or a hook cautery. In this case, care should be exercised to avoid damage to the underlying periosteum, as this can cause severe discomfort and sunburn-like pain in the postoperative period. One can carefully dissect off the parietal pleura first and perform the sympathectomy or cauterize right through to the over the rib head. If resection is used, the chain generally is mobilized at the upper and lower level, and then the collateral branches are transected in turn as the dissection proceeds. Great care should be exercised to use short bursts of cautery current in any type of dissection to minimize the chance of arcing, which can injure the stellate ganglion. Likewise, one should be careful of the adjacent vessels, especially the veins at the R3 to R4 levels, as these branches drain directly into the azygos arch and can cause significant bleeding if avulsed.

General anesthesia is used to achieve the safest procedure. The author and colleagues prefer a technique using one-lung ventilation with a double-lumen endobronchial tube, as this assures the best possible visibility. Many authors, however, prefer using a standard single lumen two-lung approach. Either way, use of CO_2 insufflation can be helpful in collapsing the lung and assisting visibility. If used, guidelines for safe CO_2 use in VATS (ie, up to 2 L/min flow and up to 10 mm Hg pressure) should be followed.[14] The author and colleagues generally recommend placing the patient in the Semi-Fowler's position to allow gravity to help pull the upper lobes out of the field of dissection.

Regarding equipment use, either an operating scope 0° 10 mm can be used or a multiple-incision technique can be done. Smaller trocars and scopes are available for smaller patients. Trocar ports can be 10 mm, 5 mm or 2 to 3 mm in size. The larger the scope, the better the view and the larger the visual field (**Figs. 2** and **3**). The sympathetic chain is identified under the overlying parietal pleura as it courses over the rib heads. The pleura are incised laterally using cutting current. The hook cautery probe then is used to encircle the sympathetic chain.

Smaller scopes can be used, but these sacrifice visual acuity for size. Hook cautery probes are available as 3 and 5 mm sizes. Bovie cautery generally is used first with cutting, then coagulation current on the divided ends. Complete division of the sympathetic chain, including the nerve of Kuntz or other parallel pathways, must be achieved to avoid a recurrence.[15] The transected ends of the sympathetic chain are separated approximately 1 cm and the ends electrocauterized. Avoiding the sympathetic chain above the level of the G1 ganglion helps to avoid a Horner syndrome postoperatively. The author and colleagues prefer cutting to clipping or coagulating the ganglia of the sympathetic trunk. The purported advantages of clipping are that the clips could be removed in case of severe adverse effects, such as compensatory hyperhydrosis and gustatory sweating, and also could avoid lesions in the adjacent intercostals structures. Unfortunately, the data for success of these reversal procedures do not exist.

POSTOPERATIVE CARE

After complete recovery from anesthesia, patients are taken to the recovery room. According to their needs, analgesic medication will be administered. They generally are able to eat 2 to 4 hours after the surgery. Usually the patients are discharged later that day. The author recommends 3 days of relative rest, and then an increase regular physical activities gradually, but patients should avoid intense physical activities within 15 days. All

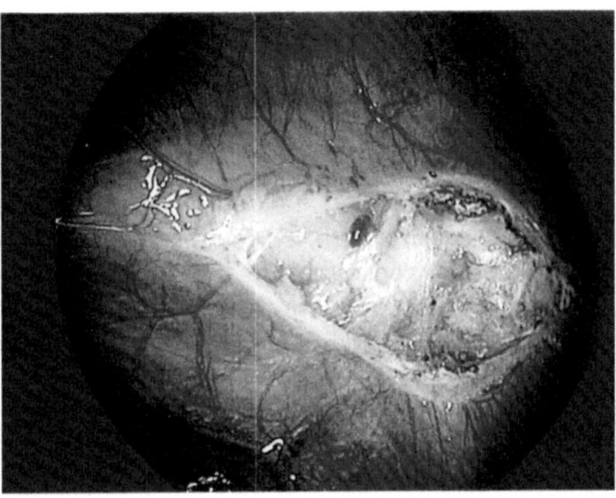

Fig. 2. Right sympathetic chain.

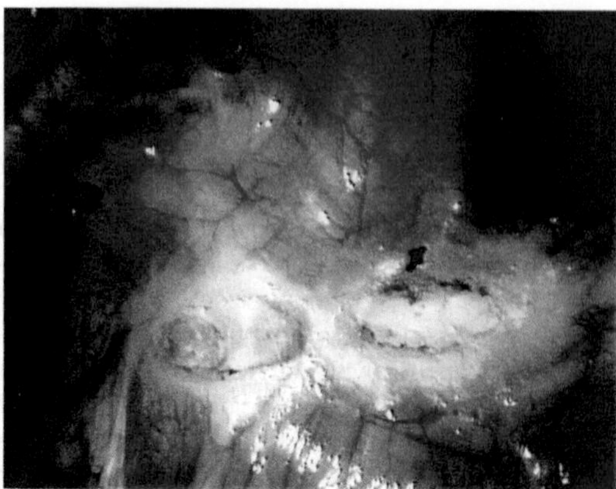

Fig. 3. Left sympathetic chain.

patients are examined before discharge for evidence of bradycardia or Horner syndrome, and a chest radiograph is done to rule out pneumothorax. Of approximately 10% of patients who get a small pneumothorax postoperatively, less than 10% require a catheter for drainage. This is generally kept in for several hours, and the patient is discharged later that day.

COMPLICATIONS

Common adverse effects include paresthesias (1%), pneumothorax (1%), bleeding and infection (1%), and incisional pain similar to post-thoracotomy pain (2%). Other rare complications reported include chylothorax and esophageal and lung injury. More unusual complications that should be discussed with the patient beforehand include Horner syndrome, which now should occur in less than 5% of patients.

In addition, compensatory sweating (CS) occurs in between 20% and 80% of cases in different series.[16–18] This, therefore, is the most common adverse effect and really should be explained to the patient almost as an expected adverse effect from this surgery. Of these patients, from 2% to 20% have severe, disabling, CS that results in their dissatisfaction to the point that they regret having the surgery.

A depression in the heart rate with resultant drop in the heart rate product and decrease in response to stress is expected to some degree in all patients. Some series have described this finding in most patients, while others report at least a 10% drop in heart rate in all patients. This is a possible major cause for postoperative dysfunction and should be cautiously sought after. Patients with resting heart rate that is below 50 to 60 beats per minute should undergo electrocardiogram (ECG). It is recommended that if the heart rate is low on subsequent ECG as well, that a tilt test should be performed to exclude patients in whom there is an inordinately high risk of postoperative bradycardia.[19,20]

RESULTS

A large number of international studies have shown that sympathectomy gives a positive result when it comes to hand perspiration and also that the adverse effects are rare. Studies by ETS surgeons have claimed a satisfaction rate around 85% to 95%[21,22] with about 2% regretting the surgery, generally because of CS. The exact results of ETS, however, are impossible to predict, because of considerable anatomic variations in sympathetic nerve distribution, and also because of variations in surgical technique used. Some reports have shown that there are clear indications for this surgery and that the adverse effects as a result of this surgery have declined and patient satisfaction has increased over time. In a recent series of 397 consecutive procedures by the author, there were 97 (48%) men and 104 (52%) women. The mean age was 29 (range 9 to 65 years). Median hospital stay was 12 hours (range 12 hours to 3 days). Median follow-up was 2.6 years (2 months to 9 years). The indications were: hyperhydrosis 174 patients; facial blushing 21; Raynaud disease in 3; digital ischemia in 2; and RSD in 1 patient. CS occurred in 40% of patients (n = 81/202).[23] In a recent series from Sao Paolo, Brazil, 378 patients were described who underwent TSSYM with excellent results in 276 patients and CS in over 60% of patients.[24]

Ramicotomy has been described by Lee[25] with a higher failure rate to stop sweating but a lower CS rate. Likewise, repeat sympathectomy either for patients who had prior other thoracic procedures or for those who had previous failed sympathectomy has been performed with low complication rates and good-to-excellent symptom relief.[26] Use of different technology for chain division or destruction includes electrocautery, harmonic scalpel, laser, and most recently clipping as originally described by Lin.[27] Reisfeld[28] has reported excellent success rates with clipping and purports a lower CS rate. No prospective data are available to support this as yet. Contentions that clip removal can improve CS are balanced by reports where this has resulted in recurrence of symptoms. Therefore, the author generally warns patients that there may only be a 20% to 50% success with reversal procedures.

Permanent adverse effects, including CS, gustatory sweating, Horner syndrome, and inability to raise the heart rate when working out physically have left a negative impact on some patients.[29,30] Recently, because of the risks and complaints by disabled patients, ETS was banned in its birthplace, Sweden, in 2003. In 2004, Taiwanese health authorities banned the procedure on patients younger than 20 years of age. The benefits of ETS to patients, however, far outweigh its disadvantages. Most surgeons still believe that ETS should be performed on certain selected patients with severe palmar hyperhydrosis and reflex sympathetic dystrophy.

SUMMARY

TSSYM is a safe procedure for the relief of hyperhydrosis and other specific indications. Patient selection and education of the patient and his or her family about the risks and adverse effects, including CS are crucial to attaining good results from this procedure. Standardization of nomenclature will allow more careful comparison of data among different trials and studies and ultimately determine the best level and technique for sympathectomy.

Thoracoscopic sympathectomy is used widely throughout the world in the management of hyperhydrosis and other medical conditions. This article proposed to explain the current indications, complications, and contraindications to the procedure. In addition, it provided an overview of the current nomenclature for describing sympathectomy and as recommendations for specific levels of destruction based on presenting diagnosis and symptoms.

REFERENCES

1. Alexander W. The treatment of epilepsy. Edinburgh (Scotland): YJ Pentland; 1889.
2. Adson AW, Brown GE. Raynaud's disease of the upper extremities: successful treatment by resection of the sympathetic cervicothoracic and second thoracic ganglions and the intervening trunk. JAMA 1929;92:444–9.
3. Kotzareff A. Resection partielle du tronc sympathique cervical droit pour hyperhidrose unilaterale. Rev Med Suisse Romande 1951;40:111–3 [in French].
4. Telford ED. The technique of sympathectomy. Br J Surg 1935;23:448–50.
5. Kux E. The endoscopic approach to the vegetative nervous system and its therapeutic possibilities. Dis Chest 1951;20:139–47.
6. Drott C, Claes G. Hyperhydrosis treated by thoracoscopic sympathicotomy. Cardiovasc Surg 1996;4: 788–90.
7. Krasna MJ, Jiao X, Sonett J, et al. Thoracoscopic sympathectomy. Surg Laparosc Endosc Percutan Tech 2000;10(5):314–8.
8. Lee DY, Yoon YH, Shin HK, et al. Needle thoracic sympathectomy for essential hyperhydrosis: intermediate-term follow-up. Ann Thorac Surg 2000; 69:251–3.
9. International Sympathetic Surgery Society. Available at: http://www.isss.net/. Accessed June 24, 2009.
10. Milanez de Campos J, Kauffman P, Wolosker N, et al. Axillary hyperhydrosis: T3/T4 versus T4 thoracic sympathectomy in a series of 276 cases. J Laparoendosc Adv Surg Tech A 2006;16(6): 598–603.
11. Schwartz PJ, Priori SG, Cerrone M, et al. Left cardiac sympathetic denervation in the management of high-risk patients affected by the long-QT syndrome. Circulation 2004;109(15):1826–33.
12. Singh B, Moodley J, Randall PK, et al. Pitfalls in thoracoscopic sympathectomy: mechanisma for failure. Surg Laparosc Endosc Percutan Tech 2001;6:364–7.
13. Chung I-H, Oh C-S, Koh K-S, et al. Anatomic variations of the T2 nerve root (including the nerve of Kuntz) and their implications for sympathectomy. J Thorac Cardiovasc Surg 2002;123:498–501.
14. Wolfer RS, Krasna MJ, Hasnain JU, et al. Hemodynamic Effects of carbon dioxide insufflation during thoracoscopy. Ann Thorac Surg 1994;58: 404–5.
15. Kuntz A. Distribution of the sympathetic rami to the brachial plexus: Its relation to sympathectomy affecting the upper extremity. Arch Surg 1927;15: 871–7.
16. Plas EG, Fugger R, Herbst F, et al. Complications of endoscopic thoracic sympathectomy. Surgery 1995; 118:493–5.
17. Shib CJ. Compensatory sweating after upper dorsal sympathectomy. J Neurosurg 1979;51:424–5.
18. Heckmann M. Complications in patients with palmar hyperhydrosis treated with transthoracic endoscopic sympathectomy. Neurosurgery 1998;42: 1403–4.
19. Papa MZ, Bass A, Schneiderman J, et al. Cardiovascular changes after bilateral upper dorsal sympathectomy. Short and long-term effects. Ann Surg 1986;204:715–8.
20. Noppen M, Dendale P, Hagers Y, et al. Changes in cardiocirculatory autonomic function after thoracoscopic upper dorsal sympathicolysis for essential hyperhydrosis. J Auton Nerv Syst 1996;60: 115–20.
21. Sung SW, Kim YT, Kim JH. Ultra-thin needle thoracoscopic surgery for hyperhydrosis with excellent

cosmetic effects. Eur J Cardiothorac Surg 2000;17: 691–6.

22. Swan MC, Paes T. Quality-of-life evaluation following endoscopic transthoracic sympathectomy for upper limb and facial hyperhydrosis. Ann Chir Gynaecol 2001;90:157–9.
23. Kwong K, Krasna M. Clinical experience in 397 consecutive thoracoscopic sympathectomies. Ann Thorac Surg 2005;80:1063–6.
24. de Campos JRM, Kauffman P, Werebe Ede C, et al. Quality of life, before and after thoracic sympathectomy: report on 378 operated patients. Ann Thorac Surg 2003;76:886–91.
25. Lee DY, Kim DY, Paik HC. Selective transaction of T3 Rami communicantes (T3 ramicotomy) in the treatment of palmar hyperhydrosis. Ann Thorac Surg 2004;78:1052–5.
26. Kim DH, Paik HC, Lee DY. Videoassisted thoracoscopic resympathetic surgery in the treatment or resweating hyperhydrosis. Eur J Cardiothorac Surg 2005;27:741–4.
27. Lin C, Mo L, Lee L, et al. Thoracoscopic T2 sympathetic block by clipping-A better and reversible operation for treatment of hyperhydrosis Palmaris: experience with 326 cases. Eur J Surg Suppl 1998;(580):13–6.
28. Reisfeld R. Video-assisted thoracic surgery sympathectomy for hyperhydrosis. Arch Surg 2005; 140(1):99.
29. Herbst F, Plas E, Fugger GR, et al. Endoscopic thoracic sympathectomy for primary hyperhydrosis of the upper limbs: a critical analysis and long-term results of 480 operations. Ann Surg 1994; 220(1):86–90.
30. Miguel A, González Ponce, Julià Serdà Gabriel, et al. Long-term pulmonary function after thoracic sympathectomy. J Thorac Cardiovasc Surg 2005; 129:1379–82.

Robotic Surgery of the Mediastinum

Annemarie Weissenbacher, MD, Johannes Bodner, MD*

KEYWORDS

- Thoracic surgery • Robotics
- Video-assisted thoracoscopic surgery
- da Vinci robotic system • Mediastinum

Approximately 25 years ago, in the late 1980s, the revolutionary era of minimally invasive video-assisted surgery began. Initially introduced for abdominal surgery, it was soon adopted for thoracic procedures, and called video-assisted thoracoscopic surgery (VATS). Early procedures were technically simple like pleural biopsies or pleurodesis for persistent pleural effusion. However, technical progress and increased experience led to rapid expansion of indications to a variety of mediastinal and pulmonary procedures.[1]

Despite the well-proved benefits regarding patient recovery and cosmetics,[2,3] VATS has encountered significant drawbacks. For technically more advanced operations, especially oncologic procedures, the VATS approach is still limited to specific centers, and has not gained general acceptance and gold standard status. The two-dimensional visualization of the operative field, limited maneuverability of the thoracoscopic instruments, and bad ergonomics make VATS procedures, at least at the beginning, technically more challenging and may suggest reduced surgical accuracy and oncologic safety.[4]

To overcome these limitations, micromechanic and robotic technology was introduced in minimally invasive surgery in the mid-1990s.[5] When operating with the da Vinci surgical system, the surgeon sits at a console distant from the patient and triggers highly sensitive motion sensors that transfer the surgeon's movements to the tip of the instruments, which are attached to the arms of a surgical arm cart next to the patient.

An early critical evaluation of the potential, benefits, and disadvantages of robotic surgery revealed coronary artery bypass surgery[6,7] and prostatectomy[8,9] as domains for this new surgical approach. Because the technical benefits have most advantage in narrowly confined and difficult-to-reach anatomic regions, thoracic surgeons' interest soon focused on the mediastinum.[10]

MATERIALS AND METHODS

Anatomy of the Mediastinum

The mediastinum is the central department of the thoracic cavity, extending from the sternum in front to the vertebral column behind; it contains all the thoracic viscera except the lungs.

For the purpose of description, the mediastinum is divided into 2 parts:

1. The upper mediastinum is bounded by the thoracic inlet and the plane from the sternal angle to the disc of T4 to T5
2. The lower mediastinum can be subdivided into 3 parts
   - anterior mediastinum in front of the pericardium
   - middle mediastinum containing the pericardium and its contents
   - posterior mediastinum behind the pericardium.

Surgery of the Mediastinum

Diseases of the thymus, the esophagus, and the lymphatic tissue are the main indications for

Department of Visceral, Transplant and Thoracic Surgery, Innsbruck Medical University, Anichstrasse 35, A-6020 Innsbruck, Austria
* Corresponding author.
E-mail address: johannes.bodner@i-med.ac.at

Thorac Surg Clin 20 (2010) 331–339
doi:10.1016/j.thorsurg.2010.01.005
1547-4127/10/$ – see front matter

surgery of the mediastinum, and, more rarely, ectopic thyroid and parathyroid glands. A variety of benign as well as primary and secondary (metastatic) malignant lesions indicate surgical biopsy or resection (**Table 1**). Although in open surgery the mediastinum is approached either transcervically or via a sternotomy, for most minimally invasive video-assisted procedures the approach is transthoracic with incision of the mediastinal pleura.

Technical Aspects

The da Vinci system allows the surgeon to maintain the skills and techniques known from open surgery. The surgeon's intuitive hand movements are transferred from the console to inside the patient. Thus, any kind of mediastinal procedure performed with the robot is similar to the corresponding open operation. Robotic pick-ups are used for tissue grasping, a cautery hook or scissors are used for dissection, a robotic needle holder for suturing. Control of major vessels is achieved either by direct ligation, by stitch tying, or with a robotic clip applier. Alternatively, conventional stapler devices can be introduced by the table-side assistant through an auxiliary port or, after intermittently removing 1 of the robotic instrument ports, through 1 of the initial incisions.

In robotic surgery, patient positioning, the placement of the robotic arm cart, and the positioning of the robotic and any eventual auxiliary trocars are crucial and procedure-specific. Poorly placed ports may cause collision of the robotic arms and thus hinder a successful operation.

Thymectomy and Thymomectomy

Robotic thymectomy has been performed from right-sided, left-sided, and bilateral approaches.[10–13] For any approach, patient positioning is incomplete (30–45°) lateral decubitus, with the approached side up; for a bilateral procedure the patient gets repositioned in the middle of the procedure.

A common position for the 0° or 30° camera is the fifth intercostal space in the midaxillary line.[10,12] Alternatively, the camera port is placed in the fourth intercostal space, anterior axillary line.[14] The robotic instrument ports are positioned in the third intercostal space, anterior to the midaxillary line, and in the fifth intercostal space, midclavicular line.[12,14] For best cosmetic results, especially in women, all 3 trocars are preferentially placed exactly along the submammary fold.[10] If necessary, auxiliary ports are introduced.[10,15,16]

The active lifting of the camera port (thoracolift)[15,16] and insufflation of CO_2 gas (6–10 mm Hg)[11] help to enlarge the space in the operative field, which improves visibility and instruments maneuverability.

An extended thymectomy with en bloc resection of the anterior mediastinal fat tissue following the rules of Masaoka and colleagues[17] is performed. The adipose tissue around the upper poles of the thymus, around both brachiocephalic veins, and on the pericardium is dissected meticulously. The resection borders are the diaphragm caudally, the thyroid gland cranially, and the phrenic nerves laterally on both sides. Smaller vessels are usually controlled by electrocautery, larger ones are ligated or clipped.[15,16]

Excision of Posterior Mediastinal Masses

Patient positioning varies from lateral decubitus[18] to supine.[19,20] Port placement depends on the position of the lesion with the camera port usually placed in the anterior axillary line, and the robotic

Table 1
Surgically relevant diseases of the mediastinum and corresponding minimally invasive procedures

Disease	Procedure
Thymoma, thymic cyst, myasthenia gravis	(Extended) thym(mom)ectomy
(Paravertebral) neurinoma	Extirpation
Lymph node metastasis	Biopsy, sampling, oncologic dissection
Foregut cyst	Extirpation
Esophageal leiomyoma	Extirpation
Esophageal cancer	Dissection, resection, reconstruction
(Ectopic) parathyroid tissue	Extirpation
(Ectopic) thyroid tissue	Extirpation
Lymphoma	Biopsy (extirpation)
Germ cell tumors including teratoma	Extirpation

instrument ports slightly anterior to the camera port.[19,20] For the resection of a paravertebral lesion, several auxiliary ports may be necessary.[21]

Dissection is performed with the cautery hook, usually without the need for ligation or clipping of any vessels.

Biopsy and Dissection of Mediastinal Lymph Nodes

In a minimally invasive esophagectomy for esophageal cancer, oncologic lymph node dissection is performed en bloc with the dissection of the thoracic esophagus.[22,23] Patient positioning is left lateral decubitus and the robot is placed dorsocranially. The 10-mm camera port is placed at the sixth intercostal space, posterior to the posterior axillary line. Two ports are placed anteriorly to the scapular rim in the fourth intercostal space and more posteriorly in the eighth intercostal space. Auxiliary thoracoscopic ports are used in the fifth and seventh intercostal spaces for assistance function. The lymph nodes from the subcarinal space (ATS7), the lower and middle paraesophageal (ATS8) lymph nodes, the nodes within the inferior pulmonary ligament (ATS9), and the paratracheal lymph nodes (ATS2,4R) are dissected with the cautery hook or a robotic harmonic scalpel. Insufflating CO_2 to 10 mm Hg of pressure helps to evacuate cautery smoke and to compress the lung away from the operative area.[11,22]

Robotic lymph node dissection as part of an oncologic pulmonary lobectomy is essentially technically the same,[24] as is diagnostic biopsy of enlarged mediastinal lymph nodes in lymphoma patients. Patient positioning and port placement depend on the exact location of the lesion. A scapular roll can be used to elevate the appropriate side of the chest.[25]

Excision of Foregut Cyst

Foregut cysts are typically located in the lower esophagus in the posterior phrenicocostal sinus and may be partially covered by the esophageal muscular layer. The robotic trocars are placed anteriorly between the midclavicular and the midaxillary line. For better exposure, the diaphragm is intermittently fixed to the thoracic wall and the pulmonary ligament is divided with the cautery hook. The cyst is removed in an endobag.[26]

Excision of Esophageal Leiomyoma

Patient positioning for robotic extirpation of an esophageal leiomyoma is (in)complete left lateral decubitus position.[24,27] Typical port positions are the sixth intercostal space posterior to the posterior axillary line for the camera and the fourth and eighth intercostal spaces for the instruments. Two auxiliary ports in the fifth and seventh intercostal spaces for suction and retraction facilitate dissection. Esophageal myotomy and enucleation of the tumor are performed bluntly and with the robotic cautery hook.

Esophagectomy for Cancer

Patient positioning for robotic dissection of the thoracic esophagus as part of a (minimally invasive or open) 3-hole esophagectomy is (overwound) left lateral decubitus.[22–24] The esophagus is circumferentially mobilized with en bloc dissection of mediastinal lymph nodes.

For transhiatal esophagectomy patients are positioned in the semilithotomy position.[28] The robot is approached from the patient's head. Dissection of the esophagus is started at the hiatus and continued in a cephalad direction.

Excision of Ectopic Parathyroid Tissue

Depending on the exact location of the lesion a right-sided or left-sided approach is chosen. Patient positioning is (in)complete lateral decubitus. The camera port is situated in the fifth/sixth intercostal space in the anterior axillary line and the 2 instrument ports are placed 1 hand breadth right and left. The lung is retracted through an auxiliary port in the midclavicular line of the sixth intercostal space. Suction is provided via a second auxiliary port, positioned more posteriorly. Enucleation starts with the incision of the mediastinal pleura covering the aortopulmonary window. Caution has to be taken to avoid injury to the vagus and recurrent laryngeal nerves. The tumor is cautiously excised using blunt dissection and the cautery hook. The vascular pedicle is controlled with clips.[16,29,30]

Excision of Germ Cell Tumors

For resection of germ cell tumors and teratomas in the anterior mediastinum, patients are placed in a lateral decubitus position. The robot cart is positioned anteriorly.[31]

RESULTS

A systematic review of the literature revealed 24 papers reporting on a total of 257 patients who underwent minimally invasive surgery with the da Vinci robot in the mediastinum (**Table 2**). The largest series are from Rueckert and colleagues (University Hospital Charitè, Berlin, Germany)[14] who performed 95 extended thymectomies and from Bodner and colleagues and Augustin and colleagues[15,16,26] (Innsbruck University Hospital,

Table 2
Summary of the literature on patients who underwent minimally invasive surgery with the da Vinci robot in the mediastinum (n = 257)

Main Author,[Ref,] Year of Publication	Procedures (n)	Diagnosis	Results
Rueckert JC,[14] 2008	Extended thymectomy (95)	Myasthenia gravis	0 intraoperative complications 2 postoperative complications 1 conversion (advanced stage thymoma) 0% perioperative mortality Mean hospital stay: no data
Bodner J,[15,16,24,26] 2004, 2005, 2006	(Extended) thymectomy (32) Esophagectomy (5), robotic dissection of thoracic esophagus in Ivor-Lewis-esophagectomy Extirpation (2) Resection of (posterior) mediastinal mass (7) Lymph node dissection (1) Resection of mediastinal lesion (2)	Different thymic pathologies Esophageal cancer, esophageal leiomyoma Ectopic parathyroid, ectopic thyroid Neurinoma, lymphoma, ectopic Cushing, carcinoid Lymph node metastases Foregut cyst, traction diverticulum	0 intraoperative complications 2 postoperative complications 2 conversions (tumor size, malignancy) 0% perioperative mortality Mean hospital stay: 10 d
Rea F,[12] 2006	(Extended) thymectomy (33)	Myasthenia gravis	0 intraoperative complications 0 postoperative complications 0 conversion 0% perioperative mortality Mean hospital stay: 2.6 d
van Hillegersberg R,[23] 2006	Esophagectomy (21): robotic dissection of thoracic esophagus in 3-hole esophagectomy (conventional laparoscopic abdominal part)	Adenocarcinoma Squamous cell carcinoma	1 intraoperative complication (bleeding) 27 postoperative complications 1 conversion (bleeding) 4.6% perioperative mortality (1 patient) Mean hospital stay: 18 d

Galvani CA,[28] 2008	Transhiatal esophagectomy (18): robotic dissection of thoracic esophagus in open 3-hole esophagectomy	Barrett esophagus (high-grade dysplasia) Adenocarcinoma	0 intraoperative complications 17 postoperative complications 0 conversions 0% perioperative mortality Mean hospital stay: no data
Savitt MA,[10] 2005	(Extended) thymectomy (18)	Different thymic pathologies	0 intraoperative complications 0 postoperative complications 0 conversions 0% perioperative mortality Mean hospital stay: 4 d
Giulianotti PC,[36] 2003	Esophagectomy (5) Resection (2)	Esophageal carcinoma Esophageal diverticulum, esophageal leiomyoma	0 intraoperative complications 2 postoperative complications 0 conversions 14.29% perioperative mortality Mean hospital stay: no data
Meehan JJ,[31] 2008	Resection of mediastinal lesion (5)	Germ cell tumor, ganglioneuroma, necrosis, ganglioneuroblastoma, mature teratoma	0 intraoperative complications 0 postoperative complications 0 conversions 0% perioperative mortality Mean hospital stay: 1,4 d
Morgan JA,[19,20] 2003	Resection of posterior mediastinal mass (2)	Neurofibroma, schwannoma	0 intraoperative complications 0 postoperative complications 0 conversions 0% perioperative mortality Mean hospital stay: 2 d
Yoshino I,[13,18] 2001, 2002	Extirpation (1) (Extended) thymectomy (1)	Bronchogenic cyst Thymoma	0 intraoperative complications 0 postoperative complications 0 conversions 0% perioperative mortality Mean hospital stay: no data
Boone J,[27] 2008	Esophagectomy (1) Robotic dissection of thoracic esophagus in open 3-hole esophagectomy	Esophageal leiomyoma	0 intraoperative complications 0 postoperative complications 0 conversions 0% perioperative mortality Hospital stay: 12 d

(*continued on next page*)

Table 2
(continued)

Main Author,[Ref,] Year of Publication	Procedures (n)	Diagnosis	Results
Brunaud L,[30] 2008	Resection (1)	Primary hyperparathyroidism (adenoma)	0 intraoperative complications 0 postoperative complications 0 conversions 0% perioperative mortality Hospital stay: no data
DeRose JJ,[25] 2003	Extirpation (1)	Diffuse B-large cell lymphoma	0 intraoperative complications 0 postoperative complications 0 conversions 0% perioperative mortality Hospital stay: 18 h
DeUgarte DA,[37] 2008	Extirpation (1)	Esophageal leiomyoma	0 intraoperative complications 0 postoperative complications 0 conversions 0% perioperative mortality Hospital stay: 5 d
Kernstine KH,[22] 2004	Robotic esophagectomy and lymph node dissection (1), complete robotic thoracic and abdominal phase in 3-hole esophagectomy	Esophageal adenocarcinoma T3 N0	0 intraoperative complications 0 postoperative complications 0 conversions 0% perioperative mortality Hospital stay: 9 d
Ruurda JP,[21] 2003	Extirpation of thoracic neurogenic tumor (1)	Ancient schwannoma	0 intraoperative complications 0 postoperative complications 0 conversions 0% perioperative mortality Hospital stay: no data
Timmermann GL,[29] 2008	Extirpation (1)	Ectopic parathyroid (hyperparathyroidism)	0 intraoperative complications 0 postoperative complications 0 conversion 0% perioperative mortality Hospital stay: <72 h

Innsbruck, Austria) who reported on 5 different mediastinal procedures in a total of 49 patients. Overall, (extended) thymectomy is the by far most frequently performed procedure, representing 69.65% of all interventions. The second most common are esophageal procedures (esophagectomy, extirpation of leiomyoma) (21.40%). However, most of these operations were hybrid procedures in which the robot was used for some steps (dissection of the intrathoracic esophagus with en bloc lymph node dissection) only. Smaller series and single case reports deal with resections of posterior mediastinal paravertebral lesions and ectopic (para)thyroids.

Overall 253 (98.44%) procedures were successfully completed with the robot. From the 4 (1.56%) conversions to an open approach, 1 (0.39%) was an emergency conversion because of major bleeding. The overall intraoperative and postoperative complication rate was 1.56% and 20.23%, respectively. The 30-day mortality rate was 0.78%.

DISCUSSION

Robotic surgery was introduced almost 15 years ago.[32] Initial reports of the few general, cardiac, and thoracic surgeons who had early access to this new technique were characterized by great enthusiasm and the strong feeling that this was the beginning of a new surgical era.[5,33,34] An early and broad spread was predicted.

However, unlike the introduction of conventional laparoscopy and thoracoscopy, the surgical community appeared reluctant to become convinced. Was it just the high costs of the robot, making it an elitist device that was adored by those who had access to it but disdained by the broad majority who did not? Or have robotic surgery and robotic surgeons failed to furnish proof of a substantial benefit over conventional minimally invasive surgery?

Which procedures cannot be performed minimally invasively except when using the robot? After which procedures are the oncologic or functional results significantly better when performed with the robot? Positive answers to these questions would justify extra costs and rapidly and efficiently convince surgeons, patients, and health care providers.

So far the gold standard approach for the mediastinum is still open surgery. The mediastinum is a delicate and difficult to reach anatomic area. Working thoracoscopically in close proximity to vulnerable large vessels and nerves poses an increased risk. There is very little space, the image of the operating field on the monitor is two-dimensional only and a surgeon's tremor is heightened by the long instruments. Of any thoracic surgery, mediastinal procedures is the one for which the robot's characteristics have a significant advantage.

This review of all published papers reporting on robotic surgery of the mediastinum proves the feasibility and safety of a variety of procedures. For extended thymectomy, especially in patients suffering from myasthenia gravis, early and midterm results suggest a benefit in the outcome when retrospectively compared with a conventional thoracoscopic or with an open approach.[10,12,14–16] Prospective randomized trials have been initiated to provide stronger evidence. Even if the results after robotic thymectomy were not better but equal to conventional VATS thymectomy, the advantage of a single-sided approach would favor the robotic technique. This is achieved by the active lifting of the robotic camera port, which augments the operative space and by the high maneuverability of the tips of the robotic instruments.[15,16] When performed by conventional VATS, complete resection of all the retrosternal tissue between both phrenic nerves nearly always requires a bilateral approach or additional subxiphoid or cervical incisions.[35]

Based on numbers, esophageal surgery seems to be another domain for the robotic approach. However, there is a broad inhomogeneity with regard to technical details and the particular application of the robot within the specific groups.[22–24,27,28,36,37] In the 2 largest published series of Hillegersberg and colleagues[23] and Galvani and colleagues[28] the robot was used only for dissection of the thoracic esophagus during 3-hole-esophagectomies. Only Kernstine and colleagues[22] performed the entire procedure (except the cervical part) with the robot. Although there are so far only 3 single case reports,[24,27,37] extirpation/enucleation of esophageal leiomyomas as well as foregut cysts[26] seem to be an ideal indication for a robotic approach. These procedures comprise delicate dissection, precise myotomy, and final closure of the esophageal muscle layer. The three-dimensional image of the operating field displayed on the robotic console, automatic tremor filtering, and the multiarticulated tips of the robotic instruments facilitate these steps significantly.[24]

Resection of ectopic (para)thyroids are rare surgical indications.[16,29,30] However, (partial) median sternotomy or thoracotomy has been the standard approach for glands displaced deep in the anterior mediastinum. A conventional VATS approach is technically challenging, especially when located within the aortopulmonary window, and has not yet been reported in the English literature. So far 3 robotic resections of ectopic (para)thyroids in the aortopulmonary window have been reported.[16,30] Although 1 patient suffered from a transient left laryngeal recurrent nerve palsy, the feasibility of these procedures represents an example where the application of the robotic technology has clearly expanded the borders of minimally invasive thoracic surgery.

A critical evaluation of any benefits or disadvantages is a precondition when a new surgical technique is being introduced. Despite the impressive potential of the da Vinci robotic system, in general thoracic surgery indications for completely robotic procedures are limited. However, this does not seem to be true for mediastinal procedures, where the available data strongly suggest a substantial benefit over conventional VATS.

SUMMARY

Several different mediastinal procedures for benign and malignant diseases have been proved to be feasible and safe when performed by a robotic minimally invasive approach. This article reviews the published data on robotic mediastinal surgery, focusing on technical aspects and perioperative outcomes. These are evaluated for differences and potential benefits over open and conventional minimally invasive techniques. Is there a need for the robot in the mediastinum? Is its application justified?

REFERENCES

1. Roviaro GC, Varoli F, Vergani C, et al. State of the art in thoracoscopic surgery. A personal experience of 2000 videothoracoscopic procedures and an overview of the literature. Surg Endosc 2002;16:881–92.
2. Nagahiro I, Andou A, Aoe M, et al. Pulmonary function, postoperative pain, and serum cytokine level after obectomy: a comparison of VATS and conventional procedure. Ann Thorac Surg 2001;72:362–5.
3. Forster R, Storck M, Schafer JR, et al. Thoracoscopy versus thoracotomy: a prospective comparison of trauma and quality of life. Langenbecks Arch Surg 2002;387:32–6.
4. Dieter RA, Kuzycz GB. Complications and contraindications of thoracoscopy. Int Surg 1997;82:232–9.
5. Schurr MO, Arezzo A, Buess GF. Robotics and systems technology for advanced endoscopic procedures: experiences in general surgery. Eur J Cardiothorac Surg 1999;16(Suppl 2):97–105.
6. Bonatti J, Schachner T, Bernecker O, et al. Robotic totally endoscopic coronary artery bypass: program development and learning curve issues. J Thorac Cardiovasc Surg 2004;127(2):504–10.
7. Bonaros N, Schachner T, Wiedemann D, et al. Quality of life improvement after robotically assisted coronary artery bypass grafting. Cardiology 2009;114(1):59–66.
8. Tewari A, Peabody J, Sarle R, et al. Technique of da Vinci robot-assisted anatomic radical prostatectomy. Urology 2002;60:569–72.
9. Murphy DG, Kerger M, Crowe H, et al. Operative details and oncological and functional outcome of robotic-assisted laparoscopic radical prostatectomy: 400 cases with a minimum of 12 months follow-up. Eur Urol 2009;55:1358–66.
10. Savitt MA, Gao G, Furnary AP, et al. Application of robotic-assisted techniques to the surgical evaluation and treatment of the anterior mediastinum. Ann Thorac Surg 2005;79:450–5.
11. Kernstine KH. Robotics in thoracic surgery. Am J Surg 2004;188:89–97.
12. Rea F, Marulli G, Bortolotti L, et al. Experience with the "da Vinci" robotic system for thymectomy in patients with myasthenia gravis: report of 33 cases. Ann Thorac Surg 2006;81:455–9.
13. Yoshino I, Hashizume M, Shimada M, et al. Thoracoscopic thymectomy with the da Vinci computer-enhanced surgical system. J Thorac Cardiovasc Surg 2001;122:783–5.
14. Rueckert JC, Ismail M, Swierzy M, et al. Thoracoscopic thymectomy with the da Vinci robotic system for myasthenia gravis. Ann NY Acad Sci 2008;1132:329–35.
15. Bodner J, Wykypiel H, Greiner A, et al. Early experience with robot-assisted surgery for mediastinal masses. Ann Thorac Surg 2004;78:259–65.
16. Bodner J, Wykypiel H, Wetscher G, et al. First experiences with the da Vinci™ operating robot in thoracic surgery. Eur J Cardiothorac Surg 2004;25:844–51.
17. Masaoka A, Yamakawa Y, Niwa H, et al. Extended thymectomy for myasthenia gravis patients: a 20-year review. Ann Thorac Surg 1996;62:853–9.
18. Yoshino I, Hashizume M, Shimada M, et al. Video-assisted thoracoscopic extirpation of a posterior mediastinal mass using the da Vinci computer enhanced surgical system. Ann Thorac Surg 2002;74:1235–7.
19. Morgan JA, Ginsburg ME, Sonett JR, et al. Advanced thoracoscopic procedures are facilitated by computer-aided robotic technology. Eur J Cardiothorac Surg 2003;23:883–7.
20. Morgan JA, Kohmoto T, Smith CR, et al. Endoscopic computer-enhanced mediastinal mass resection using robotic technology. Heart Surg Forum 2003;6(6):E164–6.
21. Ruurda JP, Hanlo PW, Hennipman A, et al. Robot-assisted thoracoscopic resection of a benign

mediastinal neurogenic tumor: technical note. Neurosurgery 2003;52(2):462–4.

22. Kernstine KH, DeArmond DT, Karimi M, et al. The robotic, 2-stage, 3-field esophagolymphadenectomy. J Thorac Cardiovasc Surg 2004;127:1847–9.
23. van Hillegersberg R, Boone J, Daaisma WA, et al. First experience with robot-assisted thoracoscopic esophagolymphadenectomy for esophageal cancer. Surg Endosc 2006;20:1435–9.
24. Bodner JC, Zitt M, Ott H, et al. Robotic-assisted thoracoscopic surgery (RATS) for benign and malignant esophageal tumors. Ann Thorac Surg 2005;80:1202–6.
25. DeRose JJ, Swistel DG, Safavi A, et al. Mediastinal mass evaluation using advanced robotic techniques. Ann Thorac Surg 2003;75:571–3.
26. Augustin F, Schmid T, Bodner J. The robotic approach for mediastinal lesions. Int J Med Robot Comput Assist Surg 2006;2:262–70.
27. Boone J, Draaisma WA, Schipper MEI, et al. Robot-assisted thoracoscopic esophagectomy for a giant upper esophageal leiomyoma. Dis Esophagus 2008;21:90–3.
28. Galvani CA, Gorodner MV, Moser F, et al. Robotically assisted laparoscopic transhiatal esophagectomy. Surg Endosc 2008;22:188–95.
29. Timmermann GL, Allard B, Lovrien F, et al. Hyperparathyroidism: robotic-assisted thoracoscopic resection of a supernumary anterior mediastinal parathyroid tumor. J Laparoendosc Adv Surg Tech A 2008;18(1):76–9.
30. Brunaud L, Ayav A, Bresler L, et al. Da Vinci robot-assisted thoracoscopy for primary hyperparathyroidism: a new application in endocrine surgery. J Chir (Paris) 2008;145(2):165–7.
31. Meehan JJ, Sandler AD. Robotic resection of mediastinal masses in children. J Laparoendosc Adv Surg Tech A 2008;18(1):114–9.
32. Himpens J, Leman G, Cadière GB. Telesurgical laparoscopic cholecystectomy [letter]. Surg Endosc 1998;12:1091.
33. Cadière GB, Himpens J, Germay O, et al. Feasibility of robotic laparoscopic surgery: 146 cases. World J Surg 2001;25:1467–77.
34. Rassweiler J, Binder J, Frede T. Robotic and telesurgery: will they change our future? Curr Opin Urol 2001;11:309–20.
35. Augustin F, Schmid T, Sieb M, et al. Video-assisted thoracoscopic surgery versus robotic-assisted thoracoscopic surgery thymectomy. Ann Thorac Surg 2008;85(2):768–71.
36. Giulianotti PC, Coratti A, Angelini M, et al. Robotica in general surgery. Personal experience in a large community hospital. Arch Surg 2003;138:777–84.
37. DeUgarte DA, Teitelbaum D, Hirschl RB, et al. Robotic extirpation of complex massive esophageal leiomyoma. J Laparoendosc Adv Surg Tech A 2008;18(2):286–9.

Index

Note: Page numbers of article titles are in **boldface** type.

Thorac Surg Clin 20 (2010) 341–344
doi:10.1016/S1547-4127(10)00063-0
1547-4127/10/$ – see front matter